Advances and Technical Standard in Neurosurgery

Volume 52

Series Editor

Concezio Di Rocco, Ist. Neurochirurgia, INI-International Neuroscience Inst, Hannover, Germany

Editorial Board

Miguel A. Arraez, Dept. of Neurosurgery Carlos Haya Univ., University of Malaga, Spain, Malaga, Spain

Frederick A. Boop, St Jude Global Program, Department of Neurosurgery, University of Tennessee Health Sciences Center, Memphis, USA

Sebastien Froelich, Department of Neurosurgery, Hôpital Lariboisière, PARIS, France

Yoko Kato, Dept.of Neurosurgery,Kutsukake, Fujita Health University, Toyoake, Aichi, Japan

Dachling Pang, NHS Trust, Great Ormond Street Hospital, London, UK

Yong-Kwang Tu, Taipei Medical University Shuang Ho Hosp, Taipei, Taiwan

This series, which has earned a reputation over the years and is considered a classic in the neurosurgical field, is now relaunched under the editorship of Professor Di Rocco, which relies on the collaboration of a renewed editorial board.

Both volumes focused on recent advances in neurosurgery and on technical standards, and monographs devoted to more specific subjects in the neurosurgical field will implement it. Written by key opinion leaders, the series volumes will be useful for young neurosurgeons in their postgraduate training but also for more experienced clinicians.

Waleed Abdelfattah Azab

Editor

Endoscope-controlled Transcranial Surgery

Advancing the Standard of Intraoperative Visualization - Vol. 52

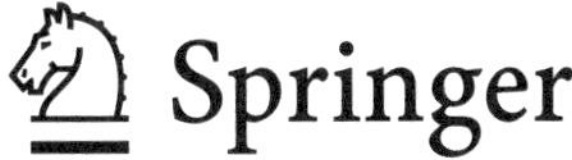

Editor
Waleed Abdelfattah Azab
Neurosurgery Department
Ibn Sina Hospital
Kuwait City, Kuwait

ISSN 0095-4829   ISSN 1869-9189   (electronic)
Advances and Technical Standards in Neurosurgery
ISBN 978-3-031-61927-4   ISBN 978-3-031-61925-0   (eBook)
https://doi.org/10.1007/978-3-031-61925-0

This Springer imprint is published by the registered company Springer Nature Switzerland AG
The registered company address is: Gewerbestrasse 11, 6330 Cham, Switzerland

If disposing of this product, please recycle the paper.

Preface

For many decades, the surgical microscope has been the gold standard for visualization in intracranial surgery. The advent of this optical device uncovered many unprecedented details of the intricate normal and pathological anatomy within the cranial cavity and paved the way for an unlimited array of new surgical horizons to be explored.

Despite the inherent drawbacks of the microscopic view, the microscope remained almost exclusively the sole method of visualization since its incorporation into brain surgery. One of the most significant disadvantages of using the surgical microscope, however, is the partial loss of light energy at the edges in those cases where brain surgery is performed through small corridors bordered by limited craniotomies, cortical incisions, and critical juxtaposed neurovascular structures. Given the lack of luxury to perform brain surgery through larger openings, most contemporary cranial microsurgical procedures are carried out through small exposures in which lower degrees of illumination and clarity are noted when surgical microscopes are used.

The use of optical devices other than the microscope during cranial microsurgery emerged out of the need to operate through limited exposures and yet obtain proper visualization and control over the structures within the surgical field. Earlier attempts demonstrated that endoscopes offered a solution to the problem of suboptimal visualization when these small exposures are used. Owing to its optical properties, design and small diameter, a rigid endoscope can be brought inside the field closer to the surgical target providing a high degree of illumination and clarity. Nevertheless, endoscope-controlled surgery did not achieve much popularity because surgeons were not accustomed to applying it, and also because using an endoscope is associated with a crowded surgical window and compromise of the space available for manipulating the instruments. An additional argument was that structures behind the endoscope lens are not visualized and are thus prone to trauma by instruments passing in and out through the surgical corridor.

Notwithstanding such arguments, this surgical philosophy is applicable and offers numerous advantages that are in my opinion indispensable to achieve a level of visualization superior to that of the surgical microscope. From this standpoint, the idea of this book arose, and I invited a group of colleague neurosurgeons who adopt this strategy to contribute, and thus get as much knowledge as possible on endoscope-controlled transcranial surgery constellated in one volume. This was geared towards demonstrating the advantages of this surgical methodology in a practical fashion that brings the idea closer to readers and practicing neurosurgeons.

The book includes a variety of chapters covering a multitude of surgical approaches in which surgery is performed under full endoscopic control, and I hope it will shed light on a different and more elegant strategy geared towards advancing the standard of intraoperative visualization in transcranial surgery.

Kuwait City, Kuwait   Waleed Abdelfattah Azab

Contents

Chapter 1
Comparative Optics of the Surgical Microscope and Rigid Endoscopes in Neurosurgery

Athary Saleem, Nathan S. Chisvo, Waleed Yousef, and Waleed Abdelfattah Azab

1.1 Surgical Microscopy

Magnification was first introduced in surgery in the form of loupe spectacles in the nineteenth century [1]. In 1921, Carl Nylen, an otolaryngologist in Stockholm, was the first to utilize a microscope during surgery for a case of chronic otitis media [2]. The first binocular microscope was developed by Gunnar Holmgren using an independent light source. Otolaryngologists continued the evolution of the microscope throughout the years [3, 4]. It was in 1952 that Zeiss developed their new microscope by Hans Littman, where the user could change the magnification of the scope without replacing the eyepieces or changing the working distance. The new microscope was OPMI 1 [3, 5].

Surgical microscopes continued to evolve and were first introduced into neurosurgery in 1957 by Theodor Kurze when he excised a facial nerve neurilemmoma in a 5-year-old child [3–5]. In 1966, Yasargil visited the microsurgical research laboratory in Burlington, where he was the first to utilize the microscope for the superficial temporal-middle cerebral artery bypass. Yasargil further developed the microscope, incorporating the ability to manually tilt the microscope's head [4]. The microscope evolved dramatically in modern times with more advanced optical technology, including clearer apochromatic lenses, automatic focus, increased depth of field, and powerful motorized zoom. Especially, magnification and focused illumination are crucial to appreciating the intricate details of the small neural and vascular structures [3]. Other advantages of the surgical microscope include providing

A. Saleem · W. Yousef · W. A. Azab (✉)
Department of Neurosurgery, Ibn Sina Hospital, Kuwait City, Kuwait

N. S. Chisvo
Barts and the London School of Medicine and Dentistry, Queen Mary University of London, London, UK

W. A. Azab (ed.), *Endoscope-controlled Transcranial Surgery*, Advances and Technical Standards in Neurosurgery 52, https://doi.org/10.1007/978-3-031-61925-0_1

magnification of anatomical details and coaxial illumination [6, 7]. Surgical microscopes have a magnification power ranging from extremely low (2–5X) to over 50X with a stereoscopic optical design. Typically, they have a large focal length that ranges from 150 to 300 mm, which is necessary to provide adequate workspace between the microscope and the surgical site [8].

1.2 Endoscopy

In 1806, Philipp Bozzini conceptualized an instrument composed of a long tube and external light source to create his "Lichtleiter" or light conductor. The Lichtleiter was a long, thin funnel with a reflecting mirror and a candle at the other end, used to look into cavities [9]. Bozzini's invention was never used in clinical practice. The earliest reported endoscope-using lens was known as the cystoscope, which was invented by Maximilian Nitze in 1877 and was used to examine the interior of the urinary bladder via the urethra. The first semiflexible gastroscope was used in 1932 by G. Wolf. In the year 1959, Harold H. Hopkins invented rod lenses for image transmission, and in 1963, Karl Storz combined rod lenses for image transmission with fiber bundles for illumination. Video endoscopes with cameras at the distal end of the endoscope saw the light in 1992. At the end of the 1990s, significant advances were seen with the endoscope that included sensors and light sources [6, 10–12]. The application of neuroendoscopy has greatly increased because of a multitude of visualization advantages, including higher intensity of the light toward the surgical target, precise close-up detail representation, and wider viewing angles [6, 7].

Optical limitations of the surgical microscope can be overcome with the endoscope's optical characteristics. Combining both visualization tools in the same procedure is termed endoscope-assisted microsurgery [6, 13, 14]. Endoscope-assisted microsurgery is an efficient way to increase illumination in the surgical area and concurrently enhance the visual representation of the pathoanatomic structures [6, 7].

The current rigid endoscopes can even be inserted through tiny surgical passages and generate clear and precise images of deep-seated pathologies. They have a diameter of roughly 2–4 mm, providing illumination of microanatomic structures [6]. When a component is zoomed, the lens scope shows more details of microscopic structures in brighter light, compared to the microscope where the focusing function causes a reduction in light intensity. The endoscope shaft and the more visible structures can both be securely manipulated while using the microscope [6]. Due to such variables, it is possible to incorporate the advantages of surgical microscopes and endoscopes so that the weaknesses of the two visual control systems are reciprocally diminished [6, 15, 16]. It is of note, however, that while angled endoscopic optics offer different viewpoints, the surgical challenge is not just to observe but also to operate on and maneuver around distant structures [17]. The current endoscopes are characterized by broad viewing angles, resulting in fish-eye phenomena that give the structures in front of the endoscope tip the appearance of being three dimensional [6].

Rigid endoscopes are used in endoscope-assisted and endoscope-controlled neurosurgical procedures since only devices with rigid shafts can have their orientation accurately determined. Endoscopic instruments with inclined shafts are also ideal for these procedures because they allow more surgical space for instrument manipulation. The front portion of the lens can be inclined to various degrees, providing angles of view of 0°, 30°, 45°, 70°, and 120° [12, 13, 18]. A summary of the optical characteristics of endoscopes versus surgical microscopes is presented in Table 1.1.

Table 1.1 Optical characteristics of endoscopes versus surgical microscopes

	Rigid endoscope	Surgical microscope
Optical design	• It uses fiber-optic or digital imaging systems to visualize the surgical field • A fiberoptic endoscope consists of thousands of glass fibers, which transmit light to illuminate the surgical site and transmit the image back to the camera • Digital endoscopes incorporate a charge-coupled device or complementary metal-oxide-semiconductor sensor to convert optical signals into digital images [18]	• Designed with a binocular viewing system, providing a stereoscopic view of the surgical field • The optical path includes an objective lens, an intermediate lens, and an eyepiece lens • The objective lens captures the image and projects it onto the intermediate lens, which then magnifies and transmits the image to the eyepiece lens for visualization by the surgeon [19]
Field of view and magnification	• Providing a wide-angle field of view, typically from 0° to 120°, to visualize the surgical field borders • The magnification is achieved digitally, enabling the surgeon to zoom in or out digitally without the need for interchangeable lenses • This flexibility enhances the surgeon's ability to adapt to varying anatomical scenarios during the procedure [20]	• They offer variable magnification options, typically ranging from 3x to 40x, allowing for the examination of the surgical site at different levels of detail • The higher magnification facilitates the precise manipulation and identification of intricate structures • Higher magnification is often associated with a narrower field of view that limits the surgeon's awareness of the surrounding anatomy [21]
Illumination	• Endoscopes utilize an integrated light source, such as LED or xenon, to illuminate • The light is transmitted through the endoscope's guide and dispersed onto the surgical field [18]	• Illumination is achieved through a coaxial light source, typically xenon or LED light • The light is transmitted through the objective lens and is focused on the surgical field • The coaxial design minimizes shadows and provides uniform illumination [22]

(continued)

Table 1.1 (continued)

Depth of field	• Endoscopes offer a greater depth of field compared to surgical microscopes • The increased depth of field allows for a broader focus range, enabling a more significant portion of the surgical area to remain in sharp focus simultaneously [20]	• The numerical aperture of the objective lens, the working distance, and the magnification affect the depth of field in surgical microscopes • Surgical microscopes offer a shallow depth of field, requiring precise focus adjustments when manipulating structures at different depths [19]

References

1. Roper-Hall MJ. Microsurgery in ophthalmology. Br J Ophthalmol. 1967;51:408–14.
2. Nylen CO. The otomicroscope and microsurgery. Acta Otolaryngol. 1972;73:453–4.
3. Uluc K, Kujoth GC, Baskaya MK. Operating microscopes: past, present, and future. Neurosurg Focus. 2009;27(3):E4.
4. Kriss TC, Kriss VM. History of the operating microscope: from magnifying glass to microneurosurgery. Neurosurgery. 1998;42:899–907.
5. Schultheiss D, Denil J. History of the microscope and development of microsurgery: a revolution for reproductive tract surgery. Andrologia. 2002;34:234–41.
6. Perneczky A, et al. Keyhole concept in neurosurgery: with endoscope-assisted microsurgery and case studies; 1999. p. 7–27.
7. Perneczky A, Fries G. Endoscope-assisted brain surgery: part 1-evolution, basic concept, and current technique. Neurosurgery. 1998;42:219–24.
8. Anbar M, Spangler R, Scott P. Clinical biophysics. W.H. Green; 1985.
9. Zada G, Liu C, Apuzzo ML. "through the looking glass": optical physics, issues, and the evolution of neuroendoscopy. World Neurosurg. 2013;79(2 Suppl):S3–13. https://doi.org/10.1016/j.wneu.2013.02.001.
10. Assina R, Rubino S, Sarris CE, et al. The history of brain retractors throughout the development of neurological surgery. Neurosurg Focus. 2014;36:E8.
11. Goodrich JT. How to get in and out of the skull: from tumi to "hammer and chisel" to the Gigli saw and the osteoplastic flap. Neurosurg Focus. 2014;36:E6.
12. Kanshepolsky J. Extracranial holder for brain retractors. Technical note. J Neurosurg. 1977;46:835–6.
13. Perneczky A, et al. Introduction. In: Keyhole approaches in neurosurgery. Vienna: Springer; 2008. p. 644. https://doi.org/10.1007/978-3-211-69501-2_1.
14. Punt J. Neuroendoscopy. In: Moore AJ, Newell DW, editors. Neurosurgery. London: Springer Specialist Surgery Series. Springer; 2005. https://doi.org/10.1007/1-84628-051-6_6.
15. Cote M, Kalra R, Wilson T, Orlandi RR, Couldwell WT. Surgical fidelity: comparing the microscope and the endoscope. Acta Neurochir. 2013;155(12):2299–303.
16. Raheja A, Kalra R, Couldwell WT. Three-dimensional versus two- dimensional neuroendoscopy: a preclinical laboratory study. World Neurosurg. 2016;92:378–85.
17. Rigante L, Borghei-Razavi H, Recinos PF, Roser F. An overview of endoscopy in neurologic surgery. Cleve Clin J Med. 2019;86(10):16ME–24ME.
18. Reisch R, Khaw AV, Dincer N, et al. 3DHD technology in neurosurgery: a review. Minim Invasive Neurosurg. 2011;54(5-6):201–6.
19. Gildenberg PL, Krauss JK. Textbook of stereotactic and functional neurosurgery. Springer Science & Business Media; 2013.

20. Zada G, Kim AH, Governale LS, Laws ER. Advances in endoscopic neurosurgery. J Neuro-Oncol. 2011;101(3):323–32.
21. Lee JY, Cho JH, Joo JD, et al. Comparative analysis of the accuracy of different minimally invasive placement techniques for freehand pedicle screw installation in the lumbar spine. J Neurosurg Spine. 2011;14(1):1–7.
22. Haque R, Sharma BS, Mathuriya SN. Microscope-integrated indocyanine green video angiography in the surgical management of cerebral arteriovenous malformations: an initial experience. Neurol India. 2011;59(3):394–8.

Chapter 2
Brain Tumor Anatomy with Tractography Fluorescence and Confocal Endoscopy

Alvaro Cordoba

Learning Objectives
- To learn the usefulness of the deep anatomy of the white matter and the brain tumor's location.
- To learn endoscopic techniques and how to combine them with histology ex vivo.
- To improve the borders of the brain tumor resection.
- To enlarge the objectives of the neurosurgical discipline.

2.1 Introduction and Historical Aspects

2.1.1 Confocal Microscope Evolution

Marvin Minsky, an American scientist and inventor, first introduced confocal microscopy in 1955 with a demonstration that it was possible to obtain optical sections via the aid of a pinhole and detector combination. Since that time, the last 60 years have seen the development of numerous confocal microscopes based on the principle that a pinhole equivalent blocks out-of-focus light.

Postoperative patient survival for brain tumor surgery is largely dependent on the extent of resection. However, surgeons continue to face challenges in the intraoperative differentiation of healthy brain parenchyma from pathologic tissue. Improvements in microscope technology, along with the development of novel fluorescent agents, are helping neurosurgeons overcome these challenges as we become

A. Cordoba (✉)
British Hospital, Montevideo, Uruguay

© The Author(s), under exclusive license to Springer Nature Switzerland AG 2024

W. A. Azab (ed.), *Endoscope-controlled Transcranial Surgery*, Advances and Technical Standards in Neurosurgery 52,
https://doi.org/10.1007/978-3-031-61925-0_2

better able to characterize these boarder zones in tumor resection. Multimodal brain navigation wide-field fluorescence image-guided surgery (FIGS) has been reported to have many benefits in glioma resection, anatomical knowledge, but it does have several challenges that limit its utility. High-resolution confocal endomicroscopy 17WFNS_17.indd has recently been introduced to the neurosurgical armamentarium and is demonstrating benefit in brain tumor resection. As this technology continues to improve and neurosurgeons become more comfortable with its incorporation into operative workflow, confocal endomicroscopy may contribute significantly to better tumor resections and patient outcomes. The reported rates of gross total tumor resection continue to remain low despite the use of imaging technologies such as intraoperative magnetic resonance imaging (MRI) and wide-field FIGS. As discussed earlier, a major reason for this is that these wide-field imaging techniques lack the resolution, and hence the sensitivity, to detect the disseminated tumor cells at the margins of such diffuse tumors. Thus, the neurosurgeon is faced with the challenge of interpreting subjective image intensities to determine an appropriate surgical margin. This process is neither quantitative nor reproducible for one surgeon or between multiple surgeons. For some extraaxial multimodal brain navigation, the gross appearance of the tumor is sufficient to establish the tumor-brain tissue planes with microdissection techniques. Other lesions, however, are less easily distinguished, particularly in the setting of prior treatment effect, cerebral edema, or microscopic infiltration. This is particularly true for gliomas and higher grade. Beyond identifying tumor margins, the opportunity to intraoperatively define tumor grade and histologic subtype is of critical importance, particularly meningiomas, where defining the extent of resection on the basis of gross tissue characteristics is insufficient and neuronavigation can be unreliable due to brain shift. Endoscopic procedures in hydrocephalus for intracranial gliomas, where tumor grade is not reliably predicted with either preoperative MRI21 or stereotactic biopsy. Some have thus advocated for the use of frozen-section pathology to confirm tissue status during glioma resection, which unfortunately is time-consuming and relies on the invasive removal of biopsies. Intraoperative frozen-section analysis can be misleading or nondiagnostic, particularly in cases of mechanical tissue disruption from the resection process. Such diagnostic unpredictability is further complicated by the inherent heterogeneity of gliomas, which can contain high-grade populations nested within a low-grade stroma. Others have suggested the need for quantitative measurements of PpIX fluorescence, such as with spectral measurement probes. To overcome these persistent challenges in the resection of complex intra- and extraaxial brain tumors, recent work has been directed toward adapting routine postoperative neuropathology methods into a real-time intraoperative technique. Overwhelmingly, this has led to the development of a potentially powerful complement to wide-field intraoperative high-resolution optical-sectioning microscopy or confocal microscopy.

2.2   Anatomical Highlights and Clinical Applications

- Deep knowledge of the white matter tracts.
- Anatomical relationships of the tracts and tumor localization.
- Multimodality approach with confocal endoscopy.
- Microanatomy of brain tumors.

Despite the enormous advances in imaging, the anatomical descriptions of the great authors of the past do not cease to be the most important source of knowledge. Our experience as a teacher in anatomy since 1982 confirms this. In 1684, Raimond Vieussens describes the brain tracts (Figs. 2.1 and 2.2), and then in 1932, Joseph Klinger confirms them by other techniques.

They are currently used as awake surgery procedures in functional and MRI to plan tumor approaches.

The combination of these techniques, together with endoscopy and endomicroscopy, allows a multidisciplinary approach to which intraoperative monitoring techniques can be associated.

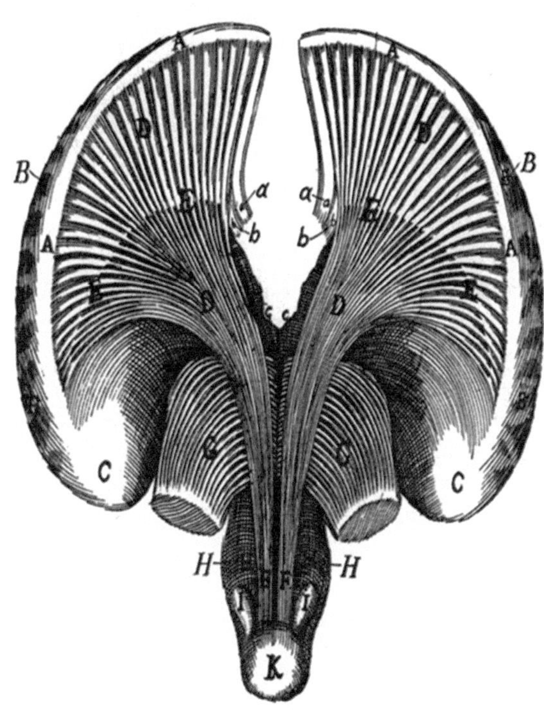

Fig. 2.1 Raymond VIEUSSENS (1641–1716), Neurographia Universalis (1684) (fixation by boiling in water/oil)

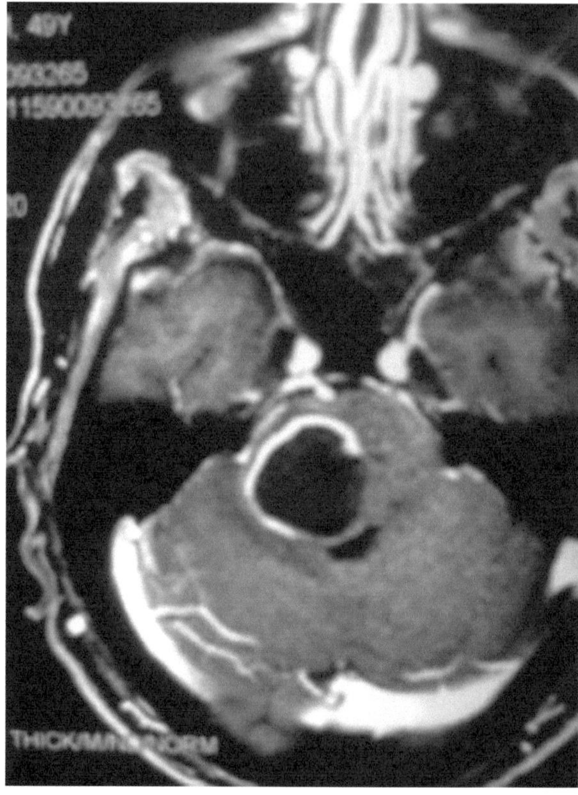

Fig. 2.2 Malignant pontine lesion with central necrosis and edema

2.3 Approach

Confocal microscopy is an optical imaging technique that uses point illumination and a spatial pinhole to eliminate out-of-focus light in specimens that are thicker than the focal plane, thereby enhancing optical resolution beyond light microscopy and detecting light produced by fluorescence very close to the focal plane. Intraoperative confocal microscopy has miniaturized this approach to enable the visualization of live tissue cytoarchitecture with spatial resolution on a cellular level. Ultimately, this allows the physician to have biopsy images displayed in real time to aid in immediate operative decision-making. This microscope can be placed directly in contact with tissues to quantify the presence of labeled cells in real time without the need for excisional biopsy and time-consuming histopathology. While late to become part of the neurosurgical armamentarium, the technology has been widely utilized and has proved feasible in various bodily regions outside the central nervous system, including the colon, pancreas, stomach, and alveoli. In neurosurgery, the ability to resolve and detect sparse subpopulations of labeled cells, such as tumors cells at the diffuse margins of a glioma, could provide a standardized quantitative metric by which neurosurgeons may eventually be able to optimize their resections as well as to objectively determine an unambiguous "extent of resection" for their surgeries. The usability of confocal endomicroscopy has been limited by instrument size and ease of surgical incorporation for the neurosurgeon (Fig. 2.3).

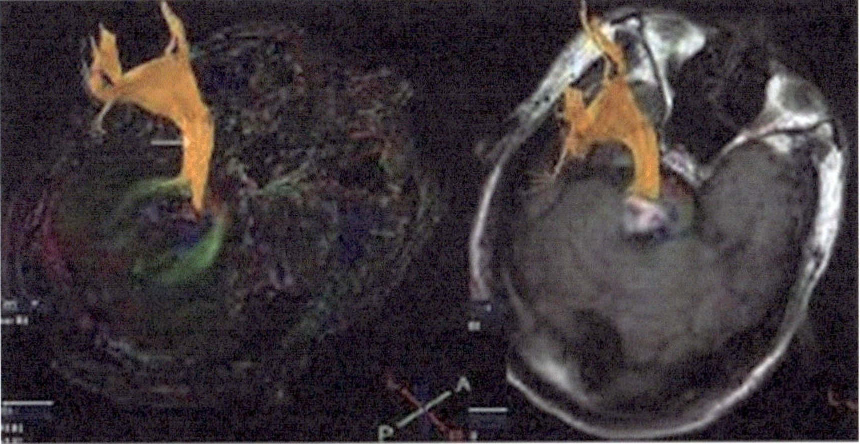

Fig. 2.3 Low-grade glioma MRI

Until recently, the size of the requisite apparatus limited the technology to the examination of excised tissue samples or isolated cells in a bench-top setting. Newer technology, however, features fiberoptic and microscopic miniaturization, substantially expanding its portability and applicability in an in vivo clinical setting. These systems now consist of a miniature handheld probe and movable workstation with an LCD screen. Using a single optical fiber as both the illumination point source and detection pinhole, high-resolution images are acquired and combined with miniaturized scanning and optical systems. Thus, the widespread use of confocal endomicroscopy in the gastrointestinal tract has been largely because of the ease of incorporating the technology into the distal tip of conventional video endoscopes. The bladder mucosa, skin, and eye have similarly been studied with in vivo confocal microscopy. Even more recently, in vivo confocal microscopy has been utilized in robotic-assisted radical prostatectomy.

Microscope designs have undergone numerous modifications to achieve optical sectioning, such as multiphoton excitation, single-axis confocal microscopy, dual-axis confocal (DAC) microscopy, and structured illumination. Designs have also differed in their scanning mechanisms, including proximally scanned coherent fiber bundles,5 distally scanned fiber tips. There are several commercially available confocal microscopy systems, including the Cellvizio (Mauna Kea Technologies, Paris, France) and Optiscan FIVE 1—both of which have been utilized in neurosurgery. The first microscope used in vivo for brain tumor resection in humans was the Optiscan system utilized by researchers at the Barrow Neurological Institute (BNI) in Phoenix. The Optiscan has a 475 × 475 μm field of view and a focal plane depth of 250 μm. As a result of the unique resonant-scanning mechanism used for imaging, this microscope is somewhat limited by a slow frame rate (0.8 frames/s) that leads to motion artifacts and makes the clinical use of the device less effective. The Cellvizio (Mauna Kea.

Technologies) is a 3 miniature microscope based on coherent fiber-bundle technologies. These confocal microscopes treat each fiber within the bundle as a separate confocal pinhole for the spatial filtering of out-of-focus and scattered light for high-contrast imaging of tissues at modest depths. Proximal scanning allows the distal tip of the device to be extremely small (0.5–3 mm) and flexible. One disadvantage of these technologies is that they often do not allow for axial adjustment of the focal plane since the mechanisms for doing so would significantly increase the size of the distal tip of these devices. While the ability to image deeply is not a fundamental necessity for intraoperative determination of tissue status, there are practical advantages for being able to adjust the focal plane of an optical-sectioning device during surgery. For example, the adjustment of the axial imaging depth allows the surgeon to search for an optimal imaging plane in which the tissues show minimal signs of surgical disruption and at which signal levels and contrast are optimal. Another limitation to fiber-bundle-based approaches is that current fiber-bundle manufacturers utilize glass fibers that create large autofluorescence backgrounds when excited at 405 nm. This is less of an issue at other excitation wavelengths, such as at 488 nm, but the autofluorescence background limits the ability of these technologies to be utilized for imaging 5-ALA-induced PpIX, in which the optimal absorption peak is at 405 nm. Both Optiscan and Cellvizio use a 488-nm excitation light, and Cellvizio additionally has a 660-nm single-band excitation light. EndoMAG1 has also been evaluated for use in neurosurgery, with a circular scanning field covering 300×300 µm and an 80 µm scanning depth. In addition to miniature optical-sectioning devices that utilize conventional single-axis confocal approaches, recent efforts have been made to develop intraoperative microscopes using an alternative confocal architecture called a DAC microscope or a divided-pupil confocal microscope. In the DAC architecture, the illumination and collection beam paths are spatially separated, as opposed to the common-path configuration of typical microscopes. Simulations and experiments have shown that the DAC configuration provides certain benefits in terms of optical sectioning contrast in tissues, including the ability to image at deeper depths compared to conventional single-axis confocal microscopes. In addition, dual-axis designs, which utilize low numerical-aperture (NA, weakly focusing) beams as opposed to high-NA beams preferred for conventional confocal microscopy, have been shown to be scalable in portable devices with diameters ranging from 3 mm to 10 mm. These devices have utilized miniature microelectronic mechanical system (MEMS) scanning mirrors to scan an image within tissues. MEMS-scanned microscopes have been shown to enable high frame rate imaging (up to 30 Hz), which is beneficial in clinical settings to reduce motion artifacts and image blur during handheld use. Handheld (i.e., the size of a pen), portable confocal laser endomicroscopy (CLE) is undergoing exploration in brain tumor [1–8] surgery because of its ability to produce the precise histopathological information of tissue with subcellular resolution in vivo in real time during tumor resection [8–13]. CLE is a fluorescence imaging technology that is used with a combination with fluorescent drugs or probes. While a wide range of fluorophores have been used for CLE in gastroenterology and other medical specialties, fluorophore options are limited for in vivo human brain use due to potential toxicity [8, 9, 11, 14]. Fluorescent dyes currently approved for use in vivo in the human brain include fluorescein sodium (FNa), indocyanine green, and 5-aminolevulinic acid (5-ALA) [9, 15, 16]. Other fluorescent dyes, such as acridine orange, acriflavine (AF), and cresyl violet, can be used on human brain tissue ex vivo [12, 17]. In neurosurgical oncology, CLE has been used to rapidly obtain optical cellular and cytoarchitectural information about tumor tissue as the resection progresses and to interrogate the resection cavity [12, 13]. The details of system operation have been previously described in detail [8, 12, 13, 18, 19]. Briefly, the neurosurgeon may hold the CLE probe by the hand, fixate it with a flexible instrument holder in place, or glide the probe across the tissue surface to obtain an "optical biopsy" with an image acquisition speed ranging between 0.8 and 20 frames per second dependent on the operation of the particular CLE system. The surgeon combining tractography may place the probe in a resting position at any time and proceed with tumor resection, then take up the probe conveniently as desired (Figs. 2.4, 2.5, and 2.6). CLE imaging is believed to be potentially advantageous for the appraisal of tumor margin regions or to examine suspected invasion into functional

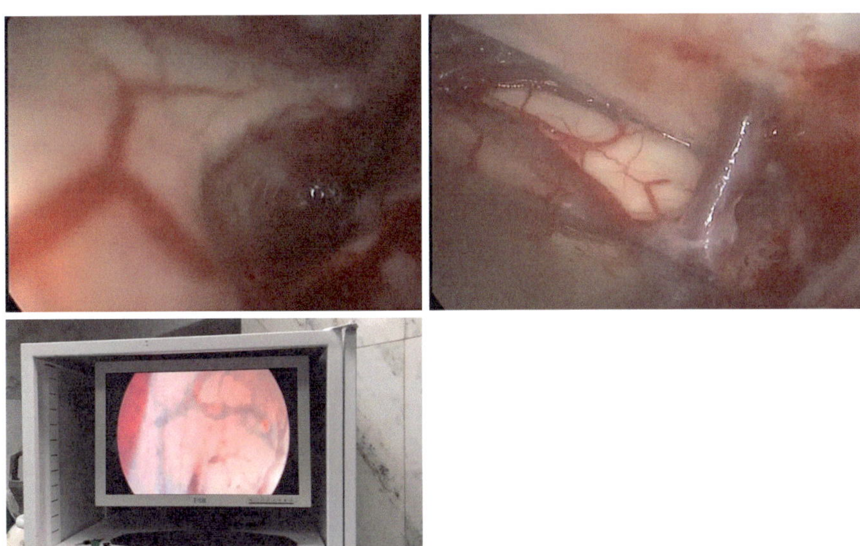

Fig. 2.4 Planning of the approach using MRI tractography and merging of navigation

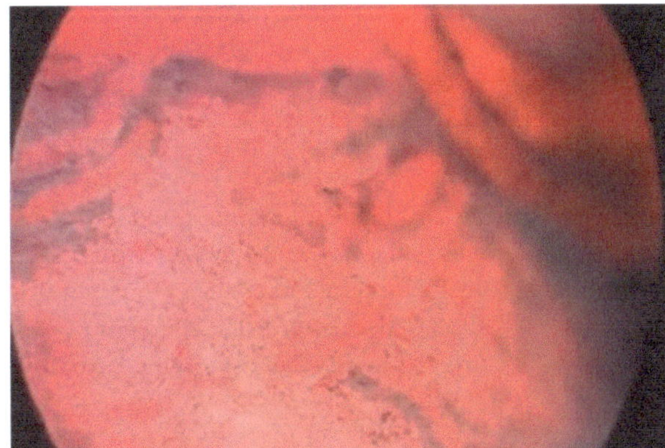

Fig. 2.5 Endoscopic images with the Andrea confocal system showing both the anatomical possibilities of use and the infiltration of the vessels

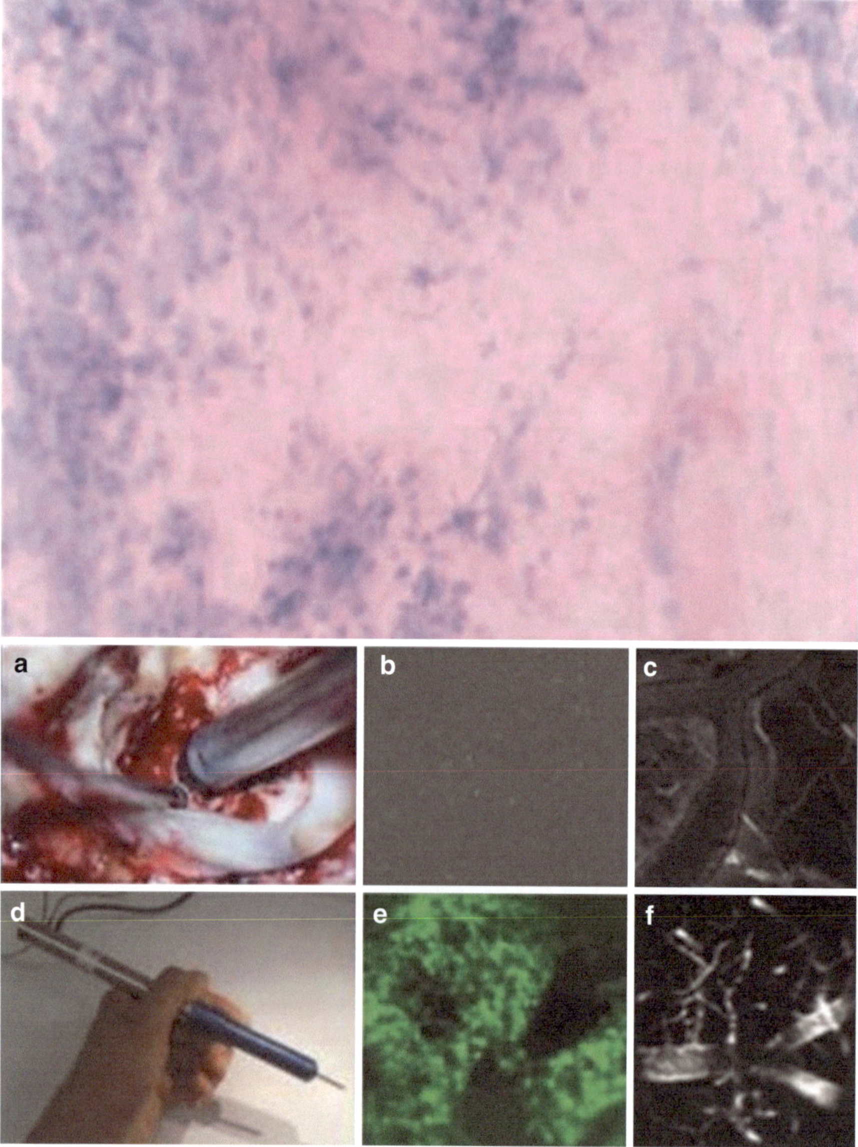

Fig. 2.6 Multimodality approach of neuronavigation with confocal endoscopy

cortex near the final phases of tumor resection. The images are displayed on a touchscreen monitor attached to the system (Figs. 2.7, 2.8, and 2.9). The neurosurgeon uses a foot pedal module to control the depth of scanning and image acquisition. An assistant can also control the acquisition of images using a touchscreen. CLE images can be processed and presented as still images, digital video loops

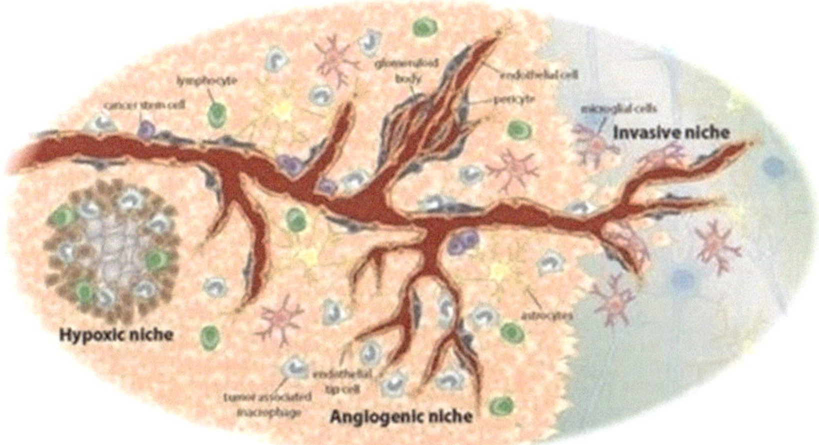

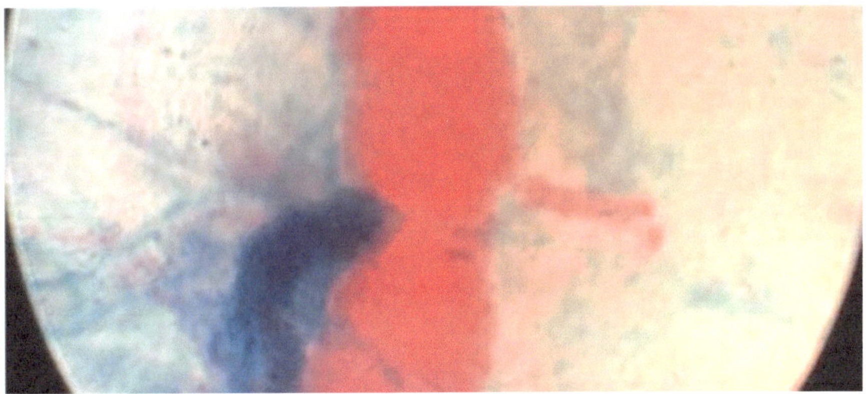

Fig. 2.7 Confocal optic image of high-grade glioma. Vascular invasion and pericytes stained along the blood vessels

showing motion, or three-dimensional digital imaging volumes. CLE is a promising technology with the strategy of optimizing or maximally increasing the resection of malignant infiltrating brain tumors and/or of increasing the positive yield of tissue biopsy. CLE may be of special value during surgery when interrogating tissue at the tumor border regions or within the surgical resection bed that may harbor a remnant malignant or spreading tumor [5], to identify all World Health Organization (WHO) microscopic criteria for glioblastoma multiforme (GBM) diagnosis (that is, cell number/density criteria, cell pleomorphism, mitotic figures, microvascular proliferation, and pseudo palisading necrosis) using LSCE ex vivo. Laser scanning confocal endomicroscopy also identified additional features seen in GBM, such as apoptotic figures in perinecrotic palisading tumor cells, giant cells, and fibrillary tumor matrix/blood vessels in select specimens.

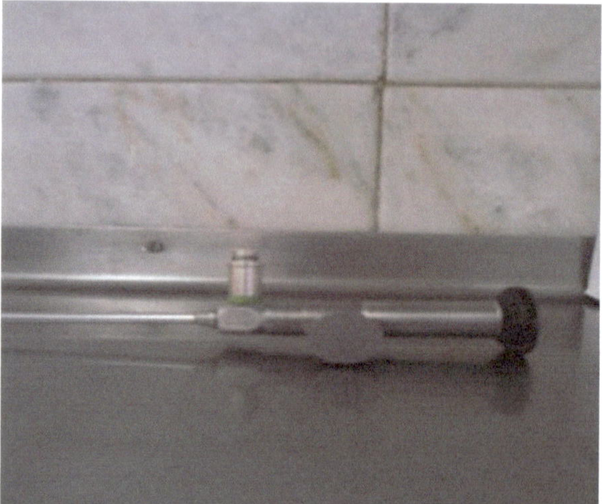

Fig. 2.8 Different techniques of confocal histology and blood vessel architecture

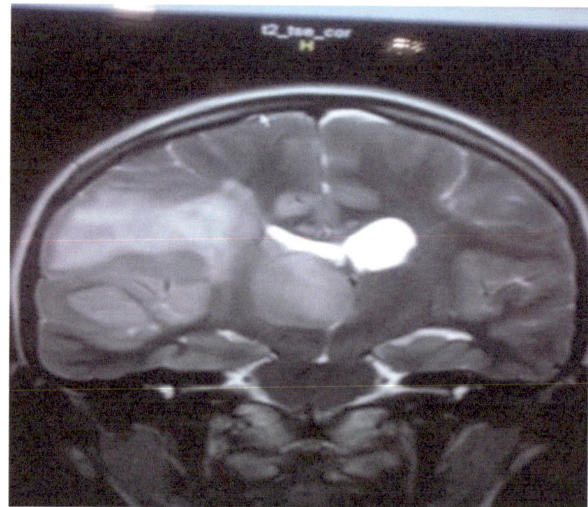

Fig. 2.9 Tumor invasion in malignant glioma. Scheme of different types of cells

2.4 Discussion

Despite the successful application of liquid single-crystal elastomer (LSCE) in vivo to date, much work remains to fully incorporate this technology into the neurosurgical operating room. We believe that future advances will come in three main realms: fluorescent and nonfluorescent technology for imaging neoplasms in vivo; confocal endoscope technology for improving imaging quality, depth, and ease of use; and improved incorporation of LSCE into the neurosurgery and neuropathology workflow. In 2010, Schlosser et al. [20] reported the first use of LSCE, which they termed neurolasermicroscopy, in human brain tissue. This study examined nine patients with glioblastoma (GBM) and compared LSCE with conventional histopathology in ex vivo brain tissue samples. LSCE was used intraoperatively immediately following the excision of the brain tumor specimen, and thereafter, the specimen was sent for conventional histopathological examination (that is, hematoxylin and eosin (H & E), periodic acidic Schiff, silver impregnation, and/or immunohistochemical staining). Acriflavine hydrochloride was applied topically to ex vivo tissue samples prior to LSCE examination. With this technique, Schlosser et al. were able Fluorescein and ICG are primarily visualized through the enhanced permeability and retention effect, which means that fluorophores are preferentially taken up by tumor tissue due to increased breakdown and leakage in the blood-brain barrier. On the other hand, 5-ALA provides the detection of neoplastic cells through intracellular fluorescence, but its ability to demarcate tumor margins is somewhat subjective, partly due to difficulty in interpreting levels of fluorescence near tumor boundaries (Fig. 2.10). All three of these currently available fluorescent agents also have limited circulation time and readily diffuse into and out of interstitial space.

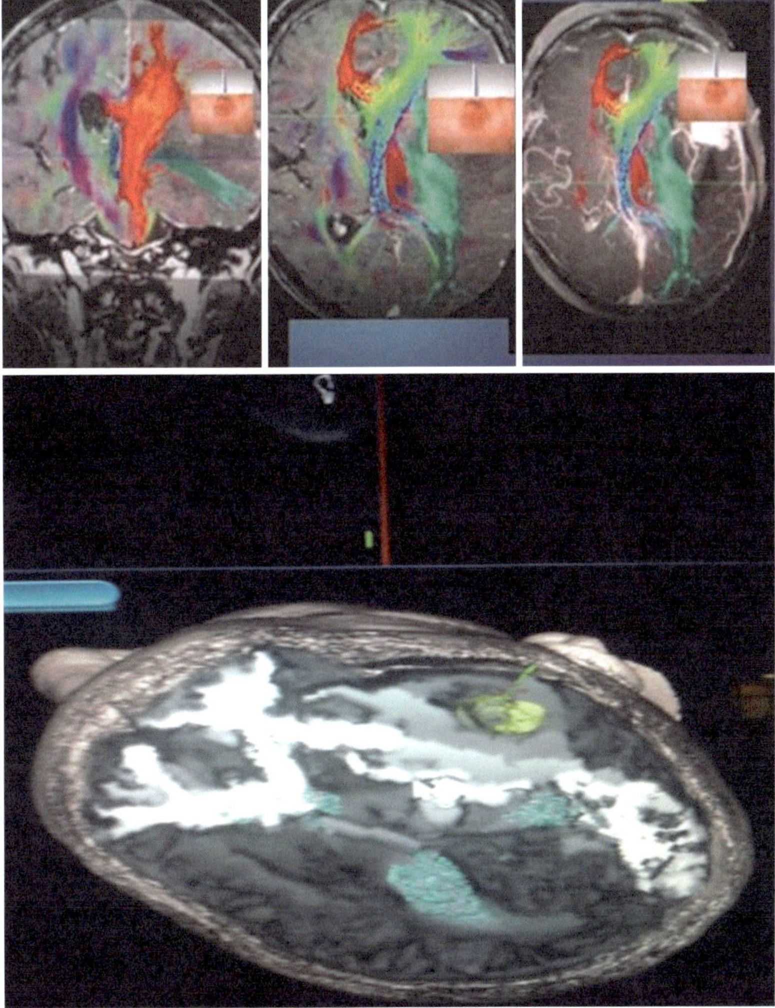

Fig. 2.10 Confocal optic model

Intraoperative confocal microscopy combined with molecular imaging probes specific for tumor biomarkers could play a significant role in future neurosurgical applications of LSCE. Molecular probes that have been investigated for use in brain neoplasms can be divided into three functional categories: peptides, antibodies, and nanoparticles. The efficacy and applicability of these probes are based on their selectiveness for tumor tissue, resistance to photobleaching and autofluorescence (by using near-infrared probes), and capacity to be safely administered to patients.

2.5 Surgical Pearls

- Multimodal approach of brain tumor resection using endoscopes like microscopes.
- Three-dimensional (3D) tracts and brain tumor reconstruction to avoid lesions in the normal areas.
- Staining of the tumor with appropriate reaction and depth.
- Appropriated check of tumor borders and supramaximal resection.

2.6 Conclusion

A multimodal approach to brain tumor surgery needs a deep knowledge of anatomy and neurosurgical techniques in order to combine all of the advantages of the technology.

The concept of supramaximal resection in brain tumor surgery should include the possibility of using confocal endoscopy at the borders of the lesion to permit a safe and true wide resection at the microscopic histologic range. Actually, with the use of modern laser devices, we can open a very interesting field in investigation and clinical applications.

References

1. Mahe E, Ara S, Bishara M, et al. Intraoperative pathology consultation: error, cause and impact. Can J Surg. 2013;56(3):E13–8. https://doi.org/10.1503/cjs.011112.
2. Paull PE, Hyatt BJ, Wassef W, Fischer AH. Confocal laser endomicroscopy: a primer for pathologists. Arch Pathol Lab Med. 2011;135(10):1343–8. https://doi.org/10.5858/arpa.2010-0264-ra.
3. Newton RC, Kemp SV, Shah PL, et al. Progress toward optical biopsy: bringing the microscope to the patient. Lung. 2011;189(2):111–9. https://doi.org/10.1007/s00408-0119282-7.
4. Tearney GJ, Brezinski ME, Bouma BE, et al. In vivo endoscopic optical biopsy with optical coherence tomography. Science. 1997;276(5321):2037–9. https://doi.org/10.1126/science.276.5321.2037.

5. Charalampaki P, Javed M, Daali S, Heiroth H, Igressa A, Weber F. Confocal laser endomicroscopy for real-time histomorphological diagnosis. Neurosurgery. 2015;62:171–6. https://doi.org/10.1227/neu.0000000000000805.
6. Kiesslich R, Neurath MF. Endoscopic confocal imaging. Clin Gastroenterol Hepatol. 2005;3(7):S58–60. https://doi.org/10.1016/S1542-3565(05)00252-1.
7. Lowe DG. Distinctive image features from scale-invariant keypoints. Int J Comput Vis. 2004;60(2):91–110. https://doi.org/10.1023/B:VISI.0000029664.99615.94.
8. Dalal N, Triggs B. Histograms of oriented gradients for human detection. In: Proceedings of the IEEE computer society conference on computer vision and pattern recognition (CVPR '05). San Diego, CA: IEEE; 2005. p. 886–93.
9. Chang C-C, Lin C-J. LIBSVM: a library for support vector machines. ACM Trans Intell Syst Technol. 2011;2(3:article 27. https://doi.org/10.1145/1961189.1961199.
10. Nister D, Stewenius H. Scalable recognition with a vocabulary tree. In: Proceedings of the IEEE computer society conference on computer vision and pattern recognition (CVPR '06). New York, NY: IEEE; 2006. p. 2161–8.
11. Gonzalez RC, Woods RE, Eddins SL. Digital image processing using MATLAB. Upper Saddle River, NJ, USA: Prentice-Hall; 2003.
12. Lowe DG. Object recognition from local scale-invariant features. In: Proceedings of the 7th IEEE international conference on computer vision (ICCV '99). IEEE; 1999. p. 1150–7.
13. Yang J, Yu K, Gong Y, Huang T. Linear spatial pyramid matching using sparse coding for image classification. In: Proceedings of the IEEE conference on computer vision and pattern recognition (CVPR '09). Miami, FL: IEEE; 2009. p. 1794–801.
14. Wang J, Yang J, Yu K, Lv F, Huang T, Gong Y. Locality-constrained linear coding for image classification. In: Proceedings of the IEEE computer society conference on computer vision and pattern recognition (CVPR '10). San Francisco, CA: IEEE; 2010. p. 3360–7.
15. Saul L. K., Roweis S. T (2000) An introduction to locally linear embedding. ; http://www.cs.toronto.edu/~roweis/lle/publications.html.
16. Boyd S, Parikh N, Chu E, Peleato B, Eckstein J. Distributed optimization and statistical learning via the alternating direction method of multipliers. Found Trends Mach Learn. 2010;3(1):1–122. https://doi.org/10.1561/2200000016.
17. Ojala T, Pietikäinen M, Mäenpää T. Multiresolution gray-scale and rotation invariant texture classification with local binary patterns. IEEE Trans Pattern Anal Mach Intell. 2002;24(7):971–87. https://doi.org/10.1109/TPAMI.2002.1017623.
18. Feichtinger HG, Strohmer T. Gabor analysis and algorithms: theory and applications. Springer; 2012.
19. Jain V, Seung HS. Natural image denoising with convolutional networks. In: Proceedings of the 22nd annual conference on neural information processing systems (NIPS '08); 2008. p. 769–76.
20. Schlosser HG, Suess O, Vajkoczy P, van Landeghem FK, Zeitz M, Bojarski C. Confocal neurolasermicroscopy in human brain—perspectives for neurosurgery on a cellular level (including additional comments to this article). Cent Eur Neurosurg. 2010;71:13–9.

Chapter 3
Fluorophores in Endoscopic Neurosurgery

Sonia Ajmera, Rachel Blue, and John Y. K. Lee

3.1 Introduction

The integration of endoscopy has transformed the landscape of anterior skull base and ventricular surgery, allowing less invasive approaches while enhancing intraoperative views. Despite the advances made by the implementation of endoscopes in various procedures, further surgical adjuncts have been sought to improve the identification of neurovascular structures and intracranial pathologies.

Two key intraoperative adjuncts are neuronavigation and Doppler ultrasound [1]. Based on advanced imaging and real-time spatial mapping, neuronavigation has improved localization and facilitated precise surgical trajectories. However, the accuracy of neuronavigation is affected once the manipulation of tissues begins, albeit more so in intrinsic surgery than skull base surgery [2]. Doppler ultrasound provides real-time feedback of vasculature but is only useful if the target areas are appropriately interrogated.

Fluorophores have gained traction as a potential solution to enhance intraoperative visualization. These agents selectively accumulate in specific tissues or structures, creating distinct visual markers during surgery. The visual contrast offered has the potential to enable the navigation of complex anatomical areas more accurately. The use of fluorophores requires appropriate intraoperative endoscopic filters, and visual feedback is combined with that offered under traditional white light. The combination of endoscopy and fluorophore use holds promise for improved intraoperative clarity and precision.

S. Ajmera (✉) · R. Blue · J. Y. K. Lee
Department of Neurosurgery, Hospital of the University of Pennsylvania, Philadelphia, PA, USA
e-mail: sonia.ajmera@pennmedicine.upenn.edu; rachel.blue@pennmedicine.upenn.edu; john.lee3@pennmedicine.upenn.edu

W. A. Azab (ed.), *Endoscope-controlled Transcranial Surgery*, Advances and Technical Standards in Neurosurgery 52, https://doi.org/10.1007/978-3-031-61925-0_3

3.2 Fluorophores Used in Endoscopic Neurosurgery

3.2.1 Five-Aminolaevulinic Acid

Five-aminolaevulinic acid (5-ALA) is a Food and Drug Administration (FDA)-approved agent for use in glioma resection, first reported by Walter Stummer in 1998 [3–5]. It is a natural building block in the heme synthesis pathway that is naturally converted to protoporphyrin IX, which is a fluorescent molecule that can accumulate in tissues in which there is blood-brain barrier disruption. Administration typically occurs around 3 h prior to anesthetic induction. Functioning as a visible light spectrum contrast agent, 5-ALA appears red within the tumor at the highest concentrations and pink at the margins. It is visible when observed under violet-blue light, with excitation wavelengths around 375–410 nm and observed red emission wavelengths from 620 to 710 nm [5]. Its application has been associated with improved glioma resection rates and progression-free survival rates [3]. Its utility has also been reported in metastatic brain tumors, malignant lymphoma, subependymomas, meningiomas, and germinomas [3, 6]. The limitations of 5-ALA include poor penetration and potential visual ambiguity due to the autofluorescence of normal brain parenchyma [7]. The adverse effects of 5-ALA include nausea, mild hypotension, and photosensitivity up to 48 h after administration [8].

3.2.2 Fluorescein

Fluorescein sodium, a nonspecific fluorescent dye, was initially utilized in ophthalmologic procedures. It excites at 465–490 nm wavelengths in cobalt blue light and fluoresces as bright green at 520–530 nm wavelengths [9]. It possesses the ability to traverse a damaged blood-brain barrier and accumulate at these sites. As such, it can accumulate not only in tumors but also beyond these boundaries into areas of surrounding edema or inflammation [10]. Fluorescein administration timing depends on clinical indication, with reported effective dosing seconds to minutes prior to desired visualization for anatomy or cerebrospinal fluid identification but earlier dosing at least 1 h before desired visualization for tumor cases [11–13]. The side effects of fluorescein include yellow urine, mucosa, and skin discoloration up to 24 h after administration, rashes, nausea, dizziness, angioedema, and abdominal and chest pains [8, 9].

3.2.3 Indocyanine Green

Indocyanine green (ICG) is a near-infrared contrast agent that binds to plasma proteins and is visible at an excitation wavelength of around 750–800 nm, with sustained visibility at longer emission wavelengths as well [1]. It has traditionally been used during intraoperative video angiography, usually administered as a 5–25 mg bolus seconds before the visualization of relevant vasculature [1, 7, 14]. Lee and colleagues recently reported an alternative technique using ICG, called the second-window ICG (SWIG), in which a 5 mg/kg dose is administered 24 h prior to operative intervention. ICG's permeability peaks at 1 h and plateaus between 7 h and 48 h; since tumors have permeable vascular endothelium, the accumulation of ICG allows sustained tumor visualization during this time frame via the enhancement permeability and retention effect (EPR) [7]. ICG has also been shown to permeate highly vascular structures, such as the pituitary gland, with an early dose of 12.5–25 mg during the opening of the sphenoid sinus during extended and standard transsphenoidal approaches [1, 15–17]. Compared to 5-ALA, ICG has been reported to have improved tissue penetration, reduced auto-fluorescence of brain parenchyma, and virtually no adverse effects [1, 7, 8, 15]. It has been shown to have particular efficacy in the visualization of commonly encountered anterior skull base pathologies, such as pituitary adenomas, craniopharyngiomas, and chordomas, while also enhancing gliomas, meningiomas, and metastases [7].

3.3 Applications of Fluorophores in Endoscopic Neurosurgery

Endoscopy has been used for skull base, ventricular, and intraaxial approaches for tumor biopsies and resections, ventriculostomies, cerebrospinal fluid leak repairs, and aneurysm treatment. The failure rates of neuroendoscopic lesion biopsies have been reported as high as 30% due to inadequate sampling [10]. The addition of fluorophores has been reported to enhance tumor identification and resection under endoscopic visualization. The combination of endoscopy and fluorophores has also been implemented to improve the resection of deep lesions that are difficult to adequately visualize using microscopy alone. Furthermore, neurovascular anatomic identification has been greatly augmented with the use of the endoscope, which allows dynamic, magnified views that are sometimes unachievable by the microscope, which is limited by direct line-of-sight viewing and a narrower visual field as operative depth increases. Fluorophore use can highlight key anatomy for the aforementioned surgical approaches that may otherwise be hidden under white light.

3.3.1 Tumor Resection: Skull Base, Ventricular, and Intraaxial

3.3.1.1 5-ala

Takeda et al. reported two cases in which intraventricular endoscopic visualization with 5-ALA allowed the safe biopsy of germinomas that otherwise looked indistinguishable from cranial tissue under white light [3]. In 2014, Cornelius and colleagues reported the endoscopic 5-ALA-guided resection of an olfactory groove meningioma resected via a trans-eyebrow approach and a clinoid meningioma with optic canal invasion resected via a frontolateral approach. These deep operative corridors limited the ability to use guidance with a conventional microscope; however, the use of endoscopy allowed residual fluorescing tumor detection and resection [18]. Similarly, Ruzevick highlighted a report of patients who went endoscopic-assisted 5-ALA-guided craniotomies for parasellar, ventricular, and cerebellopontine angle tumors, in which blue light endoscopy allowed further tumor identification and resection under fluoroscopy [19]. Strickland used 5-ALA and endoscopy for the resection of a deep frontal glioblastoma [20].

3.3.1.2   Fluorescein

Fluorescein has been used in conjunction with endoscopy for the resection of deep malignant intraaxial tumors, particularly high-grade gliomas with disrupted blood-brain barriers [12]. Some prefer its use for its cost-effectiveness compared with that of 5-ALA. Of note, low-grade glioma does not enhance well with the use of fluorescein, likely due to maintenance of the blood-brain barrier [10]. Alessando and colleagues reported a case series using fluorescein for the biopsy of intraventricular pathologies, both oncologic and inflammatory [10]. The application of fluorescein for inflammatory pathologies such as histiocytosis and granulomatosis is unique, taking advantage of fluorescein's nonspecificity.

3.3.1.3   ICG

ICG's ability to highlight intraoperative vasculature has been taken advantage of in anterior skull base surgery, particularly in visualizing the internal carotid arteries during pituitary surgery [1, 17, 21, 22]. ICG allows carotid identification before and after drilling bones [22]. In extended endoscopic endonasal approaches, a two-injection method has been reported. The first 12.5 mg dose allows the identification of the sphenopalatine artery during nasoseptal flap harvesting and the localization of the ICAs and epidural arteries; the second dose was injected during tumor removal, allowing the localization of intradural arteries [17, 21]. It has also been used to identify peritumoral and tumoral vessels during open craniotomies with endoscopic assistance [14]. Furthermore, its affinity for highly vascular tissues has allowed the visualization of the pituitary gland itself, allowing preservation during tumor removal [1, 17].

The use of ICG was applied by Fong to resect highly vascular lesions such as an orbital apex cavernous hemangioma, which was more easily contrasted to intraconal recti muscles with the use of ICG [23]. Lee has reported the improved visualization of tumors using SWIG, particularly in pituitary adenomas, craniopharyngiomas, and chordomas, in which 5-ALA has been reported to have poor uptake [7, 15–17]. Near-infrared imaging using SWIG had 100% sensitivity, which combined with the 100% specificity of trained neurosurgical eyes, resulted in increased rates of gross total resection [7]. Multiple groups have also reported the dissemination of ICG at the margins of intraventricular lesions, although more work is needed to study its selective accumulation and ability to accurately highlight the correct biopsy site [14, 24].

3.3.2 Intraoperative Anatomy

3.3.2.1 Fluorescein

The use of fluorescein has been implemented to study the extension of circumventricular organs, including the choroid plexus, median-eminence-tuber cinereum complex, lamina terminalis, and area postrema [11]. These structures are highly vascular and lack an intact blood-brain barrier; they are typically identified under white light endoscopy. Fluorescein injection has also been shown to reveal ventricular microvasculature, which may be helpful in avoiding bleeding during endoscopic procedures [25].

Fluorescein is also the commonly used fluorophore in the identification of spontaneous, iatrogenic, or traumatic skull base defects that result in cerebrospinal fluid leaks. Fluorescein is typically injected via a lumbar drain and circulates in the patient's cerebrospinal fluid. The endoscopic visualization of fluorescein-tinged cerebrospinal fluid can target the defect area that requires repair [26, 27].

3.3.2.2 ICG

ICG has been used during endoscopic ventricular procedures, i.e., endoscopic third ventriculostomies, to better visualize the basilar artery through even opaque third ventricular floors and identify a safe fenestration site [14, 28]. It has also been implemented as a surgical adjunct to assess vascular anatomy prior to and after aneurysm clipping, with one study reporting additional information provided in 42% of cases performed with endoscopic ICG as opposed to microscopic ICG alone. A key benefit of endoscopy is the ability of fluorescence to be visualized ten times longer than under the microscope alone [29]. The endoscope can be used for the dynamic visualization of various angles of the aneurysm-arterial complex, including the identification of nearby perforating arteries that need protection but are unable to be adequately visualized under the microscope due to limited angles and amplification. Once the clip is applied, endoscopic ICG can be used to confirm appropriate clip placement without compromising the parent arteries or perforators; alternatively, endoscopic ICG can also highlight residual aneurysm filling and the need to adjust a clip to trap the aneurysm [29–31].

3.4 Conclusion

The integration of endoscopy and fluorophores as surgical adjuncts has resulted in significant opportunities for improving surgical accuracy and finesse. Noteworthy among fluorophores are five-aminolevulinic acid, fluorescein, and indocyanine green. 5-ALA has exhibited effectiveness in glioma resection and other tumor types, with better visual augmentation in deep lesions using the endoscope as opposed to the microscope. Fluorescein's ability to cross the blood-brain barrier makes it a unique option for the sampling of both oncologic and inflammatory pathologies. It is also an accessible and cost-effective tool in the identification and repair of skull base defects. ICG's accumulation in vascular tissues lends its broad applicability in the identification of vasculature during multiple endoscopic approaches and the augmentation of the understanding of arterial-aneurysm complexes. Its improved tumor penetration has been applied in the resection of various pathologies, especially pituitary adenomas, craniopharyngiomas, and chordomas, in which 5-ALA has poorer uptake. The visualization of all these fluorophores is enhanced with the use of endoscopy, and these tools combined represent a promising avenue for the advancement of endoscopic neurosurgery.

References

1. de Notaris M, Sacco M, Corrivetti F, Dallan I, Cavallo LM, Somma T, Parbonetti G, Colamaria A, Solari D. Indocyanine green endoscopy for pituitary adenomas with Parasellar extension: results from a preliminary case series. World Neurosurg. 2022;166:e692–702. https://doi.org/10.1016/j.wneu.2022.07.081.
2. Sefcik RK, Rasouli J, Bederson JB, Shrivastava RK. Three-dimensional, computer simulated navigation in endoscopic neurosurgery. Interdiscip Neurosurg. 2017;8:17–22. https://doi.org/10.1016/j.inat.2017.01.003.
3. Takeda J, Nonaka M, Li Y, Komori Y, Kamei T, Iwata R, Hashiba T, Yoshimura K, Asai A. 5-ALA fluorescence-guided endoscopic surgery for mixed germ cell tumors. J Neuro-Oncol. 2017;134(1):119–24. https://doi.org/10.1007/s11060-017-2494-9.
4. Stummer W, Pichlmeier U, Meinel T, Wiestler OD, Zanella F, Reulen HJ, ALA-Glioma Study Group. Fluorescence-guided surgery with 5-aminolevulinic acid for resection of malignant glioma: a randomised controlled multicentre phase III trial. Lancet Oncol. 2006;7(5):392–401. https://doi.org/10.1016/S1470-2045(06)70665-9.
5. Orillac C, Stummer W, Orringer DA. Fluorescence guidance and intraoperative adjuvants to maximize extent of resection. Neurosurgery. 2021;89(5):727–36. https://doi.org/10.1093/neuros/nyaa475.
6. Marbacher S, Klinger E, Schwyzer L, Fischer I, Nevzati E, Diepers M, Roelcke U, Fathi AR, Coluccia D, Fandino J. Use of fluorescence to guide resection or biopsy of primary brain tumors and brain metastases. Neurosurg Focus. 2014;36(2):E10. https://doi.org/10.3171/2013.12.FOCUS13464.
7. Jeon JW, Cho SS, Nag S, Buch L, Pierce J, Su YS, Adappa ND, Palmer JN, Newman JG, Singhal S, Lee JYK. Near-infrared optical contrast of Skull Base tumors during endoscopic Endonasal surgery. Oper Neurosurg (Hagerstown). 2019;17(1):32–42. https://doi.org/10.1093/ons/opy213.

8. Senders JT, Muskens IS, Schnoor R, et al. Agents for fluorescence-guided glioma surgery: a systematic review of preclinical and clinical results. Acta Neurochir. 2017;159:151–67. https://doi.org/10.1007/s00701-016-3028-5.

9. Pothen AG, Parmar M. Fluorescein. In: StatPearls. Treasure Island (FL): StatPearls Publishing; 2023. https://www.ncbi.nlm.nih.gov/books/NBK555957/.

10. Fiorindi A, Boaro A, Del Moro G, Longatti P. Fluorescein-guided Neuroendoscopy for intraventricular lesions: a case series. Oper Neurosurg (Hagerstown). 2017;13(2):173–81. https://doi.org/10.1093/ons/opw008.

11. Longatti P, Basaldella L, Sammartino F, Boaro A, Fiorindi A. Fluorescein-enhanced characterization of additional anatomical landmarks in cerebral ventricular endoscopy. Neurosurgery. 2013;72(5):855–60. https://doi.org/10.1227/NEU.0b013e3182889e27.

12. Kutlay M, Durmaz O, Ozer İ, Kırık A, Yasar S, Kural C, Temiz Ç, Tehli Ö, Ezgu MC, Daneyemez M, Izci Y. Fluorescein sodium-guided Neuroendoscopic resection of deep-seated malignant brain tumors: preliminary results of 18 patients. Oper Neurosurg (Hagerstown). 2021;20(2):206–18. https://doi.org/10.1093/ons/opaa313.

13. Acerbi F, Broggi M, Broggi G, Ferroli P. What is the best timing for fluorescein injection during surgical removal of high-grade gliomas? Acta Neurochir. 2015;157(8):1377–8. https://doi.org/10.1007/s00701-015-2455-z.

14. Catapano G, Sgulò F, Laleva L, Columbano L, Dallan I, de Notaris M. Multimodal use of indocyanine green endoscopy in neurosurgery: a single-center experience and review of the literature. Neurosurg Rev. 2018;41(4):985–98. https://doi.org/10.1007/s10143-017-0858-4.

15. Litvack ZN, Zada G, Laws ER Jr. Indocyanine green fluorescence endoscopy for visual differentiation of pituitary tumor from surrounding structures. J Neurosurg. 2012;116(5):935–41. https://doi.org/10.3171/2012.1.JNS11601.

16. Amano K, Aihara Y, Tsuzuki S, Okada Y, Kawamata T. Application of indocyanine green fluorescence endoscopic system in transsphenoidal surgery for pituitary tumors. Acta Neurochir. 2019;161(4):695–706. https://doi.org/10.1007/s00701-018-03778-0.

17. Inoue A, Kohno S, Ohnishi T, Nishida N, Suehiro S, Nakamura Y, Matsumoto S, Nishikawa M, Ozaki S, Shigekawa S, Watanabe H, Senba H, Nakaguchi H, Taniwaki M, Matsuura B, Kitazawa R, Kunieda T. Tricks and traps of ICG endoscopy for effectively applying endoscopic transsphenoidal surgery to pituitary adenoma. Neurosurg Rev. 2021;44(4):2133–43. https://doi.org/10.1007/s10143-020-01382-4.

18. Cornelius JF, Kamp MA, Tortora A, Knipps J, Krause-Molle Z, Beez T, Petridis AK, Sabel M, Schipper J, Steiger HJ. Surgery of small anterior Skull Base Meningiomas by endoscopic 5-Aminolevulinic acid fluorescence guidance: first clinical experience. World Neurosurg. 2019;122:e890–5. https://doi.org/10.1016/j.wneu.2018.10.171.

19. Ruzevick J, Cardinal T, Pangal DJ, Bove I, Strickland B, Zada G. From white to blue light: evolution of endoscope-assisted intracranial tumor neurosurgery and expansion to intraaxial tumors. J Neurosurg. 2022;139(1):59–64. https://doi.org/10.3171/2022.10.JNS22489.

20. Strickland BA, Zada G. 5-ALA enhanced fluorescence-guided microscopic to endoscopic resection of deep frontal subcortical glioblastoma Multiforme. World Neurosurg. 2021;148:65. https://doi.org/10.1016/j.wneu.2020.12.168.

21. Hide T, Yano S, Shinojima N, Kuratsu J. Usefulness of the indocyanine green fluorescence endoscope in endonasal transsphenoidal surgery. J Neurosurg. 2015;122(5):1185–92. https://doi.org/10.3171/2014.9.JNS14599.

22. Simal Julián JA, Sanromán Álvarez P, Miranda Lloret P, Botella AC. Endo ICG videoangiography: localizing the carotid artery in skull-base endonasal approaches. Acta Neurochir. 2016;158(7):1351–3. https://doi.org/10.1007/s00701-016-2830-4.

23. Fong Ng BC, Kwan Mak CH, Chan NL, Lam CW, Yuen HK, Poon TL. Indocyanine green-assisted endoscopic Transorbital excision of lateral orbital apex cavernous hemangioma. World Neurosurg. 2022;158:167. https://doi.org/10.1016/j.wneu.2021.11.060.

24. Tsuzuki S, Aihara Y, Eguchi S, Amano K, Kawamata T, Okada Y. Application of indocyanine green (ICG) fluorescence for endoscopic biopsy of intraventricular tumors. Childs Nerv Syst. 2014;30(4):723–6. https://doi.org/10.1007/s00381-013-2266-6.
25. Longatti P, Boaro A, Canova G, Fiorindi A. The subependymal microvascular network revealed by endoscopic fluorescence angiography. J Neurosurg Sci. 2020;64(4):347–52. https://doi.org/10.23736/S0390-5616.17.04098-X.
26. Locatelli D, Rampa F, Acchiardi I, Bignami M, Pistochini A, Castelnuovo P. Endoscopic endonasal approaches to anterior skull base defects in pediatric patients. Childs Nerv Syst. 2006;22(11):1411–8. https://doi.org/10.1007/s00381-006-0114-7.
27. Marton E, Billeci D, Schiesari E, Longatti P. Transnasal endoscopic repair of cerebrospinal fluid fistulas and encephaloceles: surgical indications and complications. Minim Invasive Neurosurg. 2005;48(3):175–81. https://doi.org/10.1055/s-2005-870904.
28. Wachter D, Behm T, von Eckardstein K, Rohde V. Indocyanine green angiography in endoscopic third ventriculostomy. Neurosurgery. 2013;73(1 Suppl Operative):ons67–72; ons72-3. https://doi.org/10.1227/NEU.0b013e318285b846.
29. Nishiyama Y, Kinouchi H, Senbokuya N, Kato T, Kanemaru K, Yoshioka H, Horikoshi T. Endoscopic indocyanine green video angiography in aneurysm surgery: an innovative method for intraoperative assessment of blood flow in vasculature hidden from microscopic view. J Neurosurg. 2012;117(2):302–8. https://doi.org/10.3171/2012.5.JNS112300.
30. Mielke D, Malinova V, Rohde V. Comparison of intraoperative microscopic and endoscopic ICG angiography in aneurysm surgery. Neurosurgery. 2014;10(Suppl 3):418–25. ; discussion 425. https://doi.org/10.1227/NEU.0000000000000345.
31. Bruneau M, Appelboom G, Rynkowski M, Van Cutsem N, Mine B, De Witte O. Endoscope-integrated ICG technology: first application during intracranial aneurysm surgery. Neurosurg Rev. 2013;36(1):77–84. ;discussion 84-5. https://doi.org/10.1007/s10143-012-0419-9.

Chapter 4
Endoscopic Anatomy of the Skull Base

Jonathan A. Tangsrivimol, Moataz D. Abouammo, and Daniel M. Prevedello

4.1 Introduction

Presently, endoscopic skull base surgery has undergone significant advancements since its inception over two decades ago [1, 2]. Following a successful endoscopic pituitary surgery, the medical team employed an endoscope to further explore and extend their examination to multiple sites within the skull base using the transsphenoidal approach [3–15]. Nevertheless, it is imperative to underscore that the fundamental basis of all surgical procedures lies in the meticulous understanding of anatomy, with particular emphasis on ventral anatomy. This facet has recently garnered increased attention.

Following the advancements in endoscopic skull base surgery techniques, this chapter will concentrate on the pertinent anatomical considerations that serve as key foundations for successful procedures. These considerations are categorized into two planes: the sagittal plane and the coronal plane.

J. A. Tangsrivimol
Department of Neurosurgery, Chulabhorn Hospital, Chulabhorn Royal Academy, Bangkok, Thailand

M. D. Abouammo
Department of Otolaryngology and Head-Neck Surgery, Faculty of Medicine, Tanta University Hospital, Tanta, Egypt
e-mail: moataz.desouky@med.tanta.edu.eg

D. M. Prevedello (✉)
Department of Neurological Surgery, The Ohio State University Wexner Medical Center and James Cancer Institute, Columbus, OH, USA
e-mail: Daniel.prevedello@osumc.edu

W. A. Azab (ed.), *Endoscope-controlled Transcranial Surgery*, Advances and Technical Standards in Neurosurgery 52,
https://doi.org/10.1007/978-3-031-61925-0_4

4.2 Sagittal Plane

The sagittal plane of the endoscopic endonasal approach to the skull base is categorized into distinct subtypes based on their respective locations and targets.

The first subtype is the *transcribriform approach*, which involves accessing more anterior regions located just behind the frontal sinus.

The second subtype is the *transplanum approach*, which traverses through the planum sphenoidale. Sometimes it is also known as the "transtuberculum sellae" approach when the surgical route lies between the sellar region and the planum sphenoidale.

The third subtype is the *transsellar approach*, which involves navigating the sphenoid sinus to reach the sellar region.

The fourth subtype is the *transclival approach,* which is employed when descending further into the clival region.

Finally, the transodontoid approach is employed in cases where pathologies extend from the foramen magnum to the C1–C2 region.

By systematically classifying the endoscopic endonasal approaches based on their specific locations and trajectories, surgical practitioners better understand each method's indications and potential applications in skull base procedures (Figs. 4.1 and 4.2).

4.2.1 Transsellar and Transplanum Approach

In optic anatomy, the *opticocarotid recess* (OCR) denotes the pneumatization of the optic strut within the optic strut, extending toward the anterior clinoid process (Fig. 4.3).

The *optic strut* serves as a separation point between the optic canal, which lies superiorly, and the superior orbital fissure, located anteriorly. This positioning places the OCR just below the optic strut and in front of the carotid artery, specifically at the level of the paraclinoid segment (Fig. 4.3).

Beneath the gland, you will observe the paraclival space or clival recess, where the paraclival carotid artery courses laterally [16]. In this region, septations are

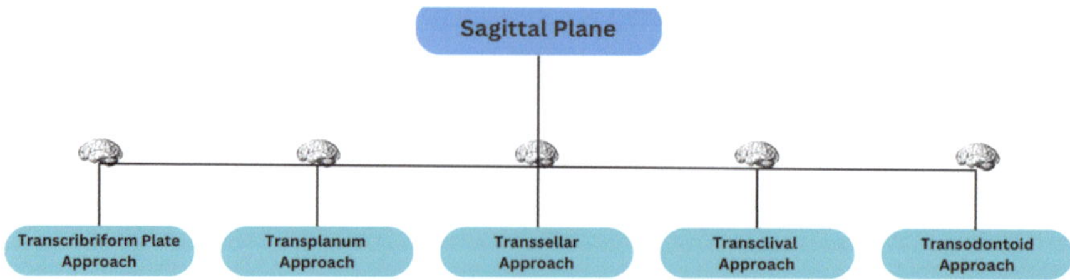

Fig. 4.1 Systematic delineation of the sagittal plane

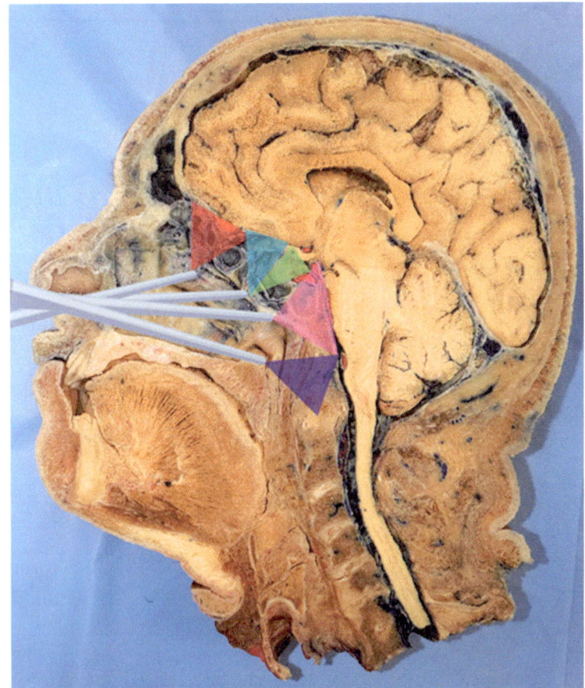

Fig. 4.2 Red: transcribriform plate approach, Blue: transplanum approach, Green: transsellar approach, Pink: transclival approach, Purple: transodontoid approach

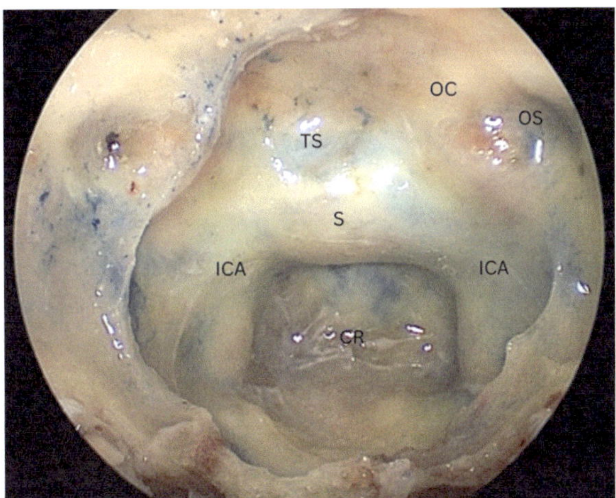

Fig. 4.3 *S* sellar, *TS* tuberculum sellae. *ON* optic nerve, *OS* optic strut, *ICA* internal carotid artery, *CR* clival recess

present, which necessitates the drilling of these structures to flatten the skull base. This process facilitates the passage of light through the area, providing better visibility of all the structures involved. Consequently, this enhanced visualization allows for the performance of an extended endoscopic endonasal approach (extended EEA) (Fig. 4.4).

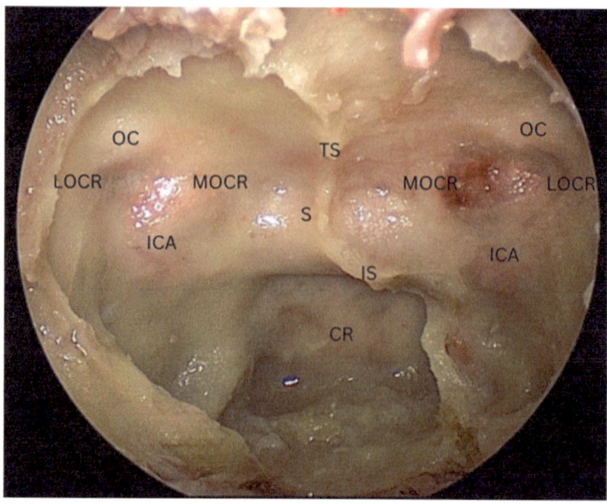

Fig. 4.4 *S* sellar, *TS* tuberculum sellae, *OC* optic canal, *MOCR* medial opticocarotid recess, *LOCR* lateral opticocarotid recess, *IS* intersphenoid septum, *ICA* internal carotid artery, *CR* clival recess

Surgical technique

When dealing with the paraclinoid segment of the internal carotid artery (ICA) dehiscence, utmost care must be exercised during the manipulation or removal of the mucosa. It is essential to avoid any damage to the carotid artery

The optic canal floor, situated between the roof of the *superior orbital fissure* (SOF), is found on the lateral wall of the sphenoid sinus. When using a speculum or cracking the side wall of the sphenoid sinus, one must be cautious not to injure the SOF as it could lead to double vision or diplopia.

The shaded area represents the region where bone removal is necessary to perform the transplanum and transtuberculum approaches. In these procedures, bone from the sellar region needs to be removed to access the area above the sellar, allowing for the retraction of the dura and pituitary gland. This enables the visualization of the back of the sellar or the suprasellar space and sometimes even the dorsal sellae.

Surgical technique

The author prefers carefully extracting the inner bone component of the lateral optic-carotid recess (LOCR) to free it from the surrounding bone, thereby providing access to the optic canal and carotid artery. This process involves meticulous skeletonization around the corner of the structure

When examining the middle clinoid region, which is located laterally to the sellar area and encompasses the carotid artery at the level of the paraclinoid segment, here we can observe the optic strut positioned below the optic nerve. In this case, it is pneumatized, allowing us to visualize the distal ring of the paraclinoid artery extending down from the optic strut into the suprasellar area. The suprasellar dura point is connected to the pituitary gland, while the internal carotid artery courses through the dura.

It is crucial to handle the bone carefully, especially the proximal ring ligament of the carotid artery, as it forms the lower portion of the optic strut, extending to the middle clinoid process (Figs. 4.5 and 4.6).

When exploring the suprasellar area, after opening the dura, one can proceed toward the optic canal direction, revealing the complete segment of the canal, spanning from the cisternal segment to the orbital portion. For tuberculum sellae meningiomas, it is often necessary to open the periosteum dura and subsequently remove the tumor from that location.

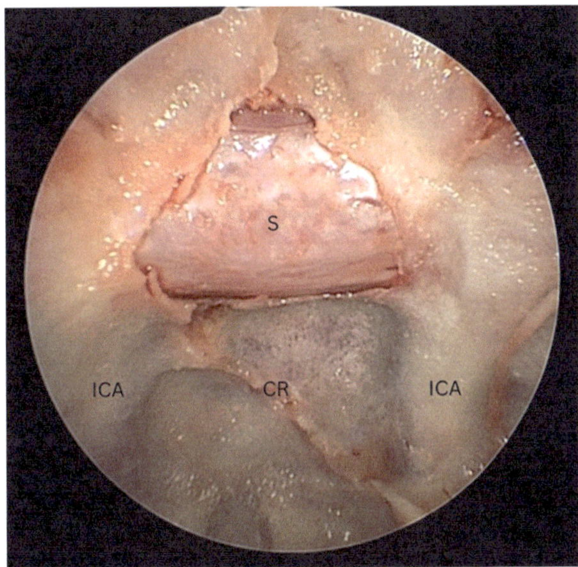

Fig. 4.5 *S* sellar, *ICA* internal carotid artery, *CR* clival recess

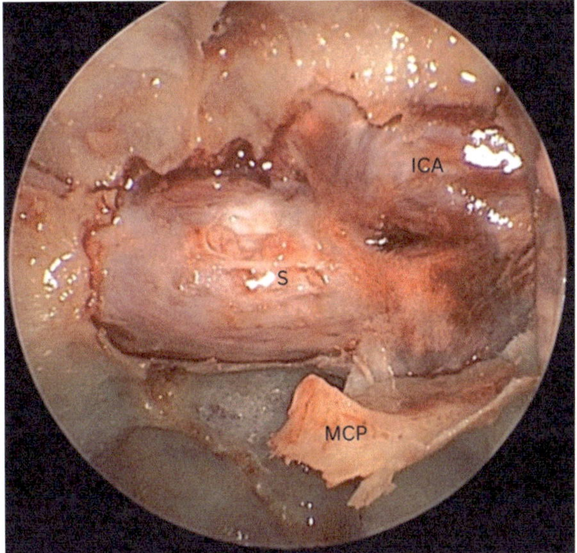

Fig. 4.6 *S* sellar, *ICA* internal carotid artery, *MCP* middle clinoid process

In normal patients, upon opening the dura at the suprasellar space, one would typically encounter the suprasellar arachnoid (Figs. 4.7 and 4.8).

Clinical application

In the case of meningiomas, the arachnoid may be pushed posteriorly due to tumor growth. During tumor removal, care should be taken to preserve the arachnoid and its associated vessels, especially the *superior hypophyseal artery* (SHA), which lies laterally to the arachnoid. It is essential to safeguard these structures during tumor resection to maintain vascular integrity (Fig. 4.9)

Craniopharyngiomas, on the other hand, tend to be located near the pituitary stalk, pushing anatomical structures against the dura. Therefore, when opening the dura in the suprasellar space for craniopharyngioma cases, one must be mindful of the SHA's location and the pituitary stalk to prevent inadvertent damage and potential risks to the patient's vision during the initial stages of the procedure

---

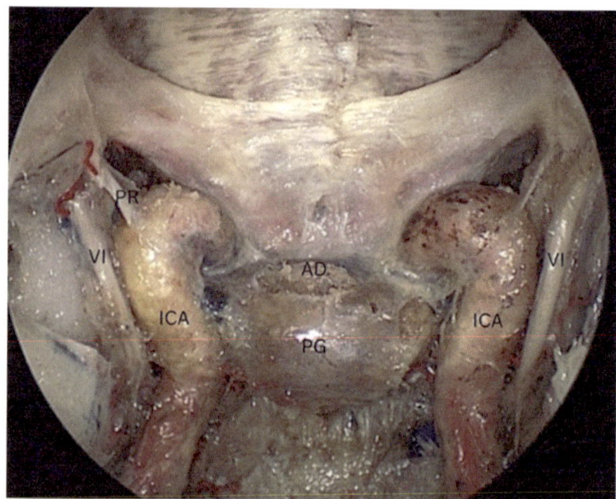

Fig. 4.7 *PR* proximal dural ring, *AD* arachnoid dura, *VI* CN VI, *PG* pituitary gland

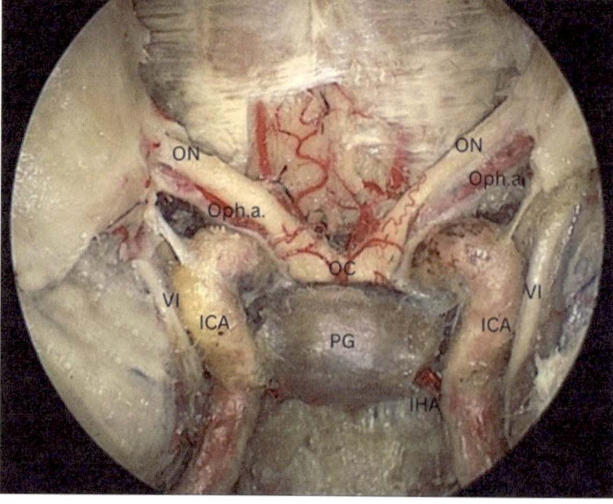

Fig. 4.8 *P* proximal dural ring, *PG* pituitary gland, *RON* rt optic nerve, *OC* optic chiasm, *LON* lt optic nerve, *Oph.a.* ophthalmic artery, *VI* CN VI, *IHA* inferior hypophyseal artery

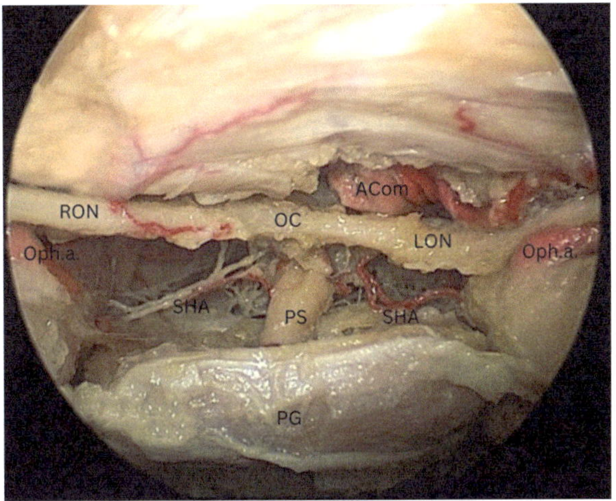

Fig. 4.9 *RON* rt optic nerve, *LON* lt optic nerve, *OC* optic chiasm, *SHA* superior hypophyseal artery, *Acom* anterior communicating aneurysm, *Oph.a* ophthalmic artery, *PG* pituitary gland

Upon opening the arachnoid, the following is the type of visualization that becomes available: the *pituitary stalk* becomes visible, and the dorsum sellae is observed with the pituitary gland being displaced downward, unobstructed by the bone in front of it. Within the corridor for the *suprasellar space*, the carotid artery can be seen, along with the ophthalmic artery arising and extending toward the *optic canal*. Both *optic nerves* and the *optic chiasm* can be observed bilaterally. Additionally, the frontal lobe and the anterior circulation, particularly the *anterior communicating artery* (ACom), are also visible (Fig. 4.9).

It is of utmost importance to note that the *superior hypophyseal artery*, the first branch of the carotid artery in the subarachnoid space, originates in the carotid cave region and extends toward the suprasellar space behind the arachnoid, subsequently supplying the pituitary stalk (Fig. 4.9). Within this region, there are chiasmatic branches that form small anastomoses to vascularize the optic chiasm. Additionally, recurrent vessels are present, coursing down toward the optic and diaphragmatic brain regions, aiding in the vascularization of the pituitary gland. This chiasmatic network, situated beneath the chiasm, is crucial for the vascular supply to the stalk as well.

Preserving the superior hypophyseal artery is of paramount importance not only for the proper functioning of the pituitary gland but also for maintaining the person's vision, ensuring visual acuity, and preventing any side-related deterioration.

4.2.2 Transcribriform Plate

In skull base anatomy, two critical structures are the *anterior ethmoidal artery (AEA)* and the *posterior ethmoidal artery (PEA)* (Fig. 4.10).

When performing a transplanum approach with the aim of preserving olfaction, it is crucial to remain posterior to the PEA. By doing so, one can effectively remove tumors from this area while avoiding damage to the olfactory function (Fig. 4.11).

Fig. 4.10 *CP* cribriform plate, *AEA* anterior ethmoidal artery, *PEA* posterior ethmoidal artery, *P* periorbita, *Pla* planum sphenoidale, *SOM* superior oblique muscle, *MRM* medial rectus muscle

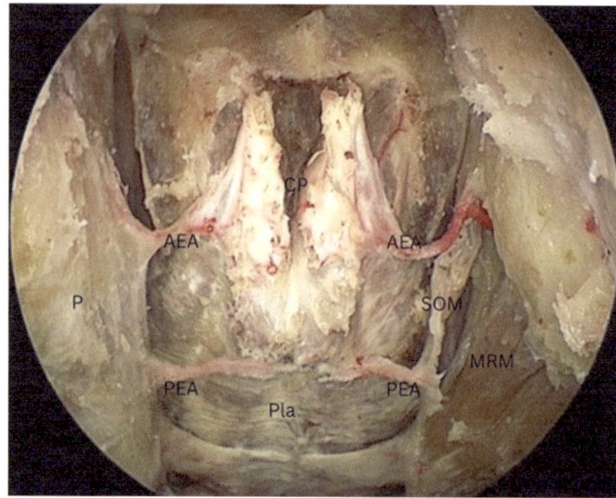

Fig. 4.11 *PEA* posterior ethmoidal artery, *Pla* planum sphenoidale, *ICA* internal carotid artery, *PG* pituitary gland

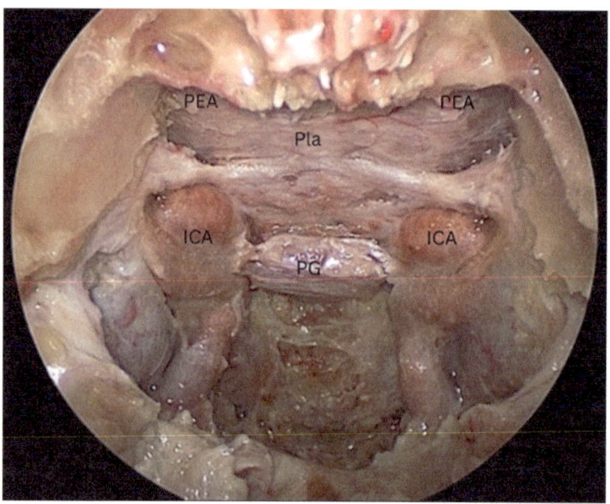

In cases where tumors involve the entire anterior skull base, such as esthesioblastoma or olfactory groove meningioma, a surgical technique involving the use of a bipolar coagulation device is employed. This method helps decrease the blood supply to the tumor before proceeding with tumor removal.

In cases where there is no intention to preserve olfactory function and the surgical approach involves accessing both sides of the anterior skull base, a procedure called Draf 3 is performed (Fig. 4.12). During this technique, the surgeon navigates around the septum and proceeds to open both frontal sinuses while communicating them with the frontal cribriform plate. Subsequently, all pieces of the frontal skull base, including the cribriform plate and crista galli, can be safely removed. With this approach, we achieve complete access to the frontal skull base, spanning from the lamina papyracea to the lamina papyracea.

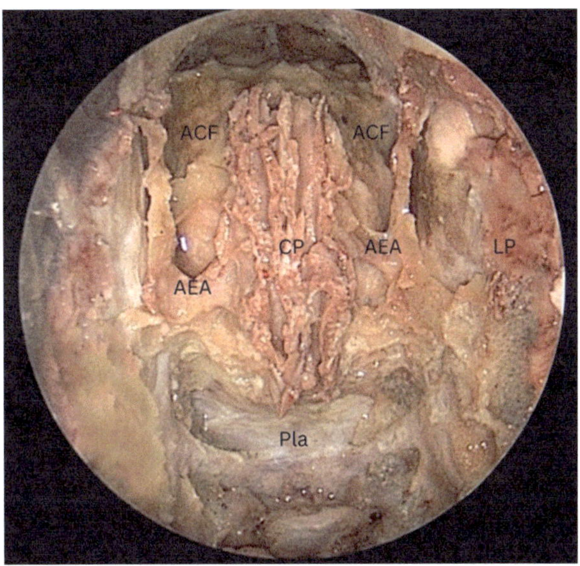

Fig. 4.12 *ACF* anterior cranial fossa, *AEA* anterior ethmoidal artery, *CP* cribriform plate, *Pla* planum sphenoidale, *LP* lamina papyracea

Surgical technique

The significance of the ethmoid artery is paramount. In the past, a double clip technique was employed to manage it. However, nowadays, a more meticulous approach involving careful bipolar coagulation is preferred. This method ensures controlled cutting, not too close to the orbit but leaving a small stump of the artery to prevent its extension into the orbit and the potential development of hematoma in the retrobulbar space. By adopting this careful bipolar coagulation and medial cutting technique, the risk of complications has been greatly minimized in recent years

4.2.2.1 Limitation

The limitations of endoscopic surgery for anterior skull base tumors are related to the extent of periorbital retraction that can be achieved [17]. Essentially, you cannot retract the periorbit more than half of its lateral aspect. As you proceed posteriorly or encounter tumors extending toward the top of the orbital apex laterally, the difficulty level increases significantly. This is due to the dense anatomical structures in the area, such as the optic nerve and the superior orbital fissure (SOF), which make it challenging to create enough space for retraction.

Moreover, when dealing with tumors that extend beyond the opposite side of the anterior clinoid process (ACP), it becomes a limitation for the endonasal approach. In such cases, accessing those regions with the endoscopic technique is not feasible.

However, in the mid-orbit region, anteriorly, you can certainly reach that level, as demonstrated by the yellow margin line. At this point, it is possible to retract the periorbit all the way, allowing for the removal of bone up to the midline or medial aspect of the orbit. Consequently, the endoscopic endonasal anterior skull base approach becomes an effective option for the removal of large tumors in this area.

It is important to note that the approach is limited to cases where the disease is situated laterally to the optic nerve. In such instances, caution must be exercised as attempting to proceed beyond this boundary would exceed the safe limits of the approach.

4.2.3   Transclival Approach

The posterior fossa can be divided into three levels: superior, medial, and inferior.

The *superior corridor* is associated with the superior turbinate and directs toward the sellar region and the pituitary gland. By passing through the dorsum sellae, access to the interpeduncular fossa is achieved. This space contains the Liliequist membrane and CN III, and its lateral limit is defined by the basilar artery, which further bifurcates into bilateral posterior cerebral arteries (PCAs) and gives rise to bilateral superior cerebellar arteries (SCAs). The mesencephalon is a part of the brainstem related to this level.

Moving on to the *medial corridor*, it involves the medial turbinate and runs from the floor of the sellar region to the curvature of the sphenoid rostrum or the roof of the choana.

The transclival approach is employed in this region, requiring the drilling of the clivus to access the dura of the posterior fossa, where the basilar plexus is situated. Upon reaching the dura, the prepontine cistern and basilar artery are encountered, with the sixth cranial nerve marking the lateral boundary. The pons itself is part of the brainstem related to this area.

It is essential to note that the medial corridor is not influenced by the pneumatization of the sphenoid as the pneumatization can vary. During a midclivectomy, one must extend the exposure down to the roof of the choana to ensure adequate visibility and freedom of movement during dissection toward the posterior fossa.

The *inferior corridor* is linked to the inferior turbinate and extends laterally toward the choana and the nasopharynx. This pathway allows access to the clivus, from the sphenoid rostrum down to the foramen magnum. Upon penetrating the dura, less blood is encountered from the basilar plexus compared to the upper portion and the retroclival area. Progressing further, the premedullary cistern is reached, where bilateral vertebral arteries and the twelfth cranial nerve are found laterally to the vertebral artery, marking the limit of this approach. The medulla itself is part of the brainstem involved at this level.

When embarking on an endonasal approach, the view encounter is critical. The superior corridor presents challenges involving the pituitary gland, which may exhibit compromised function. In such cases, the decision must be made whether to remove it entirely or opt for preservation while transposing the gland to a different location.

The middle transclival approach entails navigating from carotid to carotid, penetrating the dura to reach the prepontine cistern and the inferior segment. Essentially, the pathway extends below the lacerum foramen, allowing the removal of bone around the foramen magnum. Additionally, lateral expansion can be achieved through the supracondylar route or even via the condyle to gain proximal control over the vertebral artery. If necessary, further lateral expansion can be performed as needed.

The transclival approach is depicted. By accessing the superior aspect of the clivus and proceeding with transdorsum surgery, the interpeduncular fossa can be reached. The lateral boundary is defined by the presence of the third cranial nerve, while the mesencephalon is visible at the back of the interpeduncular fossa. The basilar artery bifurcates into the posterior cerebral artery and gives rise to the superior cerebellar artery. Depending on the specific case, lesions within this interpeduncular fossa can be approached by dissecting the pituitary gland, if needed.

During a midclivectomy, the lateral limit shifts to CN VI. Access to the prepontine cistern and the central region of the basilar artery becomes possible. It is crucial to optimize the opening by drilling and exposing the internal carotid artery at the paraclival area to achieve full access to the cistern posteriorly. Ensuring there is no residual bone left in the corridor helps maintain sufficient space for posterior dissection.

Proceeding inferiorly in the transclival approach, the visualization of the vertebral artery becomes evident, particularly at the vertebrobasilar junction (VBJ). CN VI lies more superiorly on the field, while CN XII is situated laterally to the vertebral artery, positioned more posteriorly. This information is essential for surgical planning.

Clinical application

When the disease is observed more laterally to the vertebral artery, it indicates a relationship with CN XII. On the other hand, cases where meningiomas are located medial to the vertebral artery can be approached using the inferior module of the transclival approach (Fig. 4.25)

Surgical technique

When performing surgery through the clivus, it is crucial to be prepared for potential findings like bleeding from the basilar plexus below the sellar region. To manage this, flowable hemostasis is used, and drilling is never performed without this precaution. Additionally, elevating the patient's head is beneficial in reducing venous pressure. This maneuver can be initiated at the beginning of the case to prevent increased pressure within the venous plexus

4.2.4 *Upper Clival Approach*

When considering the anatomy of the superior corridor, it is closely related to the pituitary gland and the sellar region. Of particular importance in this corridor are the OCR, the optic canal, and the paraclinoid segment of the internal carotid artery. Care must be taken with the paraclinoid artery due to the potential for dehiscence, and injuries can frequently occur in this region.

During the transclival to transdorsum approach for posterior fossa procedures, it is necessary to remove all the bone in this region to achieve optimal exposure posteriorly. Additionally, the middle clinoid process lies laterally to the sellar area. At the same time, the lateral portion of the tuberculum sellae is referred to as the medial opticocarotid recess (MOCR) (Fig. 4.4), located in a superior position [18].

Overall, understanding the anatomical structures and being cautious in these regions are vital when navigating the superior corridor. This approach allows for the excellent visualization of the pituitary gland and the surrounding sellar region, facilitating safe and effective surgical procedures.

4.3   Pituitary Transposition

In every instance of performing a posterior fossa approach through the dorsum sellae, the plan includes transposing the pituitary gland. To facilitate this, the bone in the planum and tuberculum regions is removed. This bone removal allows for the upward movement of the pituitary gland, creating the necessary space to navigate through the dorsum sellae and reach the interpeduncular fossa.

In this case, a series of bone removals were conducted to achieve exposure of the superior intercavernous sinus and the dura in the suprasellar area. The entire sellar region was thoroughly exposed, including the removal of the middle clinoid process dorsally to the carotid siphon at the paraclinoid area. It is essential to exercise caution throughout this process as the middle clinoid process can sometimes extend all the way around and form a ring encircling the internal carotid artery, potentially causing complications.

To avoid such issues, a preoperative evaluation using CTA (computed tomography angiography) is performed to ensure the absence of a ring-like formation. In approximately 4% of cases, such a ring may be present, and it is vital to identify this beforehand to prevent inadvertent carotid injury [19]. However, in most cases (96%), the projection of the middle clinoid process is limited to the dorsal aspect of the siphon, and with proper drilling and manipulation, it can be safely removed, leading to optimal exposure. This approach is also utilized during the exploration of the lateral cavernous sinus, where an endoscopic endonasal approach is employed.

Understanding the anatomy during the transposition of the pituitary gland is crucial. In this region, there are two layers of dura mater surrounding the pituitary gland. The meningeal layer of dura encases the gland, while the periosteal layer covers the lateral aspect of the sphenoid bone and extends into the sellar region, where it meets with the meningeal layer (Fig. 4.13).

Between these two layers lies the venous lake or intercavernous sinus, including the superior, inferior, and posterior cavernous sinuses. During the procedure, when opening the dura for pituitary transposition, one needs to carefully work between the tunica of the gland and the two layers of the dura in this area. Dissecting at this level, a conjunctiva-like tissue, known as the pituitary ligament, is encountered,

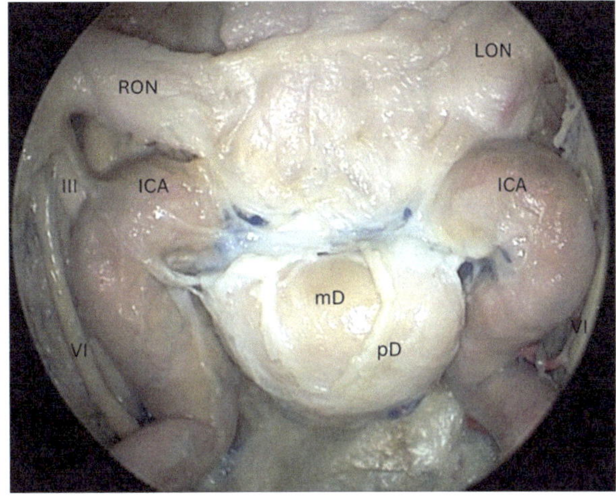

Fig. 4.13 *RON* rt optic nerve, *LON* lt optic nerve, *ICA* internal carotid artery, *mD* meningeal dura, *pD* periosteal dura, *III* cranial nerve III, *VI* cranial nerve VI

allowing dissection without entering the cavernous sinus and risking bleeding from that level.

Surgical technique

If bleeding occurs between the two dural layers, it is crucial not to use bipolar coagulation randomly. Instead, it is preferable to carefully collapse the two layers together, gently compressing and sealing them to prevent blood leakage from the cavernous sinus. Understanding this anatomical arrangement is essential for a successful pituitary gland transposition while minimizing the risk of complications during the procedure

---

Another important consideration during the process of moving the pituitary gland is to preserve the posterior pituitary gland's connection to the dura in the posterior part of the sellar region. By maintaining this connection, we aim to keep the posterior gland functional and reduce the likelihood of causing diabetes insipidus (DI) as a complication

In the provided anatomical image, you can observe the connective tissue known as the *pituitary ligament*, which is a meningeal layer closely associated with the pituitary gland. Additionally, you can see the periosteal layer in contact with the bone. A gap exists between these layers, providing access to the cavernous sinus (Fig. 4.14).

If bleeding occurs from this area, it is important to address it effectively. This can be achieved by collapsing the two layers together using bipolar coagulation or employing flowable hemostasis to fill the gap.

During the dissection, the author carefully works around the pituitary gland, ensuring both layers are kept intact. Once the floor is cut with the two layers together, the pituitary gland can be gently moved posteriorly, allowing for the preservation of the posterior dura, along with the gland. This approach aims to safeguard the posterior pituitary function and minimize the risk of postoperative complications, leading to more successful outcomes for the patient.

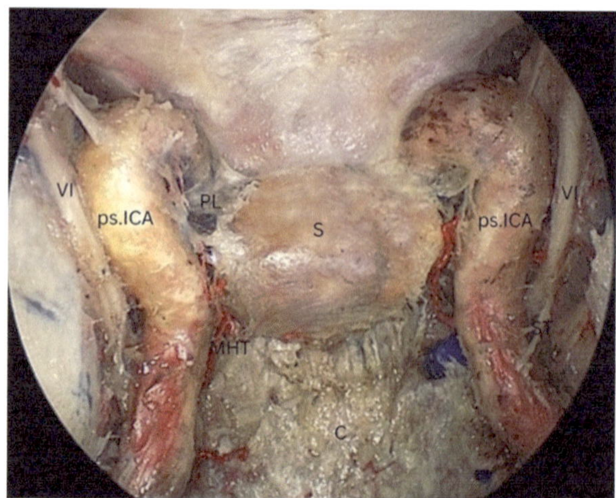

Fig. 4.14 *psICA* parasellar ICA, *VI* cranial nerve VI, *PL* pituitary ligament, *S* sellar, *MHT* meningohypophyseal, runk, *C* clivus

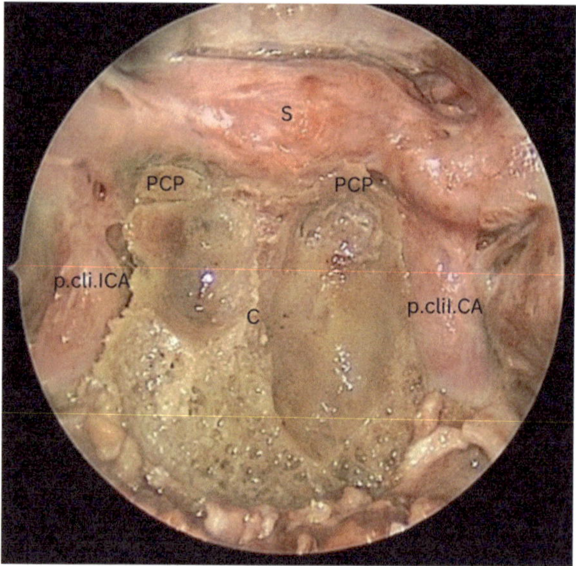

Fig. 4.15 *S* sellar, *PCP* posterior clinoid process, *p.cli.ICA* paraclival ICA, *C* clivus

Finally, the technique to elevate and fully expose the dorsum sellae is executed. At this stage, the posterior clinoid process is reached, and after removing the dorsum sellae, the posterior clinoid process can also be excised (Figs. 4.15, 4.16, 4.17, and 4.18).

Fig. 4.16 *Lat.CS* lateral cavernous sinus, *Med.CS* medial cavernous sinus, *S* sellar, *PCP* posterior clinoid process

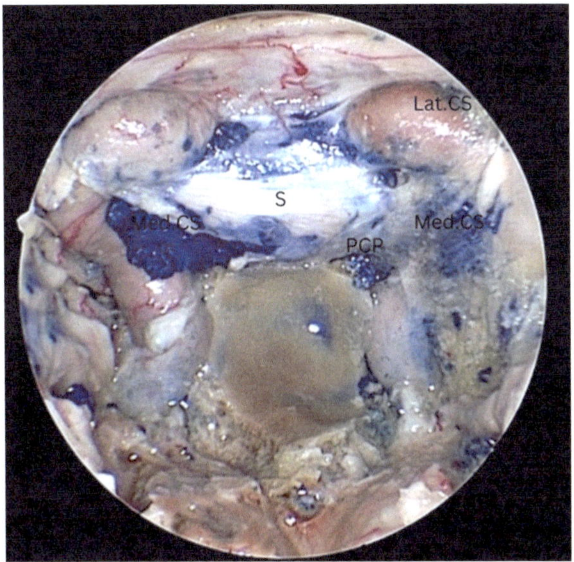

Fig. 4.17 *S* sellar, *PCP* posterior clinoid process, *ICA* internal carotid artery, *DS* dorsum sellae, *Med.CS* medial cavernous sinus

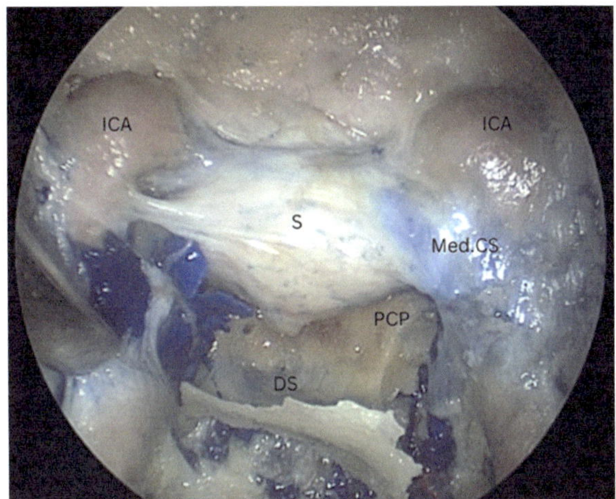

Surgical technique

It is essential to approach the removal of the dorsum sellae with a specific technique, avoiding attempting to remove it en bloc. Instead, the preferred method involves breaking it into at least two pieces. This is achieved through a dissection movement from lateral to medial while simultaneously moving the posterior clinoid process away from the carotid artery and CN III, which courses toward the cavernous sinus immediately lateral to the apex of the posterior clinoid process. Once the dorsum sellae is successfully divided into two pieces, internal mobilization is performed, allowing for the opening of the dura to access the interpeduncular fossa. This approach ensures a controlled and safe procedure while achieving complete exposure to the target area

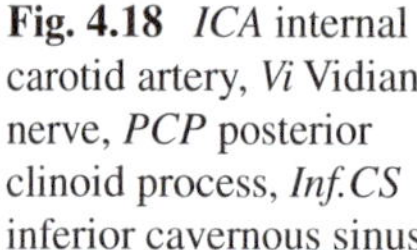

Fig. 4.18 *ICA* internal carotid artery, *Vi* Vidian nerve, *PCP* posterior clinoid process, *Inf.CS* inferior cavernous sinus

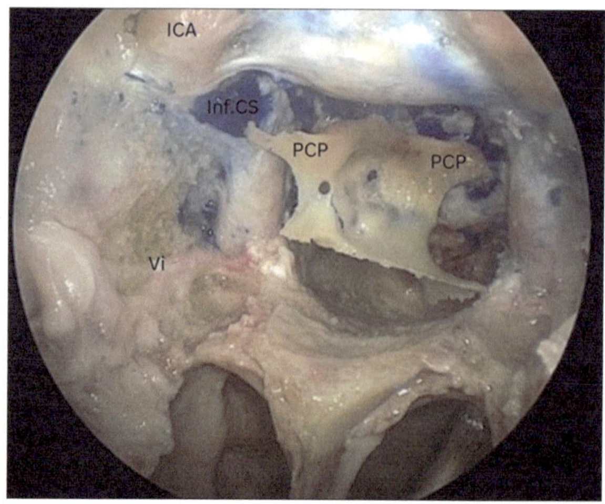

This visualization provides a clear view of CN III laterally, along with the basilar artery ascending, the superior cerebellar arteries (SCA) on both sides, and the P1 segment of the posterior cerebral artery (PCA). Additionally, a normal posterior communicating artery (Pcom) is observed parallel to the third cranial nerve, while the fetal variant of the left P1 segment is evident in the specimen. Furthermore, the P2 segment extends laterally in the view. This perspective offers a glimpse of the mammillary body of the mesencephalon and the perforator branches above the basilar artery, a crucial and noteworthy region.

This corridor provides one of the finest approaches to visualizing this region, particularly the mammillary body. It offers an advantageous angle to address and resect tumors that may be attached to highly delicate structures with direct and optimal visualization.

Right now, surgeons often prefer using a method called pituitary hemitransposition. This method is favored because there have been reports of complications when both sides of the inferior hypophyseal artery are treated with coagulation [20] (Fig. 4.19).

4.3.1 Middle Clival Approach

The crucial aspect of the anatomy in this context is the carotid artery, and the goal is to navigate between the ICA (Fig. 4.20). Achieving a comprehensive exposure becomes essential, and thus, we proceed to skeletonize the carotid artery to remove any residual bone hindering the optimal visibility of the posterior fossa. The lateral boundary is determined by *CN VI*, and any pathology within the interpeduncular fossa can be accessed through this approach.

Fig. 4.19 *PG* pituitary gland, *VI* cranial nerve VI, *IHA* inferior hypophyseal artery

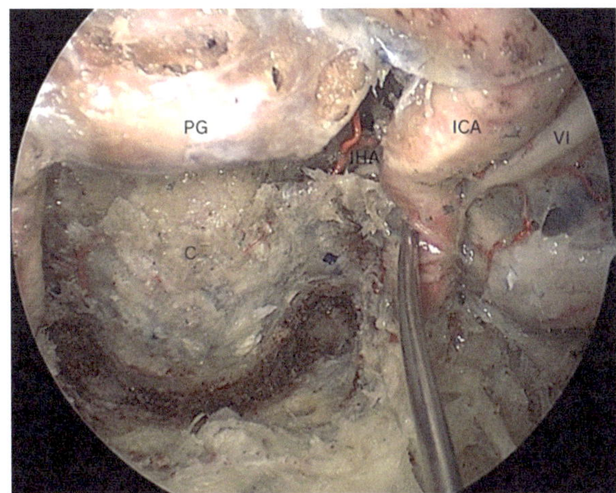

Fig. 4.20 *PG* pituitary gland, *pcli.ICA* paraclival ICA, *med.C* medial clivus, *low.C* lower clivus

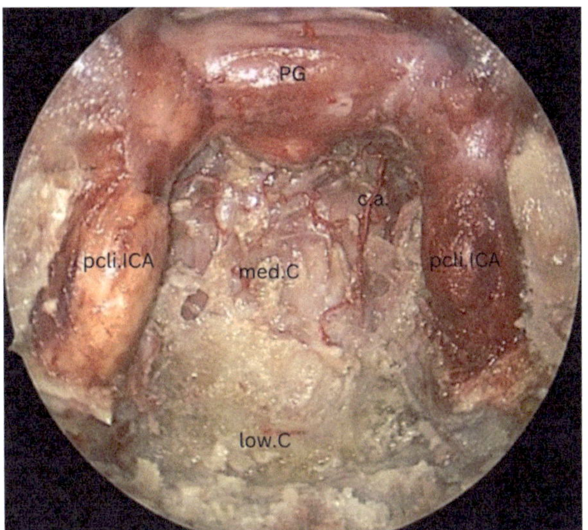

The author always prioritizes paying close attention to CN VI during procedures. CN VI can sometimes be located slightly more medial as it courses through the medial meningeal layer of the dura and enters the intradural space. In certain cases, it may extend and travel near the inferior petrosal sinus before passing through Dorello's canal (Figs. 4.21 and 4.22).

To locate CN VI, the author relies on anatomical knowledge as the primary guide. Additionally, we meticulously open the area in a progressive and medial direction. This allows us to gain a comprehensive understanding of the disease process, which may lead to the compression and displacement of CN VI toward the midline. By adopting this approach, the author aims to avoid any potential complications in this sensitive region.

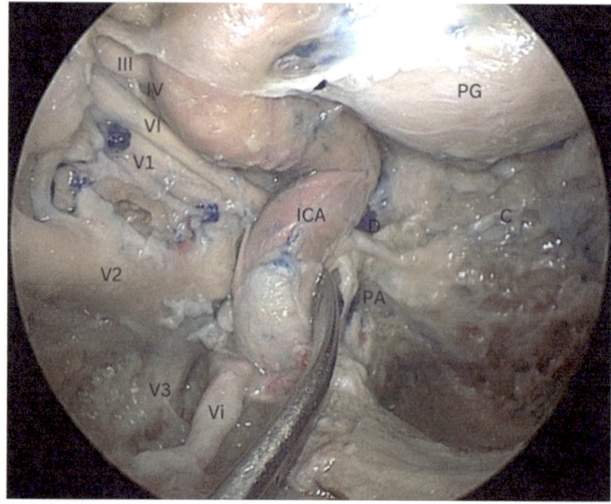

Fig. 4.21 *PG* pituitary gland, *PA* petrous apex, *D* dorello's canal, *ICA* internal carotid artery, *C* clivus

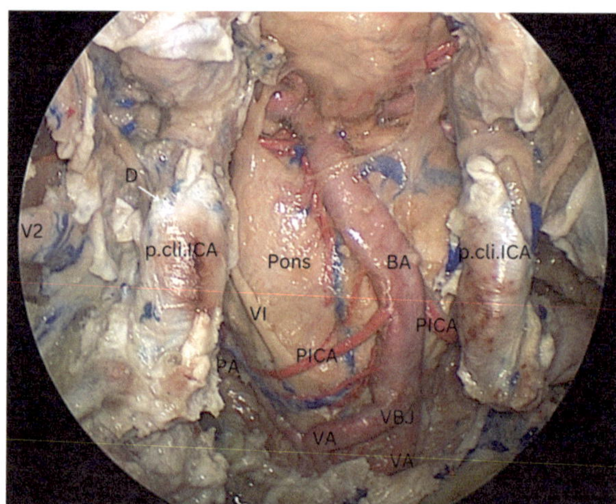

Fig. 4.22 *BA* basilar artery, *D* dorello's canal, *p.cli.ICA* paraclival ICA, *VBJ* vertebrobasilar junction, *VA* vertebral artery

Surgical technique

During procedures, the author employs dural stimulation and monitors CN VI closely. This is particularly important in transclival approaches as the most medial nerve is at risk. By using stimulation, the author can identify the region where no response is elicited before opening the dura

In terms of anatomy, when observing the basilar artery, the sixth cranial nerve lies above the vertebrobasilar junction (VBJ). When continuing to drill the bone and opening the dura, the author aims to reach as low as possible below the VBJ. In this process, the author utilizes imaging guidance, such as CTA (computed tomography angiography), to pinpoint the precise location to safely perform the procedure, minimizing the risk of damaging the sixth cranial nerve. This careful approach ensures the preservation of crucial neural structures and contributes to the overall success and safety of the surgery

4.3.2   Inferior Clival Approach and Craniocervical Junction

When conducting the inferior third of the approach, it is important to navigate through the choana. On occasion, patients may exhibit an enlarged tonsil barrier, which could impede lateral space and hinder access to the posterior fossa. In such instances, a minor shaving of the tonsil barrier might become necessary to establish adequate lateral space. Nevertheless, in the majority of patients, there exists ample space between the tonsil barrier and the target area in the posterior fossa, thereby facilitating a seamless passage. Furthermore, the presence of the inferior turbinate serves as a valuable landmark to direct you toward your intended area of focus.

One important consideration during this stage is to be cautious of a normal anatomical tendency. As you drill in a southward direction toward the foramen magnum, there is a natural inclination for the drilling to move anteriorly. This occurs due to the occipital condyle at the anterior portion of the foramen magnum. The condyles start in the middle or midway of the foramen magnum and almost meet each other anteriorly, leaving only a small space between them (Figs. 4.23 and 4.24).

Fig. 4.23 *fl* foramen lacerum, *PM* prevertebral muscle

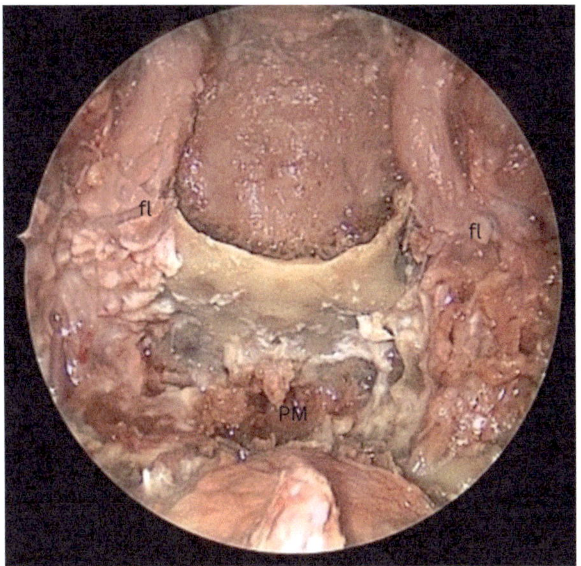

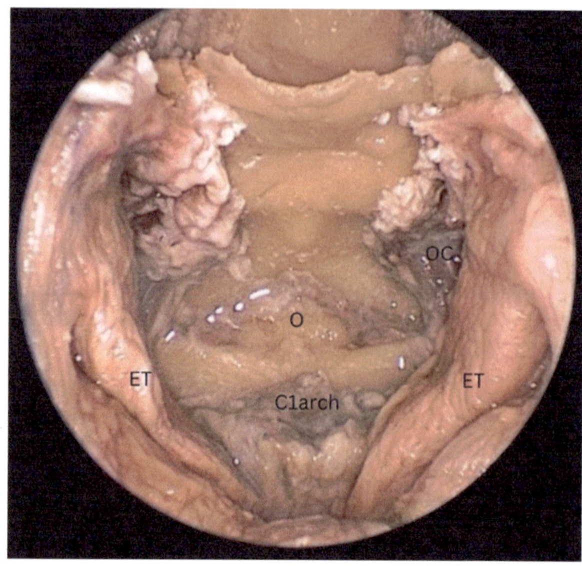

Fig. 4.24 *ET* eustachian tube, *O* odontoid, *OC* occipital condyle

Surgical technique

To avoid any complications, we aim not to enter the capsule in between the first cervical vertebra (C1) and the occipital condyle. Instead, we carefully drill in a manner that avoids this region while ensuring safe and effective progress. However, in some instances, the proximal control of the vertebral artery becomes necessary, requiring further drilling laterally into the occipital bone. This procedure is referred to as supracondylectomy

In other situations, there may be a need to take out the condyle itself, known as medial condylectomy. This involves entering the space between the occipital condyle and drilling through the bone in this area. Special care is taken to avoid drilling articularly, termed supraarticular condylectomy, preserving the jugular vein while removing a portion of the bone. By employing these precise techniques, we can safely access and address the target area while preserving vital structures and ensuring favorable outcomes.

This approach provides complete exposure, allowing us to visualize the target area, extending posteriorly through the hypoglossal canal (Fig. 4.25). By including the supracondylar region, we also gain access to the jugular tubercle. This expanded view lets us visualize CN VII and CN VIII as they enter the internal acoustic canal. Additionally, the anterior inferior cerebellar artery (AICA) can be observed in this region. Overall, this approach provides an excellent visualization of the anatomy in the inferior portion of the ventral posterior fossa, offering a comprehensive view of surgical procedures.

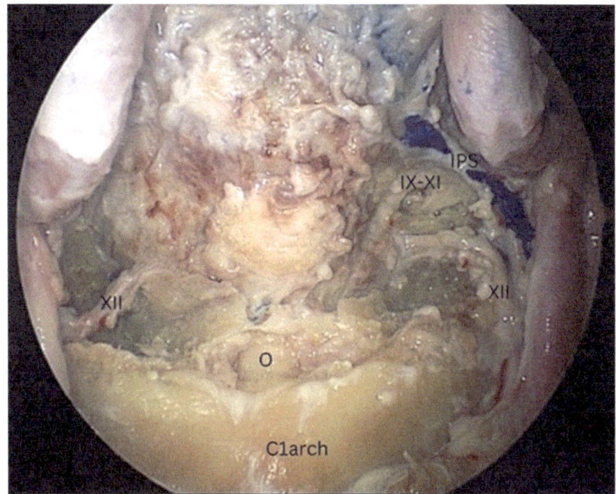

Fig. 4.25 *IPS* inferior petrosal sinus, *IX-XI* CN IX, X, XI, *XII* CN XII (hypoglossal nerve), *O* odontoid

4.3.3 Transodontoid Approach

This technique is employed in cases of rheumatoid arthritis, basilar invagination, or foramen magnum meningioma, involving the removal of nasopharyngeal mucosa from the spheno-clival junction to the soft palate level. A navigator positioned medially to the eustachian tube, due to the posterolateral location of the parapharyngeal artery, can provide assistance. Occasionally, an enlarged carotid artery might be encountered in the nasopharynx. The extent of bone removal depends on the specific pathology and necessitates an evaluation of craniocervical stability. Additionally, an endoscopic view can be utilized to approach down to the level of C2 (Fig. 4.24).

The anatomy and limitations for EEA to sagittal plane skull base are summarized in Table 4.1.

Table 4.1 Summary of anatomy and indications for EEA to the sagittal plane of skull base

Approach	Bone	Cistern	Brain	Cranial nerve	Vessel	Common pathologies
Cribriform	Cribriform plate, crista galli	Interhemispheric fissure	Gyrus rectus, Orbitofrontal gyrus	Olfactory	A2, Frontopolar, orbitofrontal artery	Olfactory groove meningiomas, esthesioblastomas, encephaloceles, CSF leaks, sinonasal tumors
Transplanum, transtuberculum	Planum sphenoidale, Tuberculum, Planum, Optic strut, Medial clinoid	Suprasellar cistern, prechiasmatic cistern	Gyrus rectus, Orbitofrontal gyrus	Optic nerve, optic chiasm	Anterior circle of Willis	Planum meningiomas, suprasellar pituitary macroadenoma, Craniopharyngioma, optic nerve gliomas
Transellar	Upper third Of clivus, Posterior clinoid, Dorsum sellae	Suprasellar cistern, anterior recess to third ventricle, basilar cistern, interpeduncular cistern	Uncus, hypothalamus, Infundibulum, mammillary body, Middle cerebral peduncles	II, III, VI	Basilar apex, P1, Pcom, P2, perforators, SCA	Retrosellar craniopharyngioma, Pituitary macroadenomas, petroclival meningiomas
Transclival and cranial-vertebral junction	Clivus, petrous apex, Dorello's canal, Foramen magnum, medial occipital condyle	Prepontine cistern, ponto-medullary cistern	Ventral pon, medulla	V, VI, VII, VIII, IX, X, XI, XII	Midbasilar, AICA, VBJ, Medullary, Perforator, Vertebral artery	Petroclival meningiomas, Chordomas, Chondrosarcomas, sinonasal tumors, Foramen magnum meningiomas
Transodontoid	Foramen magnum, Ring of C1, Odontoid, Upper body of C2	Caudal, Extension of ponto-medullary cistern	Cervico-medullary junction, Vertebral cervical spinal cord at C1 and C2	XI	Vertebral artery at intradural insertion, anterior spinal arteries	Rheumatoid arthritis/ basilar invagination, foramen magnum meningioma

4.4 Coronal Plane

Understanding the segmentation of the carotid artery is crucial for precise anatomical localization [21] (Fig. 4.26). Several landmarks play a significant role in identifying different segments:

1. In the ascend carotid, parasagittal, and parapharyngeal areas, *the eustachian tube* is the primary landmark. It not only provides orientation but also protects the carotid artery at this level.
2. The *vidian nerve* marks the level of the horizontal portion of the carotid artery. It is essential to differentiate between the vidian nerve and the Paraclival Carotid Artery as the vidian nerve indicates the position of the carotid artery concealed within the petrous bone [22] (Figs. 4.27 and 4.28).
3. The *medial pterygoid muscle* serves as a key reference point for the vertical position of the paraclival carotid artery. By drawing a vertical line, the position of the paraclival carotid artery and the anterior genu of the internal carotid artery, along with the location of the lacerum foramen, can be determined.
4. The *MOCR* serves as a marker for the location of the paraclinoid carotid artery. Familiarity with these landmarks aids in precisely locating and navigating the carotid artery in various segments of the anatomy [18].

The relationship between anatomical landmarks and segments of ICA were summarized in Table 4.2.

All of these approaches necessitate a broader lateral extension. To facilitate this, it is essential to carry out antrostomy, which involves creating an opening in the maxillary sinus. This allows for easier access to the posterior wall of the maxilla and provides a more extensive surgical field for the procedures.

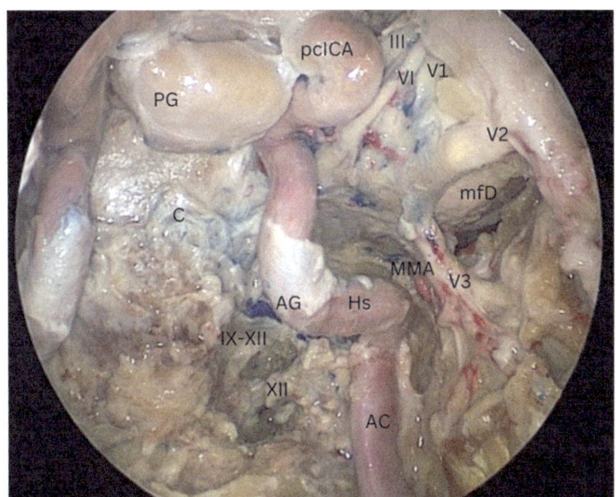

Fig. 4.26 *PG* pituitary gland, *C* clivus, *pcICA* paraclinoid ICA, *AG* anterior genu, *HS* horizontal petrous segment, *AC* ascending carotid, *mfD* middle fossa dura, *MMA* middle meningeal artery, *III* CN III, *IV* CN IV, *V1*: CN V1, *V2* CN V2, *V3* CN V3, *VI* CN VI, *IX–XI* CN IX, X, XI, *XII* CN XII

Fig. 4.27 *fl* foramen lacerum, *Vi* vidian nerve, *V2* CN V2

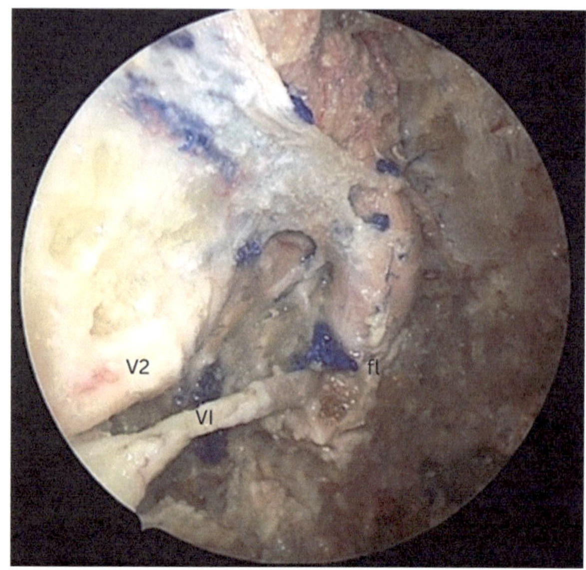

Fig. 4.28 *PG* pituitary gland, *ICA* internal carotid artery, *ST* sympathetic trunk, *Vi* vidian nerve

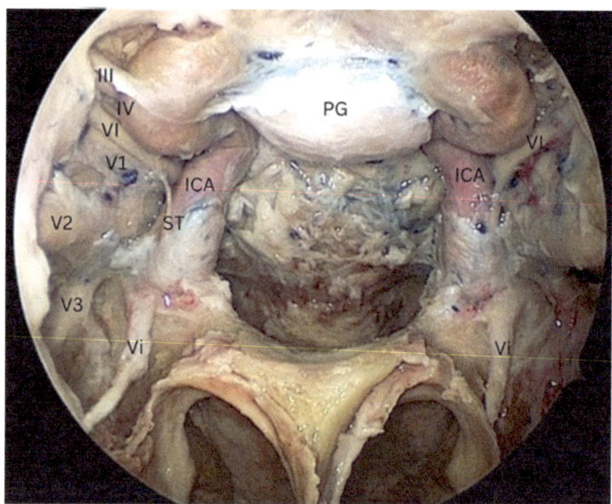

Table 4.2 The relationship between anatomical landmarks and segments of ICA

Segment	Anatomic landmark
Paraclinoid	Medial OCR
Anterior genu	Medial pterygoid
Horizontal petrous segment	Vidian nerve
Ascending carotid	Eustachian tube

To access the pterygoid area, the *pterygopalatine fossa* is a crucial landmark for this approach [10]. Therefore, we utilize the transpterygoid approach to access the lateral skull base. Within the pterygopalatine fossa, it is essential to note that the internal maxillary artery (Fig. 4.34) is located more superficially and internally than the nerve and ganglion, which are situated posteriorly. During this procedure, we carefully cut the palatine artery and nerve more medially as these structures lead to the roof of the choana. By doing so, we can effectively lateralize the contents of the pterygopalatine fossa and attain a clear view of the vidian nerve positioned more posteriorly.

This view provides a comprehensive look at the area beneath the vidian nerve, observed from an inferior perspective (Fig. 4.27). The vidian nerve can be seen as it courses toward the carotid artery, serving as a landmark for the horizontal segment of the artery. Additionally, V3 can be observed traversing through the foramen ovale, while V2 takes an anterior path toward the rotundum. There is a smaller nerve next to the palatinovaginal artery known as the palatinovaginal nerve, which we carefully cut to expose the pterygopalatine fossa (Fig. 4.29). This clear visualization showcases the vidian nerve, with the palatine vaginal nerve situated just adjacent to it on the right side. On occasion, vidian transposition may be considered as a viable option, contingent upon its necessity [23].

When approaching this area through the nostril, it is crucial to have a clear understanding of the vidian nerve's position. As the nerve travels more posteriorly, it tends to shift laterally, marking the position of the horizontal carotid artery. This region is often referred to as the "wedge" (Fig. 4.30). Awareness of this anatomical arrangement is essential for a safe and effective endonasal approach.

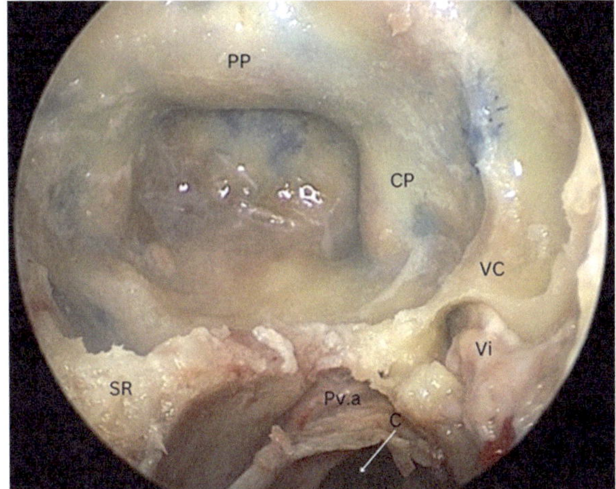

Fig. 4.29 *SR* sphenoid rostrum, *PP* pituitary protuberance, *CP* carotid protuberance, *VC* vidian canal, *Vi* vidian nerve, *Pv.a*: palatovaginal artery

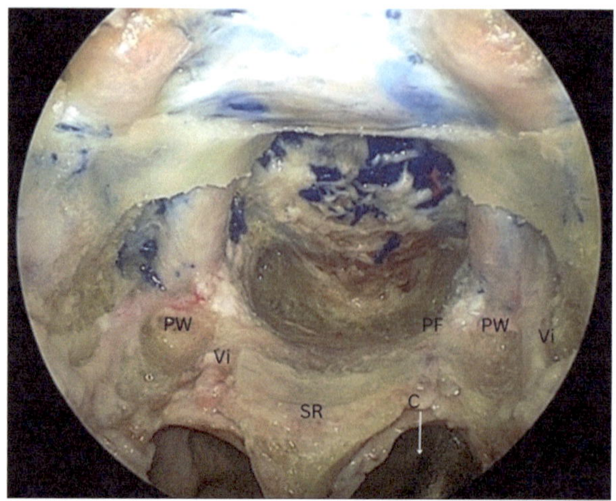

Fig. 4.30 *PW* pterygoid wedge, *Vi* vidian nerve, SP: sphenoid rostrum, *C* choana, *PF* pharyngobasilar fascia

---

Surgical technique

Once the position of the vidian nerve is identified, the drilling is carried out from the lower aspect of the nerve, roughly from 3 to 9 o'clock. This approach allows for the preservation of the undersurface of the petrous area while facilitating the detection of the lacerum foramen. Additionally, we utilize the base of the pharyngeal fascia, which is attached to the bone, to guide our path toward the lacerum foramen. This combined approach, following the course of the vidian nerve and the fascia, provides the precise localization of the lacerum foramen, enabling a safe and effective resection procedure related to the petrous apex

---

The coronal plane is delineated into seven specific zones to facilitate comprehension and potential applications: (1) petrous apex approach, (2) intrapetrous approach, (3) suprapetrous approach, (4) cavernous sinus approach, (5) infratemporal approach, (6) medial condyle approach, (7) jugular foramen approach (Fig. 4.31).

4.4.1 Zone I Petrous Apex Approach

The petrous apex approach is a unique method that allows access to the area without necessarily requiring the transposition or cutting of the vidian nerve. While it shares some aspects with the transsphenoidal approach, it extends posteriorly to reach the carotid artery and can proceed laterally behind this vessel. To achieve this, precise drilling is essential to locate the lacerum foramen, after which the drilling is extended posteriorly to reach the area behind the carotid artery. This approach offers a valuable alternative for accessing the petrous apex region with minimized disruption to the vidian nerve.

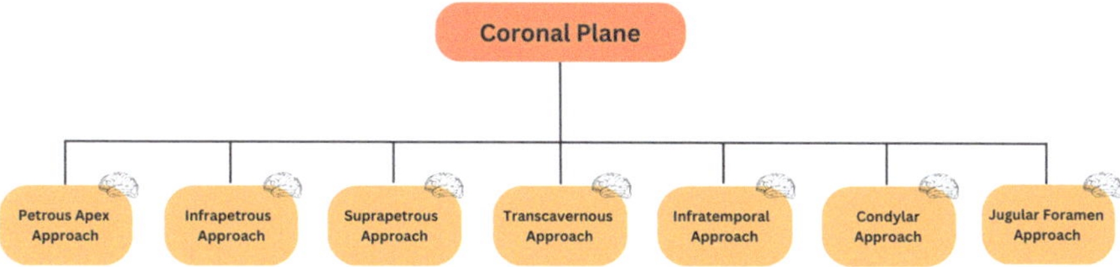

Fig. 4.31 Systematic delineation of the coronal plane

Fig. 4.32 *ICA* internal carotid artery, *VI* CN VI, *Q* Quadrangular space

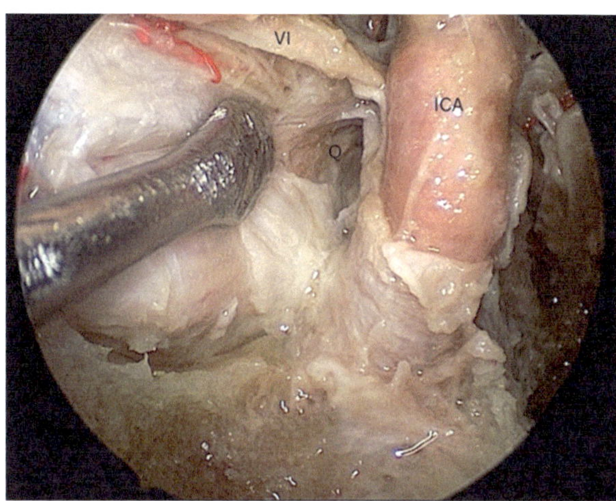

4.4.2 Zone II Infrapetrous Approach

The intrapetrous approach involves addressing the inferior petrous artery. It is crucial to precisely drill the petrous clivus, paying attention to areas affected by chondrosis.

4.4.3 Zone III Suprapetrous Approach

The suprapetrous approach is also known as *the quadrangular space* or the front door of Meckel's cave [24, 25] (Figs. 4.32 and 4.33).

The quadrangular space, also known as the anterolateral triangle of the skull base, is located between the paraclival carotid artery, the petrous carotid artery, and the medial aspect of the gasserian ganglion, typically at the level of V2 or V3. By accessing this space, you can be medial to the gasserian ganglion or utilize the area between V2 and V3 to reach the anterolateral triangle of the skull base. Additionally,

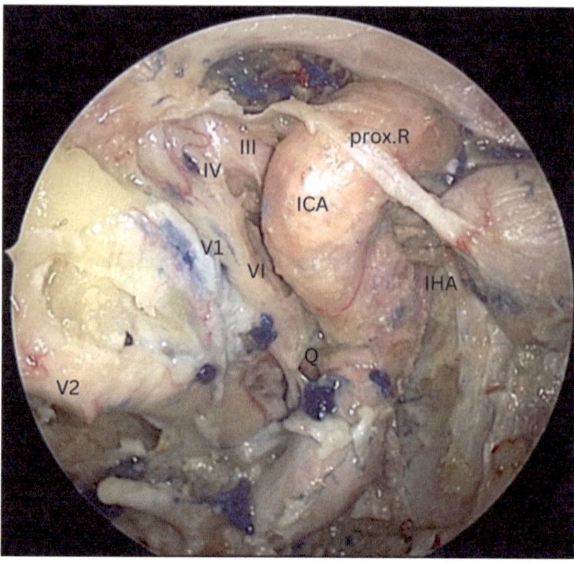

Fig. 4.33 *Prox.R* proximal dural ring, *IHA* inferior hypophyseal artery, *Q* quadrangular space, *III* CN III, *IV* CN IV, *VI* CN VI, *V1* CN V1, *V2* CN V2

you can also utilize the space between V2 and V1, known as the anteromedial triangle, and expand the dissection into the middle cranial fossa. This approach allows for effective access to various structures within the skull base.

4.4.4 Zone IV Cavernous Sinus Approach

This area is closely related to the cavernous sinus, and direct dissection within the cavernous sinus is a rare procedure. However, in certain situations, it might be necessary to approach the region above CN VI to access specific pathologies located within the cavernous sinus. When attempting to navigate the narrow space lateral to the carotid artery and above CN VI, pathology within the cavernous sinus becomes essential to justify such an approach [26].

The medial compartment of the cavernous sinus is characterized by its spaciousness, positioned medially to the carotid artery, and remarkably lacks cranial nerves. In contrast, the cranial nerves, including CN III, IV, VI, V1, and V2, are situated more laterally within the lateral compartment of the cavernous sinus (Fig. 4.33). Owing to its considerable dimensions, the medial compartment frequently becomes a target for tumor invasion, particularly when tumors originate from the pituitary region. Consequently, this presents an exceptional opportunity for performing dissection in this region, especially for the purpose of tumor removal and exploration.

The carotid artery exhibits a lateral curvature prior to its entry into the intracranial region through its distal ring. Within the medial expanse of the cavernous sinus, the sole significant anatomical structure observed is the inferior hypophyseal artery. Originating from the meningohypophyseal trunk (MHT) (Fig. 4.14), this artery courses toward the pituitary gland. The clinical relevance of this area becomes evident in cases involving tumors situated in this region. Such tumors can lead to the lateral expansion of the carotid artery, necessitating a cautious approach during surgical maneuvers.

It is of utmost importance to avoid blind grasping in this region as it could pose the risk of avulsing the meningohypophyseal trunk or creating an opening in the internal carotid artery. However, in cases where the tumor can be safely suctioned, a precise pathway can be followed into the space, ensuring a secure procedure.

Clinical application

When dealing with a tumor that significantly expands the medial compartment of the cavernous sinus, it can lead to the exposure of CN VI at the posterior region. A clear example of this is seen in the picture of Dorello's canal, where the sixth cranial nerve runs just inferior to the group of ligaments. In cases of very large tumors that extensively involve the medial compartment of the cavernous sinus, CN VI can become vulnerable in this area. As a precautionary measure, it is essential to be cautious about the inferior and lateral aspects of the surgical field to avoid compromising CN VI. For this reason, monitoring CN VI becomes crucial during the surgical planning process, especially when approaching closer to the cavernous sinus

---

4.4.5   Zone V Infratemporal Approach

The temporal access or infratemporal access is a surgical approach utilized through the endonasal approach (Fig. 4.34).

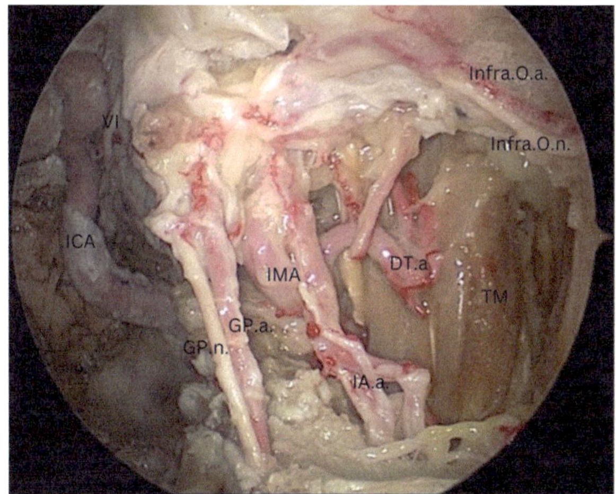

Fig. 4.34 *GP.a.* greater palatine artery, *GP.n.* greater palatine nerve, *IMA* internal maxillary artery, *IA.a.* internal alveolar artery, *DT.a.* deep temporal artery, *TM* temporalis muscle, *Infra.O.a.* infraorbital artery, *Infra.O.a.* infraorbital nerve

4.4.6   Zone VI Condylar Approach

Medial condylectomy, a surgical procedure, is employed under specific circumstances to achieve access to or the proximal control of the vertebral artery.

Surgical technique

In cases involving foramen magnum meningioma, where the proximal control of both vertebral arteries is required, a strategic approach involves the meticulous drilling of the medial aspects of both condyles. This meticulous approach enhances exposure and facilitates complete access to the foramen magnum, particularly for the purpose of proximal vertebral artery control. It is imperative to exercise caution as neglecting this facet of the procedure may inadvertently result in drilling that veers toward the fundal direction. Such an outcome could potentially lead to narrowing when progressing inferiorly in the direction of the foramen magnum. Therefore, it is crucial to extend the drilling procedure toward the medial aspect of the condyle to prevent this occurrence

---

4.4.7   Zone VII Jugular Foramen Approach

Upon directing our focus toward the jugular foramen, this approach strategically facilitates ingress into the cervical region.

Chondrosarcoma tumor, for instance, characterized by its expansion originating from the petroclival synchondrosis toward the cervical area and following ICA to the jugular vein, this technique offers a means to pursue this trajectory effectively, ultimately enabling access to the cervical compartment.

The indication and limitation for EEA to the coronal plane skull base are summarized in Table 4.3.

Table 4.3 Summary of indications and limitations for EEA to the coronal plane of the skull base

Approach	Anatomical landmark	Limitation	Pathologies
Petrous apex	Vidian nerve, foramen lacerum	CN V, VI, ICA	Cholesterol granuloma
Infrapetrous	Inferior petrous artery, petroclival region	CN V, VI, ICA	Chondrosarcoma, chordoma, Meningioma
Suprapetrous	Quadrangular space, anteromedial triangle	CN V, VI, ICA	Schwannoma
Transcavernous	Posterior ethmoid sinus LOCR, carotid protuberance	CN III, IV, V, VI, ICA	Cavernous sinus tumor
Infratemporal	Lateral pterygoid plate, foramen ovale	Lateral pterygoid muscle, levator veli palatini muscle, Cervical carotid artery	Infratemporal fossa tumor
Condylar	Medial condyle	XII, vertebral artery	Foramen magnum meningioma
Jugular foramen	Jugular foramen, Eustachian tube	IX, X, XI, vertebral artery, jugular vein	Chordoma, chondrosarcoma

4.5 Conclusion

The transsellar approach allows access to the OCR for extended EEA, preserving critical structures, and the SHA for pituitary function and vision protection. The transcribriform plate is crucial for olfaction preservation during the transplanum approach, while the Draft 3 approach provides access to both sides of the anterior skull base. The transclival approach involves navigating between the ICA and basilar artery for interventions in the ventral posterior fossa. The transodontoid approach is employed in cases where pathologies extend from the foramen magnum to the C1–C2 region. The petrous apex approach reaches the carotid artery with precise drilling, and the intrapetrous and suprapetrous approaches offer access to specific areas of the skull base. The cavernous sinus approach targets pathologies above the sixth cranial nerve, while the infratemporal approach utilizes the endonasal approach for surgeries. Medial condylectomy is used in certain situations to access or control the vertebral artery. The jugular foramen approach strategically enables entry into the cervical region by targeting the jugular foramen.

References

1. Carrau RL, Jho HD, Ko Y. Transnasal-transsphenoidal endoscopic surgery of the pituitary gland. Laryngoscope. 1996;106(7):914–8. https://doi.org/10.1097/00005537-199607000-00025.
2. Jho HD, Carrau RL. Endoscopy assisted transsphenoidal surgery for pituitary adenoma. Technical note. Acta Neurochir. 1996;138(12):1416–25. https://doi.org/10.1007/BF01411120.
3. Kassam A, Snyderman CH, Mintz A, Gardner P, Carrau RL. Expanded endonasal approach: the rostrocaudal axis. Part I. Crista galli to the Sella turcica. Neurosurg Focus. 2005a;19(1):E3.
4. Kassam A, Snyderman CH, Mintz A, Gardner P, Carrau RL. Expanded endonasal approach: the rostrocaudal axis. Part II. Posterior clinoids to the foramen magnum. Neurosurg Focus. 2005b;19(1):E4.
5. Kassam A, Snyderman CH, Mintz A, Gardner P, Carrau RL. Expanded endonasal approach: the rostrocaudal axis. Part II. Posterior clinoids to the foramen magnum. Neurosurg Focus. 2005c;19(1):E4.
6. Kassam AB, Gardner P, Snyderman C, Mintz A, Carrau R. Expanded endonasal approach: fully endoscopic, completely transnasal approach to the middle third of the clivus, petrous bone, middle cranial fossa, and infratemporal fossa. Neurosurg Focus. 2005d;19(1):E6.
7. Dm P, Doglietto F, Ja J, Jagannathan J, Han J, Er L. History of endoscopic skull base surgery: its evolution and current reality. J Neurosurg. 2007;107:206–13.
8. Cavallo LM, Messina A, Gardner P, Esposito F, Kassam AB, Cappabianca P, et al. Extended endoscopic endonasal approach to the pterygopalatine fossa: anatomical study and clinical considerations. Neurosurg Focus. 2005;19(1):E5.
9. de Lara D, Ditzel Filho LF, Prevedello DM, Carrau RL, Kasemsiri P, Otto BA, et al. Endonasal endoscopic approaches to the paramedian skull base. World Neurosurg. 2014;82(6 Suppl):S121–9. https://doi.org/10.1016/j.wneu.2014.07.036.
10. Kasemsiri P, Solares CA, Carrau RL, Prosser JD, Prevedello DM, Otto BA, et al. Endoscopic endonasal transpterygoid approaches: anatomical landmarks for planning the surgical corridor. Laryngoscope. 2013;123(4):811–5. https://doi.org/10.1002/lary.23697.

11. Prevedello DM, Ditzel Filho LF, Solari D, Carrau RL, Kassam AB. Expanded endonasal approaches to middle cranial fossa and posterior fossa tumors. Neurosurg Clin N Am. 2010a;21(4):621–35. https://doi.org/10.1016/j.nec.2010.07.003.

12. Magro F, Solari D, Cavallo LM, Samii A, Cappabianca P, Paternò V, et al. The endoscopic endonasal approach to the lateral recess of the sphenoid sinus via the pterygopalatine fossa: comparison of endoscopic and radiological landmarks. Neurosurgery. 2006;59(4 Suppl 2):ONS237–42; discussion ONS242-3. https://doi.org/10.1227/01.NEU.0000233977.79721.17.

13. Xu Y, Asmaro K, Mohyeldin A, Zhang M, Nunez MA, Mao Y, et al. The Pterygosphenoidal triangle: surgical anatomy and case series in endoscopic Endonasal Skull Base surgery. Oper Neurosurg (Hagerstown). 2023;24(6):619–29. https://doi.org/10.1227/ons.0000000000000627.

14. Oyama K, Tahara S, Hirohata T, Ishii Y, Prevedello DM, Carrau RL, Froelich S, Teramoto A, Morita A, Matsuno A. Surgical anatomy for the endoscopic Endonasal approach to the ventrolateral Skull Base. Neurol Med Chir (Tokyo). 2017;57(10):534–41. https://doi.org/10.2176/nmc.ra.2017-0039.

15. Kitano M, Taneda M. Extended transsphenoidal approach with submucosal posterior ethmoidectomy for parasellar tumors. Technical note J Neurosurg. 2001;94(6):999–1004. https://doi.org/10.3171/jns.2001.94.6.0999.

16. Low CM, Vigo V, Nunez M, Fernández-Miranda JC, Patel ZM. Anatomic considerations in endoscopic pituitary surgery. Otolaryngol Clin N Am. 2022;55(2):223–32. https://doi.org/10.1016/j.otc.2021.12.014.

17. Snyderman CH, Pant H, Carrau RL, Prevedello D, Gardner P, Kassam AB. What are the limits of endoscopic sinus surgery?: the expanded endonasal approach to the skull base. Keio J Med. 2009;58(3):152–60. https://doi.org/10.2302/kjm.58.152.

18. Labib MA, Prevedello DM, Fernandez-Miranda JC, Sivakanthan S, Benet A, Morera V, et al. The medial opticocarotid recess: an anatomic study of an endoscopic "key landmark" for the ventral cranial base. Neurosurgery. 2013;72(1 Suppl Operative):66–76; discussion 76. https://doi.org/10.1227/NEU.0b013e318271f614.

19. Sharma A, Rieth GE, Tanenbaum JE, Williams JS, Ota N, Chakravarthi S, et al. A morphometric survey of the parasellar region in more than 2700 skulls: emphasis on the middle clinoid process variants and implications in endoscopic and microsurgical approaches. J Neurosurg. 2018;129(1):60–70. https://doi.org/10.3171/2017.2.JNS162114.

20. Truong HQ, Borghei-Razavi H, Najera E, Igami Nakassa AC, Wang EW, Snyderman CH, et al. Bilateral coagulation of inferior hypophyseal artery and pituitary transposition during endoscopic endonasal interdural posterior clinoidectomy: do they affect pituitary function? J Neurosurg. 2018a;131(1):141–6. https://doi.org/10.3171/2018.2.JNS173126.

21. Labib MA, Prevedello DM, Carrau R, Kerr EE, Naudy C, Abou Al-Shaar H, et al. A road map to the internal carotid artery in expanded endoscopic endonasal approaches to the ventral cranial base. Neurosurgery. 2014;10 Suppl 3:448–71. ; discussion 471. https://doi.org/10.1227/NEU.0000000000000362.

22. Kassam AB, Vescan AD, Carrau RL, Prevedello DM, Gardner P, Mintz AH, et al. Expanded endonasal approach: vidian canal as a landmark to the petrous internal carotid artery. J Neurosurg. 2008;108(1):177–83. https://doi.org/10.3171/JNS/2008/108/01/0177.

23. Prevedello DM, Pinheiro-Neto CD, Fernandez-Miranda JC, Carrau RL, Snyderman CH, Gardner PA, et al. Vidian nerve transposition for endoscopic endonasal middle fossa approaches. Neurosurgery. 2010b;67(2 Suppl Operative):478–84. https://doi.org/10.1227/NEU.0b013e3181faaa70.

24. Kassam AB, Prevedello DM, Carrau RL, Snyderman CH, Gardner P, Osawa S, et al. The front door to Meckel's cave: an anteromedial corridor via expanded endoscopic endonasal approach-technical considerations and clinical series. Neurosurgery. 2009;64(3 Suppl):ons71–82. ;discussion ons82-3. https://doi.org/10.1227/01.NEU.0000335162.36862.54.

25. Dolci RLL, Ditzel Filho LFS, Goulart CR, et al. Anatomical nuances of the internal carotid artery in relation to the quadrangular space. J Neurosurg. 2018;128(1):174–81. https://doi.org/10.3171/2016.10.JNS16381.
26. Truong HQ, Lieber S, Najera E, Alves-Belo JT, Gardner PA, Fernandez-Miranda JC. The medial wall of the cavernous sinus. Part 1: surgical anatomy, ligaments, and surgical technique for its mobilization and/or resection. J Neurosurg. 2018b;131(1):122–30. https://doi.org/10.3171/2018.3.JNS18596.

Chapter 5
Endoport-Guided Endoscopic Excision of Intraaxial Brain Tumors

Suresh K. Sankhla, Anshu Warade, and G. M. Khan

5.1 Introduction

The surgical treatment of deep-seated intraaxial brain lesions continues to pose serious challenges because of their critical location and difficult surgical access. Although conventional microsurgery with traditional spatula-based brain retractors remains the mainstay in the surgical management of these lesions, retraction injury to the brain is common and may lead to serious consequences, including seizures, focal neurological deficits, and vascular disturbances [1–9]. Advances in preoperative imaging (magnetic resonance (MR) and diffusion tensor imaging (DTI)) and the availability of modern intraoperative technologies like neurophysiological monitoring, image guidance, and neuroendoscopy have been found to have reduced complication rates and improved surgical outcomes. Improvement in brain retraction techniques, especially the use of retractors with tubular configuration, seems to have resulted in reduced trauma to the surrounding normal brain parenchyma [10–13]. The recent introduction of tubular retractors, combined with modern neuroendoscopic techniques, in brain surgery has added new dimensions to the operative approaches to a variety of deeper intraaxial brain lesions [4, 7, 13–32].

In this chapter, we describe the surgical technique of endoscopic-assisted resection of deeper brain parenchymal and intraventricular tumors using a transparent plastic tubular port and discuss the advantages and limitations of this technique with a review of the literature.

S. K. Sankhla (✉) · A. Warade · G. M. Khan
Department of Neurosurgery, Global Hospital, Mumbai, Maharashtra, India

© The Author(s), under exclusive license to Springer Nature
Switzerland AG 2024
W. A. Azab (ed.), *Endoscope-controlled Transcranial Surgery*, Advances and
Technical Standards in Neurosurgery 52,
https://doi.org/10.1007/978-3-031-61925-0_5

5.2 Advantages of the Tubular Retractor System

Tubular retractors were introduced in neurosurgery to provide a stable working channel for tumor removal and to avoid brain-retraction-related complications associated with the traditional rigid retractor system. Unlike the flat brain spatula, the cylindrical configuration of the retractors distributes retraction forces evenly over a larger surface area around the tube. The concept was proposed first in the 1980s by Kelly and colleagues [33] for the stereotactic removal of deep-seated brain tumors. The authors used a hollow cylinder of 20–30 mm in diameter for the removal of deep brain lesions [33–35]. Since then, a large number of studies on endoport-controlled resection of parenchymal and intraventricular brain tumors using different port devices and technical modifications have been published in the literature with improved efficacy and better postoperative outcomes [10, 36–42].

The soft tubular ports tend to displace rather than transact the white matter fibers and dissipate retraction pressure homogenously over a larger surface area of the brain [10–13]. An intraparenchymal corridor is created by the gradual widening of the interfascicular space using blunt and round port obturators or dilators. A transparent endoport tube allows the maintenance of a safe passage into the brain, protects the tissue against instrument manipulation, and prevents inadvertent expansion of the corticotomy and fasciculotomy incisions during surgery. A 4-mm rigid telescope and two to three surgical instruments can be easily passed through the port simultaneously without any obstruction (Fig. 5.1). The endoport approach also provides a broader fluid-free surgical corridor and enables the surgeon to perform tumor resection using standard bimanual microsurgical techniques without making any compromise in the surgical trajectory or instrument manipulation [7, 43].

The use of endoscopy with its panoramic vision has become a widely accepted technology in brain surgery in the last few decades [16, 17, 19–23, 41, 42, 44]. In 2008, Akai et al. [19] described the endoscopic resection of intrinsic brain tumors in three patients using a transparent tubular retractor. Kassam and coworkers [24], in 2009, developed a fully endoscopic system for intraaxial tumor resection through a dilatable conduit and elaborated their technique of endoport-assisted removal of intraparenchymal and intraventricular tumors using pure endoscope in 2013 [43]. Several authors in the last few decades have described the technique of endoport-controlled endoscopic resection of parenchymal and intraventricular brain tumors using different port devices and technical modifications with improved surgical results [10, 36–42, 44].

Two technological advances, endoport and endoscope, are complementary to each other when used in combination and provide full advantages of both minimally invasive access and enhanced panoramic vision to deep brain lesions [13, 14, 18, 19, 24, 32, 44–52]. The technique of endoscopic tumor removal via a single-channel endoport is unique and different from both conventional channel endoscopy and standard microsurgery in many tways. The endoscope does not provide binocular three-dimensional (3D) vision like a microscope, but with experience, the surgeon develops 3D perception based on the proprioceptive feedback through the dynamic

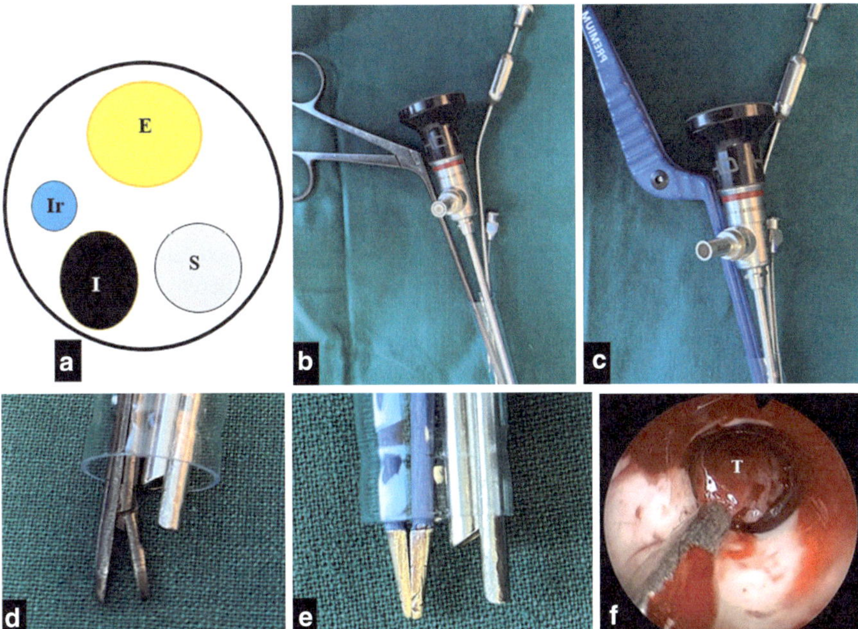

Fig. 5.1 Position of the instruments in the endoport tube (**a**). Instrument insertion at the upper end (**b** and **c**) and lower end (**d** and **e**). Intraoperative endoscopic photograph showing tumor projecting into the lumen of endoport (**f**). Abbreviations: *E* endoscope, *S* suction, *I* instrument, *Ir* irrigation cannula, *T* tumor

movements of the endoscope. The angulation, trajectory, and depth of the port can be manipulated during surgery as often as necessary to obtain enhanced illumination and optimal visualization of deep-seated lesions in all corners. Additionally, endoport-assisted endoscopic surgery can be managed with ports that are much smaller in size than those used commonly with a microscope. This is because the focused endoscopic light is projected like an inverted cone toward the lesions, whereas in a microscope, the light beam tapers gradually toward the target, thus requiring a larger corridor.

In contrast to conventional channel endoscopy, which demands working through a narrow and rigid channel system with limited maneuvering, the flexible endoport allows unrestricted instrument manipulations during surgery and permits a bimanual microsurgical technique for tumor removal [7, 43]. In addition, the endoport-assisted endoscopic technique permits the surgeon to shift the operative corridor freely and safely by changing the angles and directions of the port and the endoscope together to improve the visibility of a much larger area in the depth of the brain. The dynamic manipulation of the port and the endoscope creates a steerable conduit that provides multiple views of the tumor from different angles and improves the surgeon's quality of vision and anatomical orientation.

5.3　Surgical Technique

The entry point into the brain remains crucial and is normally chosen at the convexity of a noneloquent gyrus, which allows a trajectory that passes through the least functional white matter tracts. For parenchymal tumors, a straight and more direct trajectory is selected, avoiding eloquent areas such as the motor strip, visual cortex, superior temporal lobe, and inferior frontal gyrus (Case 1, Fig. 5.2). Tumors within the frontal horn and body of the lateral ventricle are approached through a standard ipsilateral precoronal mini-craniotomy (Case 2, Fig. 5.3), whereas lesions that are located in the atrium and occipital horns can be accessed via lateral parietal and occipital openings (>3.0 cm from the midline). To approach third ventricular tumors, the side with a more dilated lateral ventricle and foramen of Monro is usually selected to avoid a potential risk of injury to the internal capsule, head of the caudate nucleus, and fornix during insertion of the tubular retractor (Case 3, Fig. 5.4).

With a curvilinear scalp incision, a small craniotomy measuring between 2.5 and 3.0 cm in diameter is performed, which is usually sufficient to expose the gyrus or sulcus required for the insertion and manipulation of the tubular retractor without any obstruction from the bone edges (Fig. 5.3d). The dura is opened in a cruciate

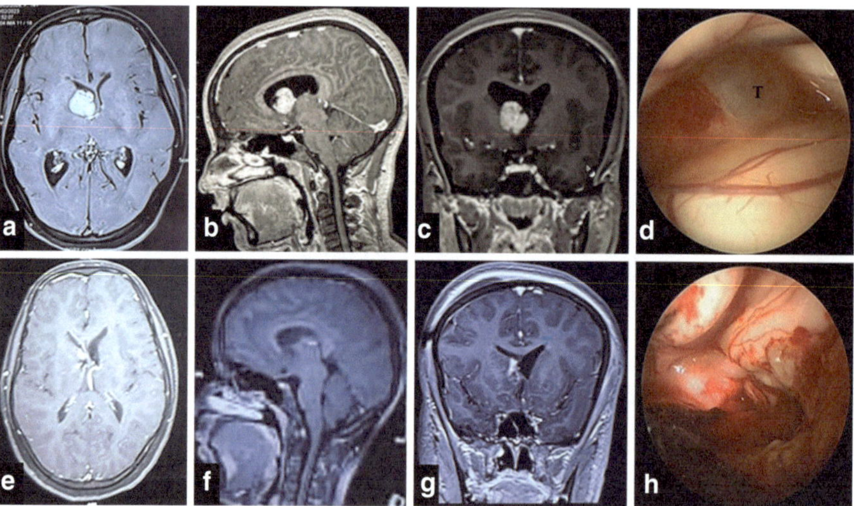

Fig. 5.2 Case 1. A 14-y.o.f. presented with generalized tonic/clonic seizures associated with a transient loss of consciousness, three episodes in the last 1 month. Contrast MR imaging in axial (**a**), sagittal (**b**), and coronal views (**c**) showing a well-enhancing tumor in the right frontal subependymal region extending into the frontal horn of the right lateral ventricle with a mild enlargement of the right lateral ventricle. Endoscopic intraoperative photograph (**d**) showing a grayish tumor in the frontal horn of the right lateral ventricle. Postoperative contrast MR images (**e–g**) and intraoperative endoscopic photograph (**h**) demonstrating complete tumor removal. Histopathology: subependymal giant cell astrocytoma. Abbreviations: *T* tumor

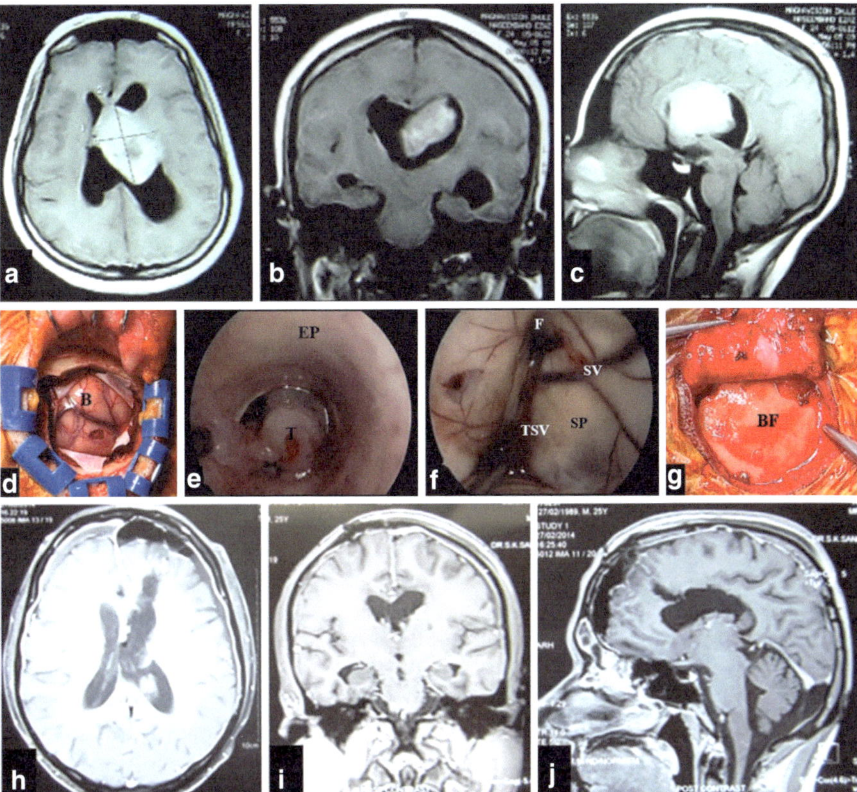

Fig. 5.3 Case 2. A 24-y.o.f. presented with headache, vomiting, and papilloedema. Her T1-weighted MR images in axial (**a**), coronal (**b**), and sagittal (**c**) views showing a well-circumscribed tumor in the left lateral ventricle, compressing the left foramen Monro and causing obstructive hydrocephalus. Intraoperative photographs showing a small left frontal craniotomy of 2.5 cm in diameter (**d**), endoscopic microphotographs (**e** and **f**) showing an intraventricular tumor protruding in the endoport lumen (e) and after removal (**f**), and photograph g showing the replacement of the bone flap and closure of the surgical wound. Postoperative contrast MR images in axial (**h**), coronal (**i**), and sagittal (**j**) views demonstrating a complete resection of the tumor. Histopathology: central neurocytoma. Abbreviations: *B* brain, *BF* bone flap, *EP* endoport, *F* foramen Monro, *SP* septum pellucidum, *SV* anterior septal vein, *T* tumor, *TSV* thalamostriate vein

fashion, large enough to allow the identification and protection of the major draining veins on the brain surface and to help achieve a water-tight dural closure at the end of the procedure. We use a transparent soft and flexible plastic tube with a diameter of 11 mm as a port to access deep brain lesions and to introduce a 4-mm rigid endoscope and three instruments, including a suction canula, bipolar forceps or a dissector, and an irrigation cannula (Fig. 5.1). A small pial incision is taken, and superficial corticotomy is performed to introduce the endoport into the brain with its obturator.

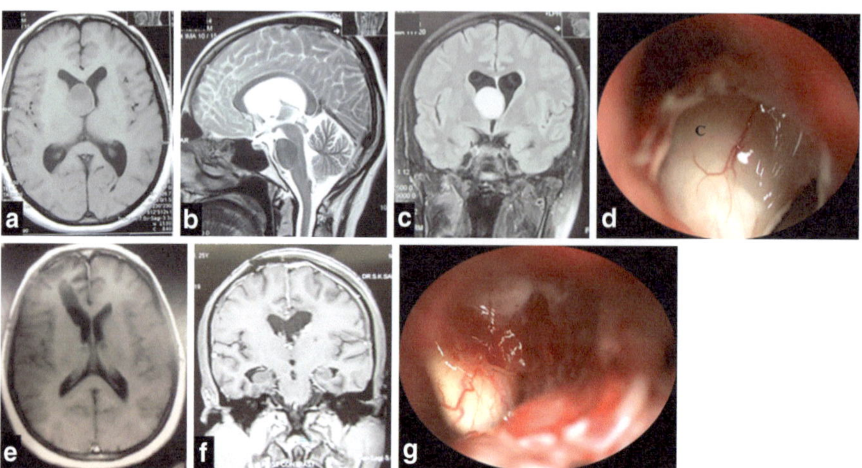

Fig. 5.4 Case 3. A 42-y.o.f. c/o intermittent severe headaches since the last 4 months, progressively increasing over the last 1 month. One episode of generalized seizure 2 weeks back. Bilateral papilloedema on fundoscopy. MR images T1 weighted in axial (**a**), T2 weighted in sagittal (**b**), and in FLAIR (**c**) showing a large cyst in the frontal horn of the right lateral ventricle compressing the foramen Monro; intraoperative endoscopic photographs before (**d**) and after (**g**) the removal of the cyst. Postoperative T1-weighted MR images in axial (**e**) and coronal (**f**) views showing a complete removal of the cyst. Histopathology: colloid cyst. Abbreviations: *C* cyst

Since the conduit is usually positioned deeper within the tumor mass, the local extracavitary tumor pressure forces it to protrude itself into the port lumen, from where it can be removed with the help of a suction canula and tumor-grasping forceps (Fig. 5.1f). The port tube is then gently withdrawn and maneuvered in different directions to continue slow and uniform tumor removal from all directions until normal brain tissue is visualized. In cases of lateral ventricular lesions, the port is initially fixed at a position in the ventricular cavity where tumor mass and intraventricular structures like choroid plexus, larger veins, septum pellucidum, and fornix are visualized clearly for initial anatomical orientation. For colloid cysts and third ventricular tumors, the endoport is positioned closer to the foramen Monro to have a clear and constant transforaminal view of the anterior third ventricular cavity and the tumor.

Tumor resection is performed in an air medium using standard bimanual microsurgical techniques in a step-by-step method that includes initial internal debulking, followed by dissection of the peripheral tumor component, and, finally, hemostasis. At the end of tumor removal, the corticotomy opening is plugged with a piece of gelfoam and the dura is closed in a water-tight fashion using a pericranial graft or any synthetic dural substitute. The bone flap and skin are closed in a standard fashion (Fig. 5.3g). An external ventricular drain is kept for 3–4 days postoperatively in cases of intraventricular tumor surgery.

5.4 Surgical Complications and Limitations

There is usually a steep learning curve for surgical techniques like endoport-guided endoscopic resection of intraaxial brain lesions. For surgeons who are used to binocular 3D microscopic vision and those who are not comfortable working in a narrow operative field, this learning curve can be longer and difficult. The key to a successful endoscopic tumor surgery is the optimal position of the endoport, and even a slight deviation in its trajectory can disturb the visualization of the operative field and can put adjacent critical neurovascular structures at a higher risk of injury. Brain shift after cerebrospinal fluid (CSF) release or tumor debulking during surgery can displace the endoport in a different direction and may transform the resection of the residual lesion into a challenging task. A large volume of CSF drainage during operation may cause the collapse of the ventricular cavity and brain tissue and may induce postoperative extraaxial hygromas or hematomas.

The majority of authors agree that tumors with a large size (>3 cm), firm or hard consistency, or the presence of heavy calcification can affect the degree of tumor removal adversely and, thereby, reduce the chances of gross total removal using this technique [36, 37, 41, 47]. Similarly, highly vascular deep-seated lesions pose a technical challenge and present as a major limiting factor with the endoport technique. Largely superficial tumors that occupy a significant portion of the pial surface relative to the whole tumor volume are mostly not suitable for endoport endoscopic surgery. These tumors can be resected more effectively via an open microsurgery, and there is no special advantage of using either the endoport or endoscope in such cases.

Surgical complications and their treatment and avoidance have been described extensively in the recent literature [13, 20, 24, 27, 40, 52–55]. Shapiro et al. [32], in 2020, reviewed the literature on the tubular retractors of the ViewSite Brain Access System (VBAS, Vycor Medical Inc.) for tumor resections, hematoma evacuations, and cyst removals, and they reported a complication rate of 2.8% in 106 patients. A retrospective analysis by Eichberg et al. [56], of ten cases in their study and 77 cases in the literature, reported an overall incidence of complications of 7.8–10%.

5.5 Conclusions

Endoscopic surgery using a transparent tubular retractor is safe and effective for the removal of deep-seated intraaxial brain lesions. As compared to conventional microsurgery, the technique of endoport-assisted endoscopic surgery is simple and minimally invasive. Using this technique, selected deep primary and metastatic brain tumors may be removed safely with smaller skull openings, short corticectomy incisions, and minimal white matter dissections. With the aid of dynamic and easily tiltable retraction during surgery, tumors much larger than the size of the endoport can be effectively removed. This endoscopic approach may be a feasible alternative for brain tumor removal in selected cases.

Disclosures None.

References

1. Andrews RJ, Bringas JR. A review of brain retraction and recommendations for minimizing intraoperative brain injury. Neurosurgery. 1993;33:1052–63; discussion 1063–1064
2. Hongo K, Kobayashi S, Yokoh A, Sugita K. Monitoring retraction pressure on the brain. An experimental and clinical study. J Neurosurg. 1987;66:270–5.
3. Rosenorn J, Diemer N. The risk of cerebral damage during graded brain retractor pressure in the rat. J Neurosurg. 1985;63:608–11.
4. Herrera SR, Shin JH, Chan M, Kouloumberis P, Goellner E, Slavin KV. Use of transparent plastic tubular retractor in surgery for deep brain lesions: a case series. Surg Technol Int. 2010;19:47–50.
5. Yokoh A, Sugita K, Kobayashi S. Intermittent versus continuous brain retraction: an experimental study. J Neurosurg. 1983;58:918–23.
6. Zhong J, Dujovny M, Perlin AR, Perez-Arjona E, Park HK, Diaz FG. Brain retraction injury. Neurol Res. 2003;25(8):831–8.
7. Jo KI, Chung SB, Jo KW, Kong DS, Seol HJ, Shin HJ. Microsurgical resection of deep-seated lesions using transparent tubular retractor: pediatric case series. Childs Nerv Syst. 2011;27(11):1989–94.
8. Rosenorn J, Diemer NH. Reduction of cerebral blood flow during brain retraction pressure in the rat. J Neurosurg. 1982;56:826–9.
9. Singh L, Agrawal N. Cylindrical channel retractor for intraventricular tumour surgery- a simple and inexpensive device. Acta Neurochir. 2009;151(11):1493–7.
10. Bander ED, Jones SH, Kovanlikaya I, Schwartz TH. Utility of tubular retractors to minimize surgical brain injury in the removal of deep intraparenchymal lesions: a quantitative analysis of FLAIR hyperintensity and apparent diffusion coefficient maps. J Neurosurg. 2016;124:1053–60.
11. Bennett MH, Albin MS, Bunegin L, Dujovny M, Hellstrom H, Jannetta PJ. Evoked potential changes during brain retraction in dogs. Stroke. 1977;8:487–92.
12. Rosenørn J, Diemer NH. The influence of intermittent versus continuous brain retractor pressure on regional cerebral blood flow and neuropathology in the rat. Acta Neurochir. 1988;Wien) 93:13–7.
13. Ogura K, Tachibana E, Aoshima C, Sumitomo M. New microsurgical technique for intraparenchymal lesions of the brain: transcylinder approach. Acta Neurochir. 2006;148:779–85; discussion 785
14. Otsuki T, Jokura H, Yoshimoto T. Stereotactic guiding tube for open-system endoscopy a new approach for the stereotactic endoscopic resection of intra-axial brain tumors. Neurosurgery. 1990;27:326–30.
15. Barlas O, Karadereler S. Stereotactically guided microsurgical removal of colloid cysts. Acta Neurochir. 2004;146(11):1119–204.
16. Jho HD, Alfieri A. Endoscopic removal of third ventricular tumors: a technical note. Minim Invasive Neurosurg. 2002;45(2):114–9.
17. Harris AE, Hadjipanayis CG, Lunsford LD, Lunsford AK, Kassam AB. Microsurgical removal of intraventricular lesions using endoscopic visualization and stereotactic guidance. Neurosurgery. 2005;56(1):125–32.

18. Greenfield JP, Cobb WS, Tsouris AJ, Schwartz TH. Stereotactic minimally invasive tubular retractor system for deep brain lesions. Neurosurgery. 2008;63(4):334–40.
19. Akai T, Shiraga S, Sasagawa Y, Okamoto K, Tachibana O, Lizuka H. Intra-parenchymal tumor biopsy using neuroendoscopy with navigation. Minim Invasive Neurosurg. 2008;51:83–6.
20. Engh JA, Lunsford LD, Amin DV, Ochalski PG, Fernandez- Miranda J, Prevedello DM, Kassam AB. Stereotactically guided endoscopic port surgery for intraventricular tumor and colloid cyst resection. Neurosurgery. 2010;67(3):198–205.
21. Fahim DK, Relyea K, Nayar VV, Fox BD, Whitehead WE, Curry DJ, Luersen TG, Jea A. Transtubular microendoscopic approach for resection of a choroidal arteriovenous malformation. J Neurosurg Pediatr. 2009;3(2):101–4.
22. Fries G, Perneczky A. Endoscope-assisted brain surgery: part 2-analysis of 380 procedures. Neurosurgery. 1998;42:226–31.
23. Perneczky A, Fries G. Endoscope-assisted brain surgery: part 1-evolution, basic concept, and current technique. Neurosurgery. 1998;42:219–24.
24. Kassam AB, Engh JA, Mintz AH, Prevede DM. Completely endoscopic resection of intraparenchymal brain tumors. J Neurosurg. 2009;110:116–23.
25. Almenawer SA, Crevier L, Naresh M, Kassam A, Reddy K. Minimal access to deep intracranial lesions using a serial dilatation technique. Neurosurg Rev. 2013;36(2):321–9.
26. Raza SM, Recinos PF, Avendano J, Adams H, Jallo GI, Quinones-Hinojosa JA. Minimally invasive trans-portal resection of deep intracranial lesions. Minim Invas Neurosurg. 2011;54:5–11.
27. Recinos PF, Raza SM, Jallo GI, Recinos VR. Use of a minimally invasive tubular retraction system for deep-seated tumors in pediatric patients. J Neurosurg Pediatrics. 2011;7(5):516–21.
28. Barber SM, Rangel-Castilla L, Baskin D. Neuroendoscopic resection of intraventricular tumors: a systematic outcomes analysis. Minim Invasive Surg. 2013;2013:898753.
29. Depreitere B, Dasi N, Rutka J, Dirks P, Drake J. Endoscopic biopsy for intraventricular tumors in children. J Neurosurg. 2007;106(5 Suppl):340–6.
30. Ibanez-Botella G, Segura M, De Miguel L, Ros B, Arraez MA. Purely neuroendoscopic resection of intraventricular tumors with an endoscopic ultrasonic aspirator. Neurosurg Rev. 2019;42:973–82.
31. Mohanty A, Thompson BJ, Patterson J. Initial experience with endoscopic side cutting aspiration system in pure neuroendoscopic excision of large intraventricular tumors. World Neurosurg. 2013;80(655):e15–21.
32. Shapiro SZ, Sabacinski KA, Mansour SA, Echeverry NB, Shah SS, Stein AA, et al. Use of vycor tubular retractors in the management of deep brain lesions: a review of current studies. World Neurosurg. 2020;133:283–90.
33. Kelly PJ, Goeres SJ, Kall BA. The stereotaxic retractor in computer assisted stereotaxic microsurgery. Technical note J Neurosurg. 1988;69:301–6.
34. Kelly PJ, Kall BA, Goerss S, Earnest F. Computer-assisted stereotaxic laser resection of intraaxial brain neoplasms. J Neurosurg. 1986;64:427–39.
35. Morita A, Kelly PJ. Resection of intraventricular tumors via a computer-assisted volumetric stereotactic approach. Neurosurgery. 1993;32:920–7.
36. Ratre S, Yadav YR, Parihar VS, Kher Y. Microendoscopic removal of deep-seated brain tumors using tubular retraction system. J Neurol Surg A. 2016;77:312–20.
37. Sihag R, Bajaj J, Yadav YR, Ratre S, Hedaoo K, Kumar A, Sinha M, Parihar VS, Swamy MN. Endoscope-controlled access to thalamic tumors using tubular brain retractor: an alternative approach to microscopic excision. J Neurol Surg A Cent Eur Neurosurg. 2022;83(2):122–8. https://doi.org/10.1055/s-0041-1722966.
38. Xie S, Xu L, Wang K, Sun FJ, Xie M-X, Wang P, Xiao SW. Endoport-assisted neuroendoscopic techniques used in the resection of intraventricular lesions. Turk Neurosurg. 2021;33:929–35. https://doi.org/10.5137/1019-5149.JTN.32824-20.5.
39. Yan C, Yan H, Jin W. Application of endoport-assisted neuroendoscopic techniques in lateral ventricular tumor surgery. Front Oncol. 2021;13:1191399. https://doi.org/10.3389/fonc.2023.1191399.

40. Takeuchi K, Ohka F, Nagata Y, Maeda S, Tanahashi K, Araki Y, Yamamoto T, Sasaki H, Mizuno A, Harada H, Saito R. Endoscopic trans-mini-cylinder biopsy for Intraparenchymal brain lesions. World Neurosurg. 2022;167:e1147–53. https://doi.org/10.1016/j.wneu.2022.08.147.
41. Sankhla SK, Warade A, Khan GM. Endoport-assisted endoscopic surgery for removal of lateral ventricular tumors: our experience and review of the literature. Neurol India. 2023;71:99–106.
42. Cappabianca P, Cavallo LM, Colao A. Del basso de Caro M, Esposito F, Cirillo S, Lombardi G, de Divitiis E: endoscopic endonasal transsphenoidal approach: outcome analysis of 100 consecutive procedures. Minim Invasive Neurosurg. 2002;45:193–200.
43. McLaughlin N, Prevedello DM, Engh JA, Kelly DF, Kassam AB. Endoneurosurgical resection of intraventricular and intraparenchymal lesions using the port technique. World Neurosurg. 2013;79(2S):S18.e1–8. https://doi.org/10.1016/j.wneu.2012.02.022.
44. Teo C, Nakaji P. Application of endoscopy to the resection of intra-axial tumors. Oper Tech Neurosurg. 2005;8:179–85.
45. Ding D, Starke RM, Crowley RW, Liu KC. Endoport-assisted microsurgical resection of cerebral cavernous malformations. J Clin Neurosci. 2015;22:1025–9.
46. Nakano T, Ohkuma H, Asano K, Ogasawara Y. Endoscopic treatment for deep-seated or multiple intraparenchymal tumors: technical note. Minim Invasive Neurosurg. 2009;52:49–52.
47. Badie B, Brooks N, Souweidane MM. Endoscopic and minimally invasive microsurgical approaches for treating brain tumor patients. J Neurooncol. 2004;69:209–19.
48. Jo KW, Shin HJ, Nam DH, Lee JI, Park K, Kim JH, Kong DS. Efficacy of endoport-guided endoscopic resection for deepseated brain lesions. Neurosurg rev. 2011;34(4):457–63.
49. Miranda JCF, Engh JA, Pathak SK, Madhok R, Boada FE, Schneider W, Kassam AB. High-definition fiber tracking guidance for intraparenchymal endoscopic port surgery. J Neurosurg. 2010;113:990–9.
50. Ochalski PG, Engh JA. Endoscopic port surgery for intraparenchymal brain tumors. In: Hayat MA, editor. Tumors of the central nervous system, vol. 3. Springer: Science+Business Media BV; 2011. p. 60–267.
51. Moosa S, Ding D, Mastorakos P, Sheehan JP, Liu KC, Starke RM. Endoport-assisted surgical evacuation of a deep-seated cerebral abscess. J Clin Neurosci. 2018;53:269–72.
52. Sujijantarat N, Tecle NE, Pierson M, Urquiaga JF, Quadri NF, Ashour AM, et al. Transsulcal endoport-assisted evacuation of supratentorial intracerebral hemorrhage: initial single-institution experience compared to matched medically managed patients and effect on 30-day mortality. Oper Neurosurg (Hagerstown). 2018;14:524–31.
53. Moshel YA, Link MJ, Kelly PJ. Stereotactic volumetric resection of thalamic pilocytic astrocytomas. Neurosurgery. 2007;61:66–75.
54. Russell SM, Kelly PJ. Volumetric stereotaxy and the supratentorial occipito-subtemporal approach in the resection of posterior hippocampus and parahippocampal gyrus lesions. Neurosurgery. 2002;50:978–88.
55. Kelly PJ. Technology in the resection of gliomas and the definition of madness. J Neurosurg. 2004;101:284–6. discussion 286
56. Eichberg DG, Buttrick SS, Sharaf JM, Snelling BM, Shah AH, Ivan ME, et al. Use of tubular retractor for resection of colloid cysts: single surgeon experience and review of the literature. Oper Neurosurg (Hagerstown). 2019;16:571–9.

Chapter 6
Fully Endoscopic Nontubular Retractor Approach for Intraaxial Tumors

Waleed Abdelfattah Azab, Mustafa Najibullah, Zafdam Shabbir, Athary Saleem, and Mohammed S. Alkhaldi

6.1 Introduction

Advances in endoscopic technology have significantly contributed to the development and refinement of minimally invasive brain surgery. As a matter of fact, minimally invasive approaches are associated with lower complication profile, comparable or even better outcomes, better cosmetic results, and faster recovery times in comparison to conventional approaches [1–3]. Fully endoscopic or endoscope-controlled approaches are essentially keyhole approaches in which rigid endoscopes are the sole visualization tools used during the whole procedure.

The term "Keyhole Surgery" was first coined in 1971 by Donald Wilson, who elaborated on a variety of approaches for supratentorial pathologies in his technical note titled "Limited Exposure in Cerebral Surgery," which was then published in the Journal of Neurosurgery. He employed small linear incisions and a 2-inch D' Errico trephine to create limited craniotomies that were yet sufficiently large to operate through. He pointed out that such an operating methodology avoided the unnecessary exposure of brain tissue and thus its potential damage [4]. Later, Axel Perneczky popularized the principle of keyhole surgery, especially the supraorbital keyhole approach, and demonstrated the importance of endoscopic assistance in these approaches through several published large series of vascular and tumor cases [1, 3, 5].

Endoscopic assistance in cranial surgery emerged out of the need to operate via small openings and yet obtain appropriate visualization and control of the structures within the field, in other words, to perform minimally invasive yet maximally

W. A. Azab (✉) · M. Najibullah · Z. Shabbir · A. Saleem · M. S. Alkhaldi
Department of Neurosurgery, Ibn Sina Hospital, Kuwait City, Kuwait

© The Author(s), under exclusive license to Springer Nature Switzerland AG 2024
W. A. Azab (ed.), *Endoscope-controlled Transcranial Surgery*, Advances and Technical Standards in Neurosurgery 52, https://doi.org/10.1007/978-3-031-61925-0_6

effective surgery. At the early attempts of endoscope-assisted cranial surgery, it was noted that rigid endoscopes enabled overcoming the problem of suboptimal visualization when small exposures are used.

In 1974, Werner Prott, working then as an otosurgeon at the University of Würzburg, used a rigid endoscope to explore and operate within the cerebellopontine angle via a transpyramidal retrolabyrinthine approach through Trautmann's triangle. After a mastoidectomy, a bone flap with a diameter of 1 cm was made, and then the endoscope was inserted through this narrow space between the sigmoid sinus, the superior petrosal sinus, the posterior semicircular canal, and the endolymphatic sac without damaging any functional structure of the inner ear or of the cerebellum [6]. In 1981, Falk Oppel and colleagues used a similar approach for sectioning the sensory root of the trigeminal nerve, the glossopharyngeal nerve, and the cranial part of the vagus nerve to treat an intractable facial pain in a patient with recurrent upper jaw carcinoma [7]. Apuzzo and colleagues in 1977 described the use of Hopkins 70° and 120° side-viewing telescopes in a variety of approaches, including intrasellar procedures by either the transsphenoidal or subfrontal routes, to assist with visualization for complete gland ablation or total tumor excision. They also employed this endoscope-assisted strategy in aneurysm surgery while working in the vicinity of the circle of Willis, with particular emphasis on the assessment of adequacy and accuracy of clip placement, especially in lesions of the apex of the basilar artery [8].

Currently, the use of endoscopes in transcranial surgery can broadly be categorized into endochannel, endoscope-assisted, and endoscope-controlled or fully endoscopic approaches. Fully endoscopic resection of intraparenchymal brain tumors is a minimally invasive approach that is not routinely practiced by neurosurgeons, with few major series published so far. Unfamiliarity with the technique, steep learning curve, and concerns about inadequate exposure and decreased visibility may explain this fact [9]. The majority of purely endoscopic resections for intraparenchymal brain lesions are performed nowadays through tubular retractor systems [10–14]. In very limited instances, however, the fully endoscopic technique is performed without tubular retractors [15].

Our technique is a balanced one, in which tubular retractors are used very frequently to gain access to the tumor and are then removed after the corridor has been established and significant debulking of the tumor has been achieved. In many cases, the brain parenchyma remains retracted despite removing the tubular retractor. Should the need arise, a handheld brain spatula or a spatula attached to a Leyla retractor is used to prevent the gravitational fall of brain tissue. This is especially true when the tumor being resected is not very deeply seated. On the contrary, the endoscope-controlled tubular retractor-based approach is far more efficient for the excision of relatively small deep tumors and is our preferred technique in these cases.

In this chapter, we describe the purely endoscopic resection of intraparenchymal brain tumors and focus mainly on its surgical technique and nuances.

6.2 Rationale for the Fully Endoscopic Technique

The technical specifications and design of the currently available rigid endoscopes are associated with a group of unique features that define the endoscopic view and lay the basis for its superiority over the microscopic view during brain surgery (Fig. 6.1).

When a rigid endoscope is inserted into the surgical field, a very highly illuminated area of interest is obtained because the light beam is completely brought inside the field without any loss of light energy at the edges of the craniotomy or cortical incision. Furthermore, the close proximity of the light source to the structures being viewed eliminates shadows within the field, adding to the extreme

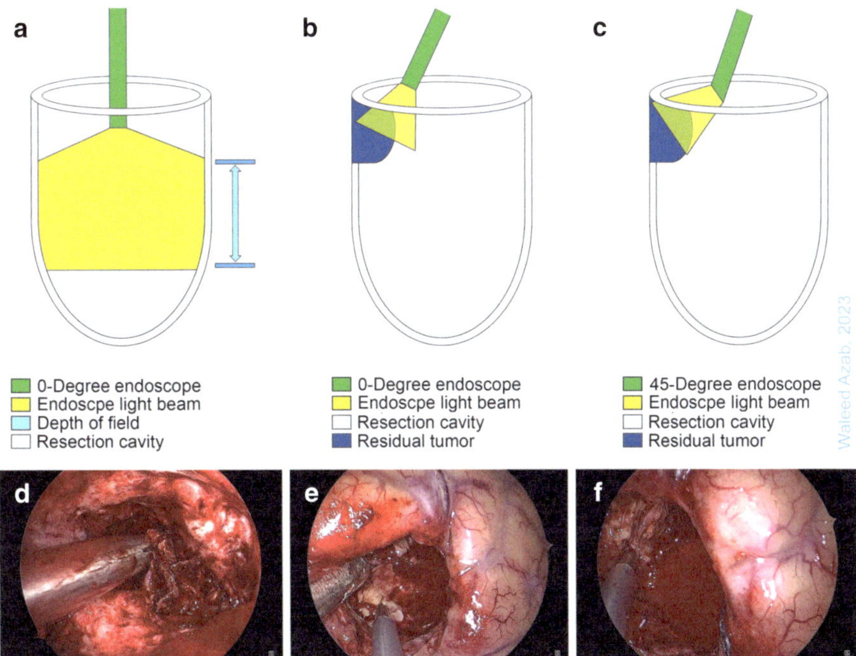

Fig. 6.1 The rationale for the purely endoscopic approach. (**a**) As the rigid endoscope is inserted into the surgical field, a very highly illuminated area of interest is obtained without any loss of light energy at the edges of the craniotomy or cortical incision. The proximity of the light source to the structures and the greater depth of field add to the extreme clarity of the endoscopic images. Angulating a 0° scope (**b**) and the use of angled scopes (**c**) brings concealed tumor remnants into view and obviates the need for the retraction of neurovascular structures. These advantages are exemplified in (**d–f**). The high depth of field and illumination can be clearly appreciated despite the very small cortical incision in (**d**). Angulation of the 0° scope in (**b**) and the use of a 30° angled scope in **c** bring concealed tumor remnants into view and subsequent resection using a CUSA

clarity of the endoscopic images. The superiority of the endoscopic view also results from the wide-angle view as well as the high color fidelity and image definition capabilities of today's state-of-the-art rigid endoscopes. In addition, rigid endoscopes are characterized by a greater depth of field. Therefore, the viewed objects remain in focus throughout a greater range of distances from the viewing lens. This means a lesser need to adjust the focus of the endoscope during the procedure and, consequently, a seamless operative workflow. The use of angled scopes also enables "looking around the corners" and, thereby, adds further to the efficacy and safety of the procedure as it brings concealed tumor remnants into view and obviates the need for the retraction of neurovascular structures. On the contrary, the microscope in keyhole surgery requires frequent changing of the viewing angle to allow the illumination and visualization of the area of interest deep in the surgical field, an inevitable consequence of the light source, and the viewing lens being located outside the craniotomy. The loss of light energy at the edges of the small craniotomy and the dropped shadows on the structures within the field further contribute to the lesser quality of the microscopic view obtained during keyhole brain surgery [16].

The frequently raised concerns of endoscopic visualization include the lack of three-dimensionality, the need for familiarity with endoscopic devices, the need to develop eye-hand coordination, and the limitation of the operating range of movement of instruments [17]. These drawbacks are easily overcome by the surgeon's experience and are largely balanced by the superb image quality, increased radicality, and lower risk of complications that this form of surgery offers. In our opinion, rigid endoscopes are indispensable components of the array of surgical tools required to perform a keyhole brain surgery, and we firmly believe that they will eventually completely replace surgical microscopes for this type of surgery.

6.3 Surgical Technique

6.3.1 Operating Room Setup

The operating room setup is illustrated in Fig. 6.2 and is geared toward achieving an unobstructed line of view of the endoscope monitor by the surgical team and ergonomically appropriate working space around the patient's head.

6.3.2 Endoscopic Equipment Setup and Ergonomics

The rigid endoscope (0, 30, or 45°) is connected to a 4 K endoscopic camera and inserted into the suction-irrigation sheath. The assembly is fixed to a holding mechanical arm (Karl Storz, Germany) or to an intuitively movable manual support arm (ENDOFIX exo, AKTORmed, Germany). The endoscope-holding arm is fixed to the side rail of the operating table to the left of the operating surgeon in cases

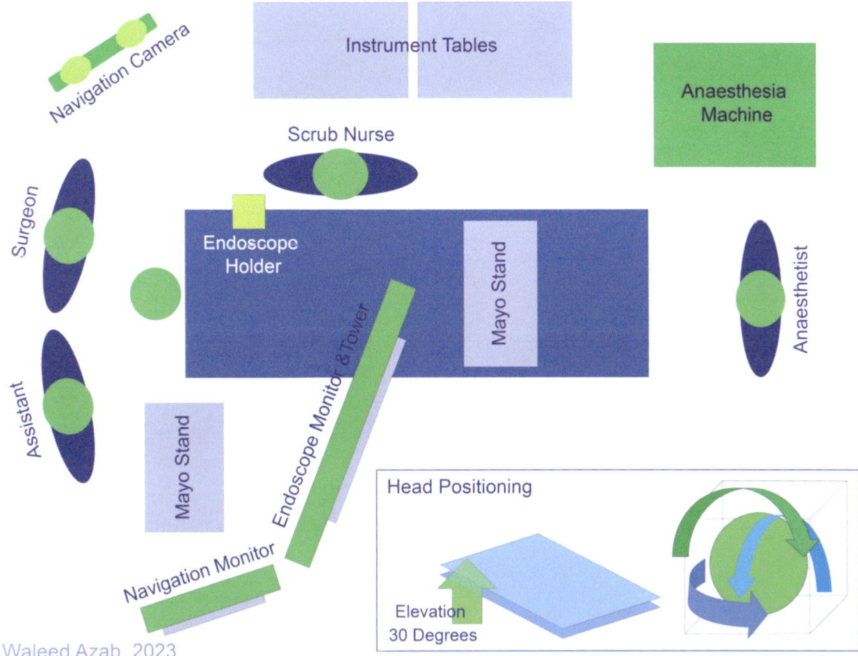

Fig. 6.2 The operating room setup for purely endoscopic resection of an intraaxial tumor. Some minor changes may be required on a case-by-case basis in order to obtain better ergonomics during the procedure

where the patient is in a supine or prone position. In cases where the patient is in the lateral position, the holding arm is fixed opposite to the surgeon across the operating table. The endoscope tower and monitor are positioned on one side of the operating table so that a straight line of view by the operating surgeon is established (Fig. 6.3). At the initial phase of the procedure, the endoscope is fixed in an exoscopic position and is later inserted through the craniotomy as tumor resection proceeds. At some point, the endoscope is held free hand by the assistant surgeon.

6.3.3   Positioning

The patient is positioned with the head elevated 30° above the level of the heart and fixed in a three-pin head clamp. The selection of the position depends on the location of the lesion; most of the time the patient is positioned supine with or without head tilt and, at times, in the lateral position with the tumor side up. The patient's head should be positioned so as to prevent the gravitational fall of the brain at the edges of the cortical incision. This helps keep the surgical field relatively open, allowing better visualization and easier instrument manipulation (Fig. 6.2, insert).

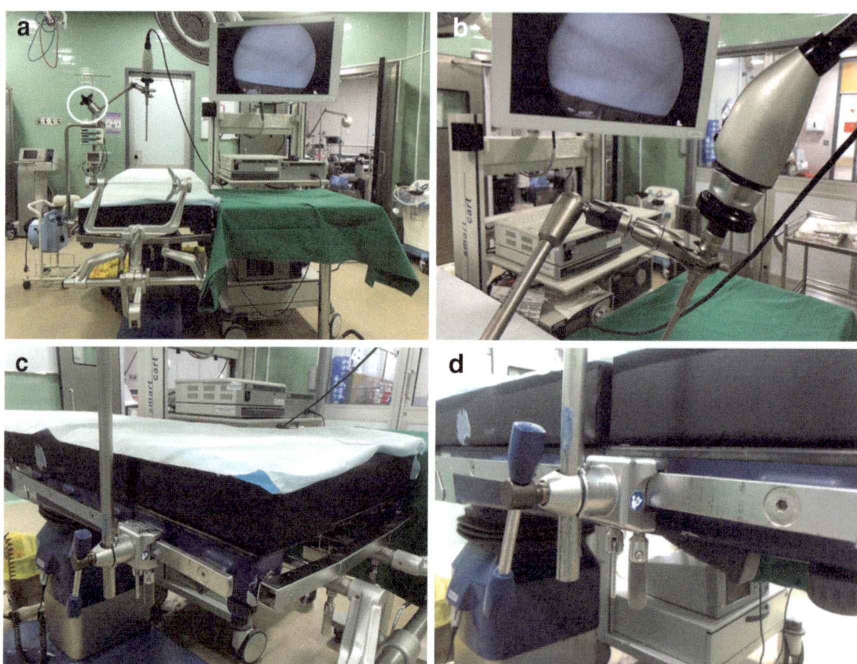

Fig. 6.3 (**a**) The rigid endoscope is connected to a 4 K endoscopic camera and inserted into the suction-irrigation sheath. The assembly is fixed to a holding mechanical arm. The position of the scope can be adjusted (white circle) according to the required position. At the initial phase of the procedure, the endoscope is fixed in an exoscopic position. (**b**) A close-up view of the clamping jaw holding the endoscope and connecting it to the mechanical holding system. (**c, d**) The rotational socket clamps the mechanical holder to the side rail of the operating table at a point around 20 cm from its end

6.3.4 Scalp Incision and Craniotomy

Neuronavigation is essential to tailor the scalp incision and the craniotomy flap and is also crucial to precisely localize the area of tumor surface presentation if present and to plan the surgical trajectory. An important technical point is to try to choose a trajectory of resection that follows the longitudinal axis of the tumor (Fig. 6.4).

A 3–5 cm scalp incision is performed down to the bone. Fishhook retractors are used to retract the scalp. The use of a fishhook is very important because of its low profile, which helps in achieving a much less crowded field and allows more space for endoscope shaft and instrument manipulation. A craniotomy flap is performed in a standard fashion, taking care to benefit maximally from the confines of the scalp incision.

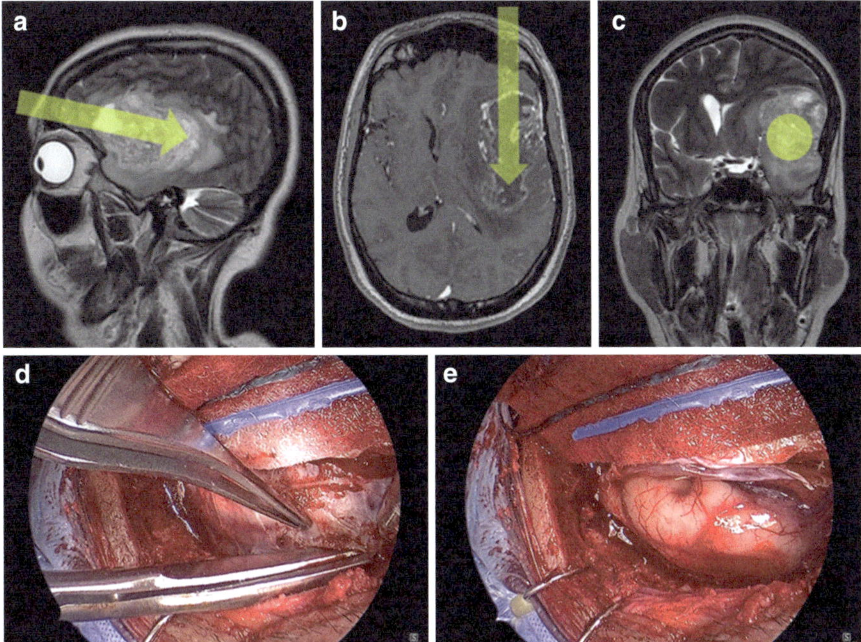

Fig. 6.4 The trajectory of resection should as possible be planned to follow the longitudinal axis of the tumor. Preoperative MR images in sagittal (**a**), axial (**b**), and coronal (**c**) planes with superimposed axis of resection represented with yellow arrows in (**a** and **b**) and a yellow circle in **c**. A left supraorbital eyebrow keyhole approach was therefore selected (**d, e**)

6.3.5 Tumor Resection

After reflecting the dural flap, if the tumor is seen presenting at the cortex, its surface is bipolar coagulated so that it is devascularized and subsequently entered. A pair of micro scissors is used to sharply open the coagulated pial surface within the confinements of the tumor cortical presentation. In tumors without cortical presentation, a neuronavigation-guided trans-sulcal insertion of a tubular retractor (ViewSite Brain Access System (VBAS™), Vycor Medical®, USA) or Leyla-retractor-mounted brain spatula is performed until the tumor is encountered (Fig. 6.5a).

An initial biopsy is taken, and tumor debulking is started using an ultrasonic surgical aspirator or two suction tubes. The endoscope shaft is advanced and angulated, and its focus is adjusted for a closer view according to the need. Aggressive tumor debulking is then undertaken. With more tumor debulking, a larger cavity within the tumor is created. All the standard technical steps for tumor removal are performed under endoscopic control and include piecemeal tumor resection, resection using a cavitron ultrasonic surgical aspirator (CUSA), developing the plane of

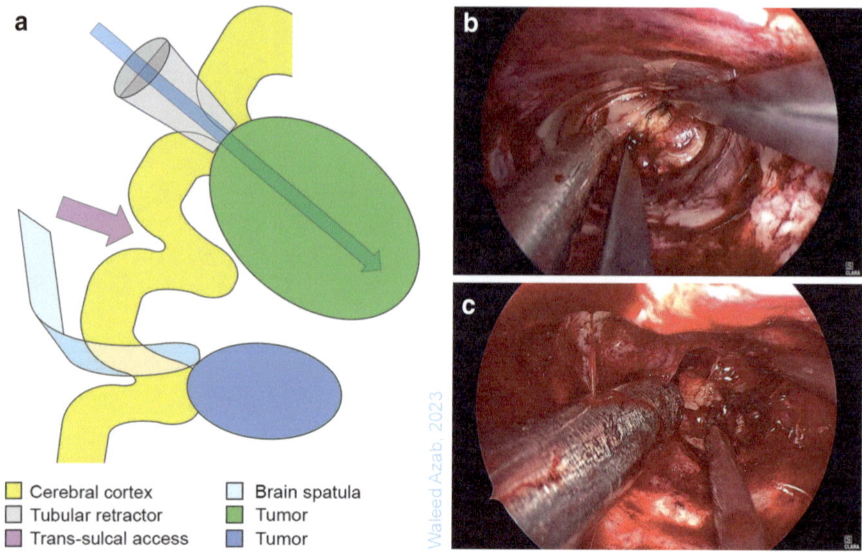

Fig. 6.5 (**a**) In tumors without cortical presentation, a trans-sulcal insertion of a tubular retractor or Leyla-retractor-mounted brain spatula is performed until the tumor is encountered. (**b**) Intraoperative endoscopic view through the tubular retractor. The tumor tissue is reached and clearly seen. (**c**) Intraoperative endoscopic view after the removal of the tubular retractor system after a significant debulking of the tumor has been achieved

cleavage around the tumor using a spreading movement of the forceps while the suction tube holds the tumor tissue, bipolar coagulation of bleeding vessels, and hemostasis.

Some important principles are of great help during the endoscope-controlled excision of intraaxial tumors. In general, angled low-profile instruments are to be used, obviously because they occupy a smaller area within the limited working space. Also, suction irrigation using a 50 ml syringe connected to the irrigation sheath and controlled by the assistant is very important for an uninterrupted seamless procedure because it enables keeping the lens clean without the need to take the scope outside the surgical field.

In addition, it is very frequently possible to remove the tubular retractor system after a significant debulking of the tumor has been achieved, and a handheld spatula is used as a dynamic retractor. The handheld spatula prevents the gravitational brain from falling and obscuring the view and is very helpful in obtaining better visualization within the small and deep surgical cavity (Fig. 6.5b, c).

Further to these technical points, the two-suction technique in which one suction gently pulls the tumor tissue while the other suction teases away the small vessels attached to the tumor capsule is a very useful maneuver in tumors with a surrounding plane of cleavage. After the confirmation of hemostasis, closure then proceeds in a standard fashion.

Many of the aforementioned steps and technical considerations are detailed in the following representative cases and their corresponding figures.

6.4   Representative Case 1

A 23-year-old male patient was presented to the emergency room with tonic-clonic seizures. He had a history of mild-to-moderate daily headaches in the previous 4 months. Neurological examination revealed bilateral papilledema and subtle left-sided lower limb weakness with exaggerated deep tendon reflexes. Magnetic resonance (MR) imaging revealed a large right parietal partially cystic mass. The details of the MRI findings are shown in Fig. 6.6. He underwent a purely endoscopic

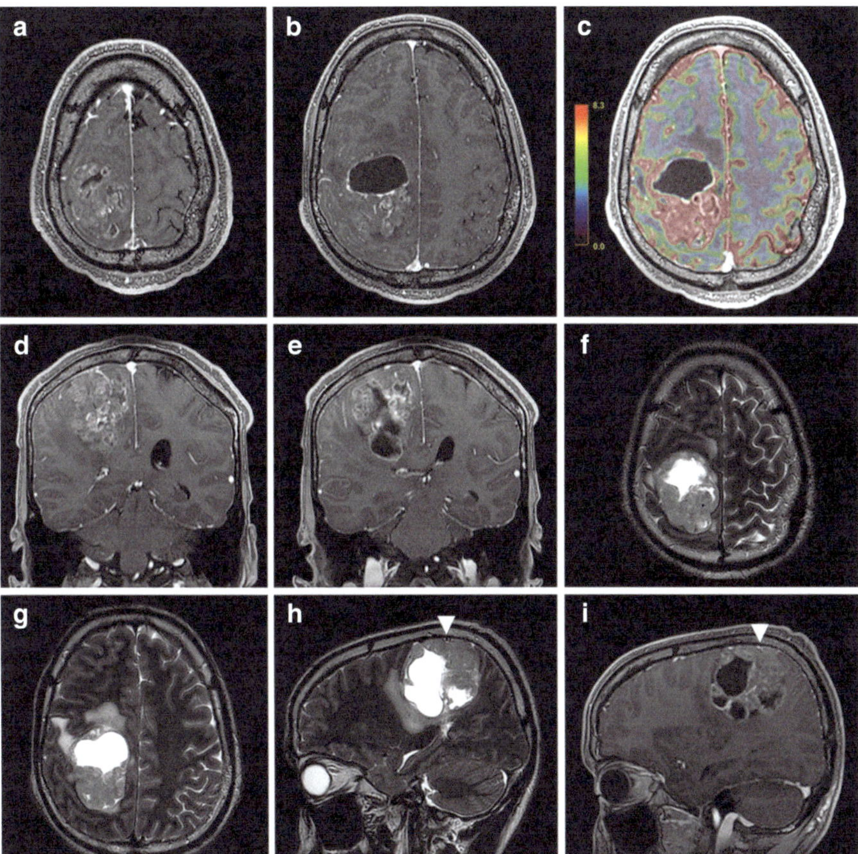

Fig. 6.6 Representative case 1. Preoperative MRI in a case of supratentorial extraventricular ependymoma. Axial T1-weighted FSPGR postcontrast MR images revealed a large right parietal partially cystic mass with a heterogeneous enhancement pattern of the solid component (**a, b**). The solid component hypervascularity is seen on the MR perfusion map superimposed on the axial MR image (**c**). On coronal T1-weighted FSPGR postcontrast MR images, the tumor is seen extending from the cortical surface through the white matter and ending short of the periventricular area of the body and atrium of the right lateral ventricle without direct communication with the ependymal surface (**d, e**). The hyperintense signal and lobulated pattern of the solid component are seen on axial (**f, g**) and sagittal (**h**) T2-weighted MR images. On the sagittal T2-weighted (**h**) and T1-weighted postcontrast (**i**) MR images, the cortical presentation of the tumor and the neighboring cortical vein (white arrowhead) are clearly seen and were used for the neuronavigation-assisted planning of the entry point on the tumor surface

excision of the tumor. The patient's positioning is demonstrated in Fig. 6.7. The operative details of the procedure are demonstrated in Figs. 6.8, 6.9, and 6.10. Postoperative MR imaging (Fig. 6.11) revealed gross total resection of the tumor. The patient did very well with the resolution of his focal deficit and was discharged 5 days after surgery. After histopathological examination, a final diagnosis of supratentorial extraventricular ependymoma was made.

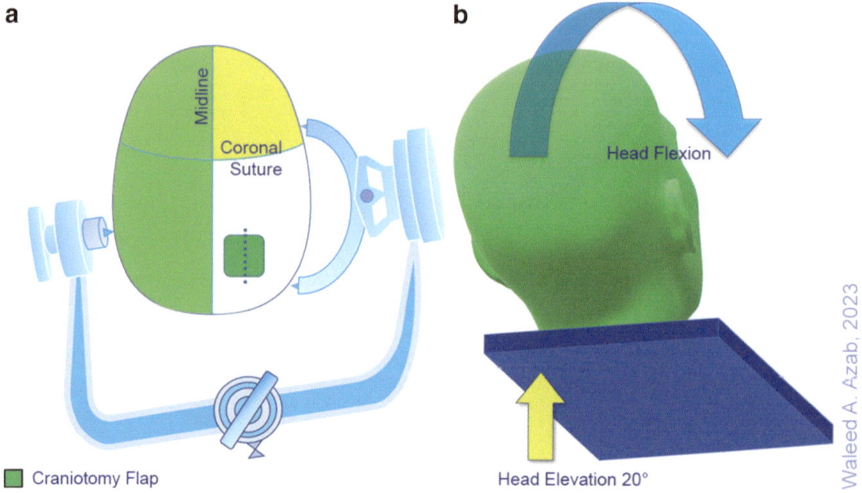

Fig. 6.7 Representative case 1. (**a**) Head fixation in the three-pin head holder is performed in a standard fashion according to the planned craniotomy. (**b**) Adjustment of the head position to avoid gravitational brain falling. Head flexion in this case was performed so that the surgical corridor remains open during the procedure

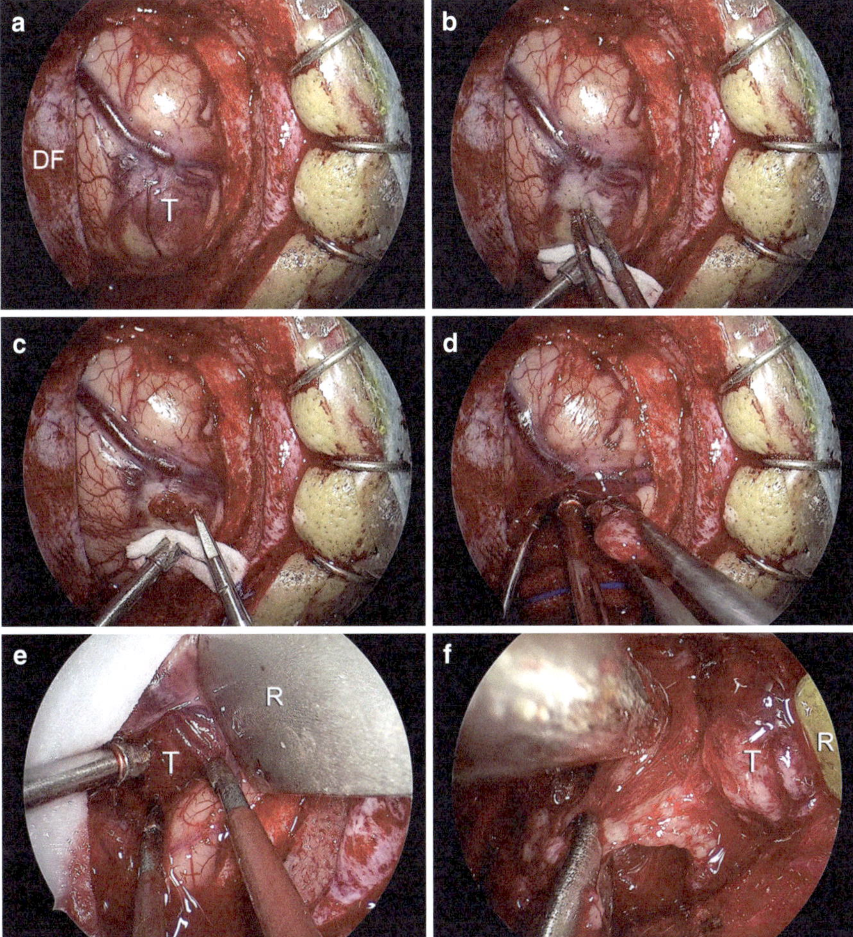

Fig. 6.8 Representative case 1. (**a**) Intraoperative view of the tumor with the endoscope held in the exoscopic position. After reflecting the dural flap (DF), the tumor cortical presentation (T) is seen. The adjacent cortical vein seen on the pre-operative MRI is clearly seen. Fishhook retractors are used for low profile reflection of the scalp incision. (**b**) Bipolar coagulation of the tumor surface is performed. The principles of microsurgery are applied with bimanual use of the instruments. (**c**) The coagulated tumor surface is sharply open with a microscissors. (**d**) Initial tumor debulking is performed using a suction and a tumor forceps is used for obtaining a biopsy. Another suction tube held by the assistant is used to help clearing the field. (**e**) The plane around the tumor is developed in the standard fashion using a mechanical spreading movement of the two shafts of the bipolar forceps. (**f**) The endoscope has been advanced deeper into the surgical field and a pituitary forceps is used to create gentle countertraction and the suction tube is used on the surface of the tumor for further dissection. The hand-held brain spatula (R) is used to gently retract the brain in (**e** and **f**)

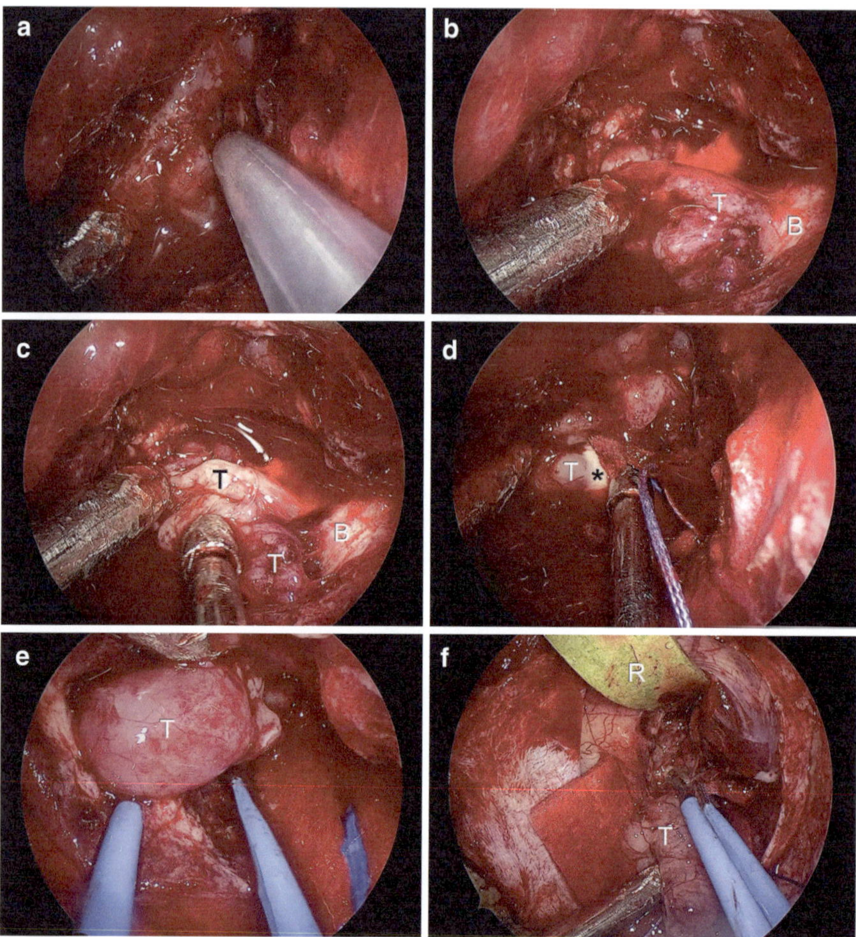

Fig. 6.9 Representative case 1. (**a**) CUSA is used for further tumor resection. (**b**) More tumor is removed and the tumor brain interface is delineated. Because of the large depth of field of the endoscope, both the normal brain deep within the field and the superficial tumor still attached to the surrounding brain tissue (B) all remain in focus. (**c**) The variable appearance of the tumor tissue (T) can be appreciated at this stage of tumor resection. (**d**)The two-suction technique is used for bimanual separation of the tumor (T) from the surrounding brain tissue (asterisk). (**e**) A tumor lobule is retrieved while held by suction and freed from attached brain tissue by spreading movements of the bipolar forceps. (f) Bipolar coagulation of a bleeding vessel as the tumor (T) is being resected. The hand-held brain spatula (R) supports the gravitational falling of the brain tissue

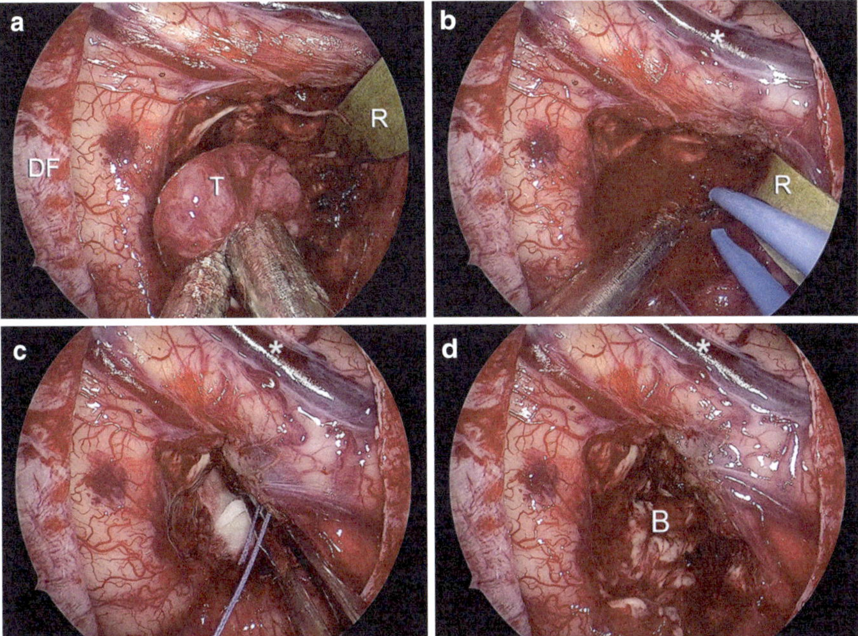

Fig. 6.10 Representative case 1. (**a**) The final part of the tumor (T) is removed while the cortex is retracted by a hand-held brain spatula (R). (**b**) Bleeding within the tumor bed is controlled and a bleeding vessel is bipolar coagulated. (**c**) Final hemostasis is performed using saline irrigation and cottonoid patties. (**d**) View of normal brain (B) within the resection cavity after tumor excision has been completed. The vein of Trolard (asterisk) is seen in (**b-d**)

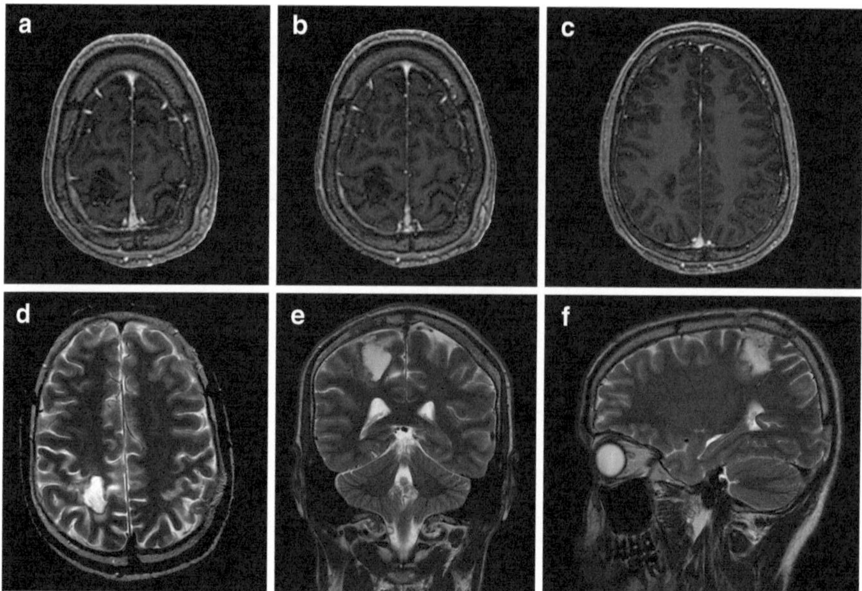

Fig. 6.11 Representative case 1. Postoperative axial T1-weighted FSPGR post-contrast (**a–c**) and T2-weighted axial (**d**), coronal (**e**), and sagittal (**f**) images demonstrating gross total resection of the tumor

6.5 Representative Case 2

A 26-year-old female patient was presented to the emergency room with a disturbed level of consciousness. Neurological examination revealed a Glasgow Coma Scale (GCS) score of 12/15. MR imaging revealed a large right frontal partially cystic mass. The details of the MRI findings are shown in Fig. 6.12. She underwent a purely endoscopic excision of the tumor. The operative details of the procedure are demonstrated in Fig. 6.13. Postoperative MR imaging (Fig. 6.14) revealed gross total resection of the tumor. The patient did very well and was discharged 4 days after surgery. Histopathological examination was consistent with pleomorphic xanthoastrocytoma with anaplastic features.

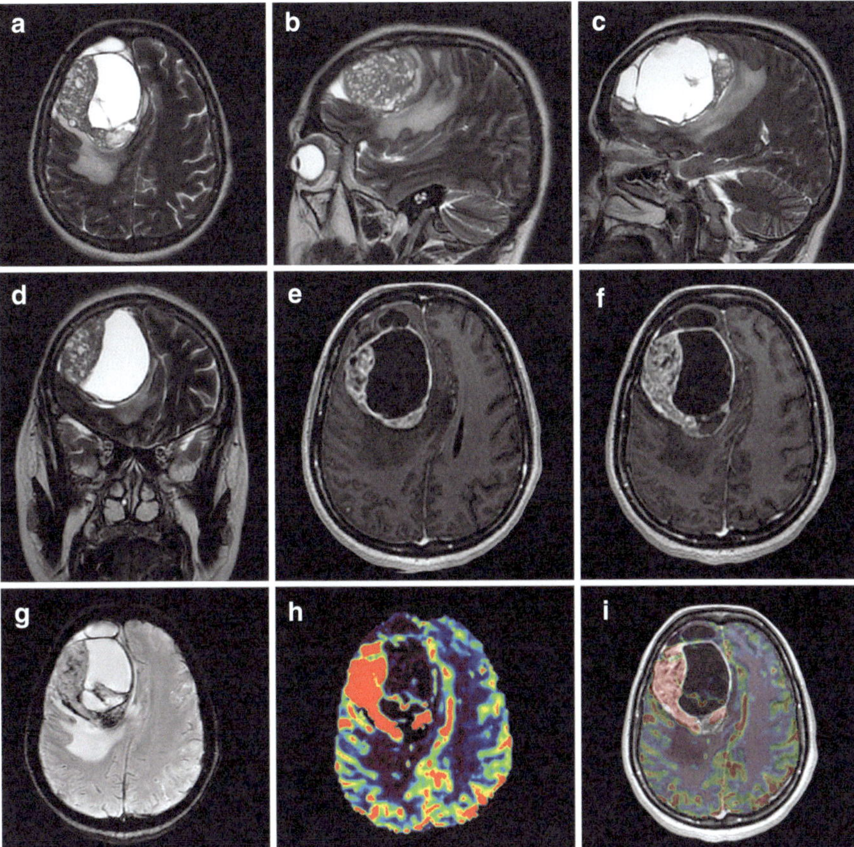

Fig. 6.12 Representative case 2. Preoperative MRI in a case of pleomorphic xanthoastrocytoma with anaplastic features. Axial (**a**), sagittal (**b, c**), and coronal (**d**) T2-weighted MR images revealed a large right frontal partially cystic mass. The solid component displayed an intermediate signal intensity. Axial T1-weighted FSPGR post-contrast MR images demonstrated avid enhancement of the solid component and cyst wall (**e, f**). On susceptibility weighted images (SWI), evidence of intratumoral hemorrhage is seen. The solid component hypervascularity is seen on the MR perfusion map (**g**). MR perfusion (**h**) superimposed on the axial MR image is seen in (**i**)

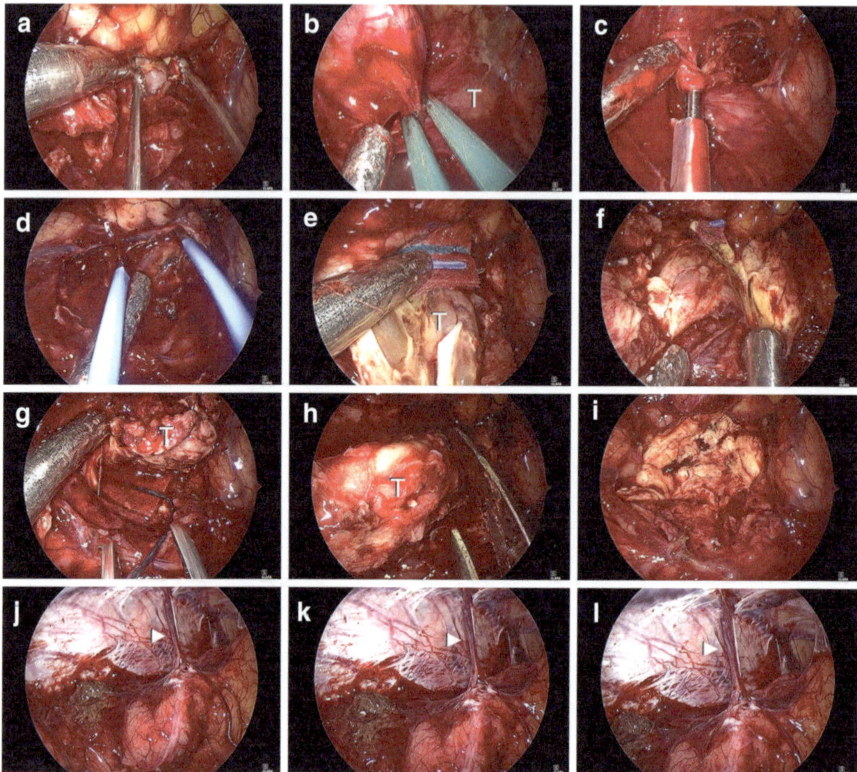

Fig. 6.13 Representative case 2. (**a**) Tumor biopsy is taken using a tumor forceps. (**b**) Bipolar coagulation of tumor vessels attached to the tumor capsule. (**c**) Tumor resection proceeds in a standard microsurgical fashion. Suction tube holds the tumor and CUSA is used to resect the tumor. Further development of the plane around the tumor capsule is undertaken using the shafts of the bipolar forceps in (**d**), and using a cottonoid patty with gentle countertraction in (**e, f**). As more tumor is freed (**g**), resection proceeds using a scissors (**h**). The final view of the resection cavity is seen in (**i**). (**j–l**) Sequential views using a 45° angled scope after some bleeding was notable to take place on the cortical surface that was followed to its origin from a small avulsion of one bridging vein. The bleeding area is seen controlled using Surgicel. The endoscopic views demonstrate how fine rotation of the endoscope shaft results in expansion of views while keeping the structures in focus. *T* Tumor, *Arrowhead* Bridging vein

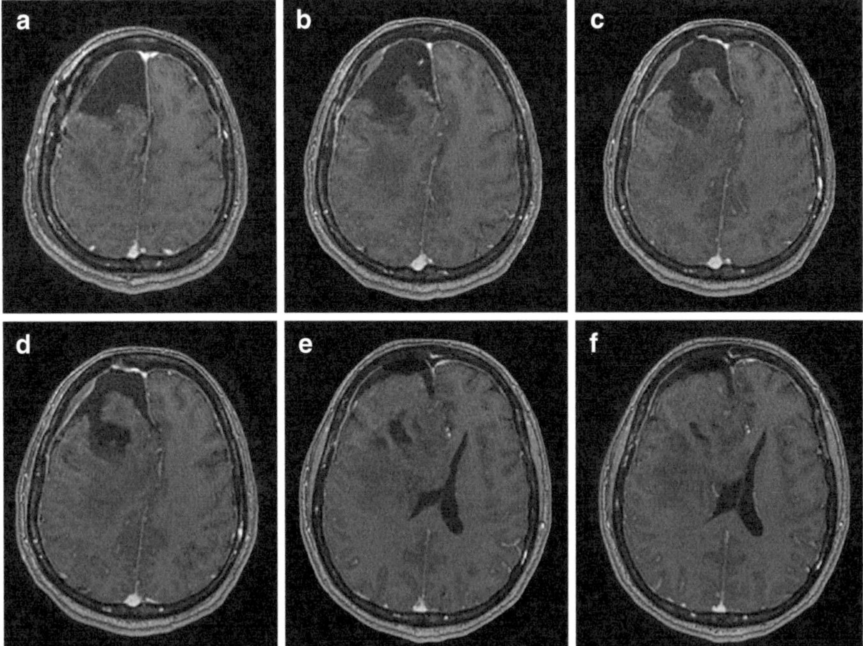

Fig. 6.14 Representative case 2. Postoperative axial T1-weighted FSPGR post-contrast images (**a–f**) demonstrating gross total resection of the tumor

References

1. van Lindert E, Perneczky A, Fries G, Pierangeli E. The supraorbital keyhole approach to supratentorial aneurysms: concept and technique. Surg Neurol. 1998;49:481–90. https://doi.org/10.1016/s0090-3019(96)00539-3.
2. Ottenhausen M, Rumalla K, Alalade AF, Nair P, La Corte E. Decision-making algorithm for minimally invasive approaches to anterior skull base meningiomas. Neurosurg Focus. 2018;44(4):E7. https://doi.org/10.3171/2018.1.FOCUS17734.
3. Perneczky A, Müller-Forell W, van Lindert E, Fries G. Keyhole concept in neurosurgery: with endoscope-assisted microsurgery and case studies. 1st ed. Stuttgart: Thieme Medical Publishers; 1999.
4. Wilson DH. Limited exposure in cerebral surgery: technical note. J Neurosurg. 1971;34:102–6. https://doi.org/10.3171/jns.1971.34.1.0102.
5. Fries G, Perneczky A. Endoscope-assisted brain surgery - part 2- analysis of 380 procedures. Neurosurgery. 1998;42(2):226–32.
6. Prott W. Cisternoscopy - endoscopy of the cerebellopontine angle. Acta Neurochir. 1974;31:105–13. https://doi.org/10.1055/s-0028-1098305.
7. Oppel F, Mulch G, Brock M. Endoscopic section of the sensory trigeminal root, the glossopharyngeal nerve, and the cranial part of the vagus for intractable facial pain caused by upper jaw carcinoma. Surg Neurol. 1981;16(2):92–5. https://doi.org/10.1016/0090-3019(81)90102-6.

8. Apuzzo ML, Heifetz MD, Weiss MH, Kurze T. Neurosurgical endoscopy using the side-viewing telescope. J Neurosurg. 1977;46(3):398–400. https://doi.org/10.3171/jns.1977.46.3.0398.
9. Budhiraja M, Pathak A, Brar H, Brar R. Pure endoscopic excision of parenchymal brain tumors: feasibility, risks, advantages and realities-a beginners perspective. Arq Bras Neurocir. 2020;39(3):201–6.
10. Jo KW, Shin HJ, Nam DH, Lee JI, Park K, Kim JH, Kong DS. Efficacy of endoport-guided endoscopic resection for deep-seated brain lesions. Neurosurg Rev. 2011;34:457–63.
11. McLaughlin N, Prevedello DM, Engh J, Kelly DF, Kassam AB. Endoneurosurgical resection of intraventricular and intraparenchymal lesions using the port technique. World Neurosurg. 2013;79(2 Suppl):S18.e1–8. https://doi.org/10.1016/j.wneu.2012.02.022.
12. Newman WC, Engh JA. Stereotactic-guided dilatable endoscopic port surgery for deep-seated brain tumors: technical report with comparative case series analysis. World Neurosurg. 2019;125:e812–9. https://doi.org/10.1016/j.wneu.2019.01.175.
13. Otsuki T, Jokura H, Yoshimoto T. Stereotactic guiding tube for open-system endoscopy: a new approach for the stereotactic endoscopic resection of intra-axial brain tumors. Neurosurgery. 1990;27:326–30.
14. Kassam AB, Engh JA, Mintz AH, Prevedello DM. Completely endoscopic resection of intra-parenchymal brain tumors. J Neurosurg. 2009;110:116–23.
15. Plaha P, Livermore LJ, Voets N, Pereira E, Cudlip S. Minimally invasive endoscopic resection of intraparenchymal brain tumors. World Neurosurg. 2014;82:1198–208.
16. Azab WA, Elmaghraby MA, Zaidan SN, Mostafa KH. Endoscope-assisted transcranial surgery for anterior skull base meningiomas. Mini-invasive. Surgery. 2020;4:88. https://doi.org/10.20517/2574-1225.2020.75.
17. Linsler S, Fischer G, Skliarenko V, Stadie A, Oertel J. Endoscopic assisted supraorbital keyhole approach or endoscopic endonasal approach in cases of tuberculum sellae meningioma: which surgical route should be favored? World Neurosurg. 2017;104:601–11. https://doi.org/10.1016/j.wneu.2017.05.023.

Chapter 7
Endoscopic Cylinder Surgery for Ventricular Lesions

Kazuhito Takeuchi

7.1 Introduction

Intraventricular tumors account for approximately 1% of primary brain tumors [1, 2]. They can arise from the brain or the ependyma of the ventricles, as well as from structures outside the brain parenchyma [1]. These tumors exhibit a wide range of characteristics, including cystic or solid lesions, requiring careful consideration of their specific nature during surgical treatment [2].

Accessing the ventricles necessitates making an incision into the healthy brain tissue. However, since the ventricles are located deep within the brain, minimizing the invasiveness of the surgical approach is crucial. Cylinder retractors are believed to reduce the risk of brain retraction injury by dispersing the retraction pressure on the brain [3, 4]. The use of cylinder retractors for the removal of deep-seated brain tumors was first reported by Kelly et al. in the 1980s [5]. Since then, various improvements have been made, leading to the development and widespread utilization of specialized cylinder retractors for brain surgery [4, 6–19].

The advantages of endoscopy include the ability to obtain a bright and wide field of view even in deep regions through narrow surgical corridors, as well as the possibility of maintaining visualization in underwater environments [20–22]. However, there are also drawbacks, such as the limited space within the cylinder, which can lead to interference between the endoscope and the instruments [18]. Overcoming these limitations and capitalizing on the benefits require innovative solutions. In this chapter, we will introduce the surgical technique using an endoscope through a port cylinder and discuss strategies to facilitate smooth surgical procedures.

K. Takeuchi (✉)
Department of Neurosurgery, Nagoya University, Nagoya, Japan
e-mail: ktakeuchi@med.nagoya-u.ac.jp

© The Author(s), under exclusive license to Springer Nature Switzerland AG 2024
W. A. Azab (ed.), *Endoscope-controlled Transcranial Surgery*, Advances and Technical Standards in Neurosurgery 52,
https://doi.org/10.1007/978-3-031-61925-0_7

7.2   Preoperative Surgical Planning and Preparation

Since the ventricles are deep structures within the brain, careful preoperative considerations are necessary. It is crucial to fully understand the shape of the ventricles and the course of the surrounding brain structures or subcortical fibers in order to develop a treatment plan [13, 23]. Computed tomography (CT) scans can provide information on features such as tumor calcification. Three-dimensional (3D) CT angiography allows the visualization of the relationship between tumor feeders and drainers, as well as provides valuable three-dimensional information about deep veins, especially in intraventricular lesions.

Magnetic resonance imaging (MRI) with and without Gd enhancement is essential for understanding tumor characteristics. It helps in assessing the spatial relationship with intraventricular structures, particularly the choroid plexus, which is useful for determining the tumor's location during surgery. In the case of lesions within the lateral ventricles, MR diffusion tensor imaging is important for understanding the course of crucial white matter fibers [24, 25].

Integrating and processing this information as three-dimensional data using simulation software like iPlan® is recommended.

Before surgery, consideration should also be given to the type and size of the cylinder to be used during the procedure. For instance, a smaller-diameter cylinder may be sufficient for general biopsy procedures, but larger-diameter cylinders are required for hemorrhagic tumors or lesions with significant calcification. Since predicting the hardness and bleeding tendency of the tumor completely before surgery is impossible, and to prepare for unexpected bleeding, it is essential to have multiple types of cylinders available.

7.3   Surgical Technique

7.3.1   Cylinder Insertion

For the proper placement of the cylinder as per the surgical plan, using navigation is recommended [8, 26]. The size of the craniotomy is adjusted based on the size of the cylinder to be used. For instance, if a 6-mm-diameter cylinder is used, a burr hole of approximately 15 mm in diameter is sufficient. However, when using a larger cylinder, a correspondingly larger craniotomy is required. A craniotomy that is too small may not allow enough range of motion for the cylinder, potentially leading to an inability to capture the tumor's edges. On the other hand, a craniotomy that is too large may result in the instability of the cylinder, and excessive movement of the cylinder during surgery can increase the retraction pressure on the brain around the surgical corridor. As a basic guideline, the authors typically employ craniotomy about twice the diameter of the cylinder. After the dural incision, the brain surface is observed, and if there is a sulcus available for cylinder insertion, the arachnoid over the sulcus is incised to allow the passage of the cylinder through it. An

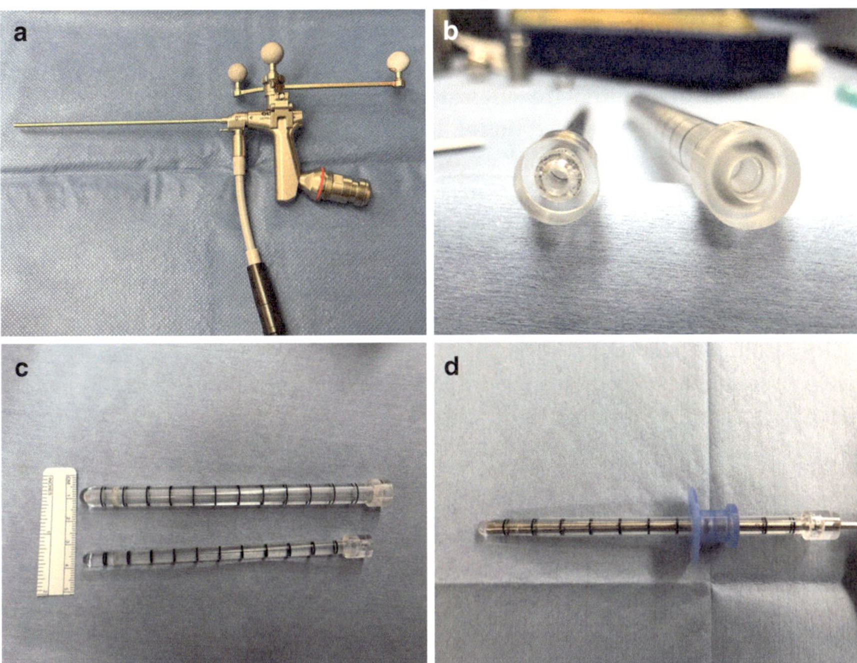

Fig. 7.1 (**a**) An instrument adapter array is attached to the endoscope, and the endoscope tip is calibrated using the navigation system. (**b, c**)Two types of transparent test tap needles with a 3-mm inner lumen. (**d**) A 2.7-mm endoscope can be inserted into the test tap needle for direct visualization during insertion

instrument adapter array is attached to the endoscope, and the endoscope tip is calibrated using the navigation system (Fig. 7.1a). A transparent test tap needle with a 3-mm inner lumen is used during the insertion of the cylinder (Fig. 7.1b and c). A 2.7-mm endoscope can be inserted into this test tap needle to visualize the tip of the needle directly during insertion (Fig. 7.1d). After reaching the ventricle, the cylinder is placed through the same tract. It is also important to observe the ventricle and gather anatomical information to ascertain the position of the cylinder tip. Since the surgical field is generally narrow in ventricular surgery and the shape of the ventricles changes as the resection progresses, it is advisable to identify the anatomical structures in the early stages of the surgery that can be used as landmarks during the surgical procedure.

7.3.2 Tumor Removal

During tumor removal, two techniques are utilized: the 'wet-field" method, where the surgical field is filled with artificial cerebrospinal fluid (CSF) or saline, and the "dry-field" method, where CSF is drained. Below are the advantages of each technique.

7.4   Wet-Field Technique

This method involves filling the surgical field with artificial CSF or saline solution, which is continuously irrigated during the tumor removal procedure. The natural water pressure prevents the shrinkage of the ventricle cavity, enabling surgery in a broader field [8]. This allows for better visualization, especially during tumor dissection from the ventricle wall. The underwater environment promotes the spontaneous hemostasis of minor bleeding, such as oozing or small vessels, by continuing irrigation with artificial CSF and applying water pressure [22]. However, excessive bleeding may reduce visibility. Additionally, finding a balance between aspiration and irrigation is sometimes difficult, especially when encountering hemorrhage, and care should be taken not to overaspirate CSF to maintain the wet-field environment [8].

7.5   Dry-Field Technique

In this method, CSF is aspirated, and the removal procedure is performed in an air-filled environment, providing a surgical field similar to microsurgery under a microscope. Blood flows downward due to gravity, improving the visibility of bleeding points. The dry-field technique also enables the use of monopolar electrocoagulation through the aspiration tube, and it can be used to coagulate the bleeding artery by aspirating the hemorrhage and can also be used to soften the tumor and aspirate the tumor with an aspiration tube simultaneously, especially in the case of glioma. However, a continuous dry-field environment may lead to a collapse of the ventricle, making it difficult to maintain a wide enough surgical field. Therefore, intermittently irrigating CSF into the surgical field (switch to the wet field) is important to minimize ventricle collapse. Alternating between wet-field and dry-field techniques can promote the natural hemostasis of small bleeding and help maintain a favorable surgical environment.

7.5.1   Wound Closure

After the tumor removal procedure, the ventricles are enlarged by filling the ventricle with fluid to ensure complete hemostasis and successful tumor removal. When withdrawing the cylinder, it is advisable to confirm that there is no bleeding in the tract while continuously irrigating with artificial CSF. If bleeding is observed, continue irrigation until hemostasis is achieved. After removing the cylinder, if possible, suture the arachnoid membrane around the surgical tract or pack the superficial layer with Surgicel® containing fibrin glue to prevent postoperative subdural fluid collection.

7.6 Surgical Treatment of Ventricular Tumors

7.6.1 Tumors Located in the Lateral Ventricle

Most of the lateral ventricular tumors are slowly growing benign or low-grade tumors. The most common tumors are ependymoma, low-grade astrocytoma, choroid plexus papilloma, meningioma, subependymoma, and central neurocytoma [27]. The most common clinical manifestations of tumors in the lateral ventricles include headaches as well as memory, cognitive, and gait disturbances [27]. Since hydrocephalus often accompanies the disease, the spinal fluid flow pathways must be secured through tumor removal. The surgical strategies for each site inside the lateral ventricle are described below.

7.6.2 Anterior Lateral Ventricle

In cases of lesions in the anterior horn of the lateral ventricles, obstructive hydrocephalus due to the obstruction of the foramen of Monro often accompanies the lesion. The surgical removal of the lesion, especially around the foramen of Monro, is required to ensure unobstructed CSF flow pathways. Microscopic surgery has utilized both transcortical and transcallosal approaches [28, 29]. For endoscopic cylinder surgery, the transcortical approach using an anterior horn tap is mainly employed. The patient is positioned supine, and the head is fixed with a head clamp. The head is elevated and inclined based on the position and angle of the cylinder to reduce the risk of postoperative air contamination. The shape of the lateral ventricles appears arched in the sagittal section, and surgical planning should consider this shape [30]. For instance, if the tumor is located near the corpus callosum, the access route should be more anterior to avoid excessive intraoperative changes to the cylinder angle. On the other hand, if the tumor protrudes toward the third ventricle, a direct approach facing the foramen of Monro is more appropriate. Therefore, the access route should be tailored according to the tumor's location and extension (Fig. 7.2).

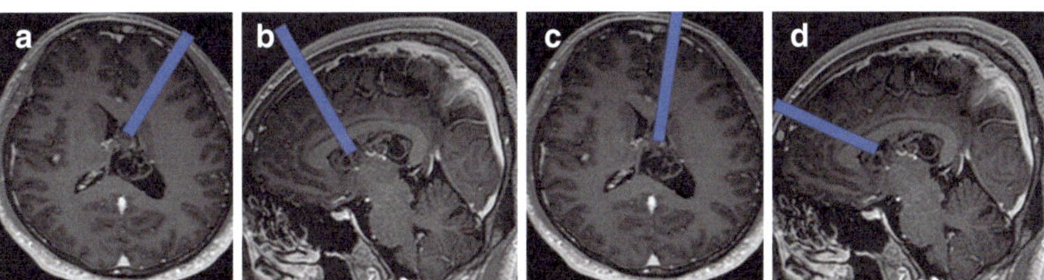

Fig. 7.2 Left intraventricular tumor extending widely in the anteroposterior direction. The access route similar to that of conventional endoscopic third ventriculostomy makes access to the posterior lesion difficult. (**a**, **b**) A more anterior and medial approach is preferable to allow linear access to the postero-lateral lesion (**c**, **d**)

The thalamostriate vein runs laterally to medially and connects with the anterior septal vein posterior to the foramen of Monro, leading to the internal cerebral vein. Injury to the thalamostriate vein can cause severe venous infarction of the basal ganglia, so careful attention should be paid to avoid injuring these veins during the removal procedure [31–33].

As the tumor removal progresses, the choroid plexus can be identified posterior to the foramen of Monro. The choroid plexus runs in the anterior-posterior direction on the mediocaudal aspect of the lateral ventricle and serves as an effective landmark even when the ventricle's shape has changed due to tumors. By following the choroid plexus posteriorly, the surgeon can reach the posterior portion of the lateral ventricle without disorientation. It is crucial to be mindful of the fornix, which runs anterior to medial on the foramen of Monro and inferior to the choroid plexus, to prevent any damage. The corpus callosum, a relatively fibrous white tissue that is easily distinguishable from the tumor, serves as an excellent landmark. After tumor removal, it is essential to ensure that the CSF pathway to the foramen of Monro is secure (Fig. 7.3).

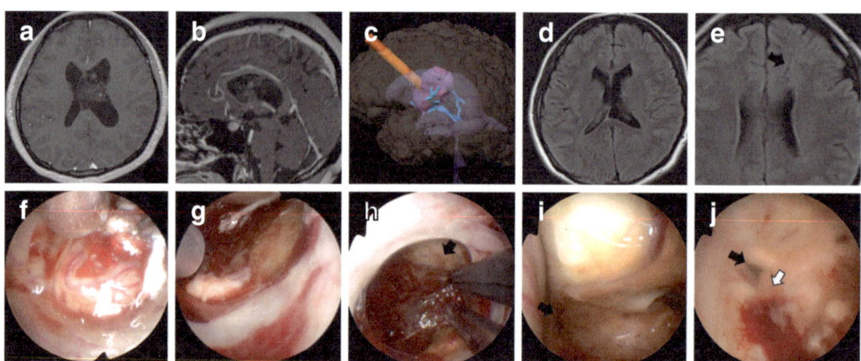

Fig. 7.3 A 46-year-old female presented with gradually worsening headaches. (**a**, **b**) Gadolinium-enhanced MR axial and sagittal images revealed a less enhancing mass in her left lateral ventricle. (**c**) Preoperative planning was performed using iPlan®, with the tumor shown in purple, the ventricles in blue, and the intraventricular veins in light blue. The orange cylinder indicates the appropriate position and angle for cylinder insertion. (**d**, **e**) MR FLAIR images taken 3 months after surgery showed the gross total removal of the tumor and a small trajectory scar (**e**, black arrow). (**f**) Intraoperative findings revealed that after inserting the cylinder, the surface of the tumor was coagulated. (**g**) Tumor debulking was performed using an ultrasound aspirator. (**h**) As internal decompression of the tumor progressed, normal anatomical structures such as the septum pellucidum (black arrow) became visible. (**i**) After tumor removal, the foramen of Monro (black arrow) was only slightly observed under dry-field conditions. (**j**) In contrast, under wet-field conditions, the foramen of Monro (black arrow) and the choroid plexus (white arrow) could be easily visualized without additional retraction

7.6.3 Trigone of the Lateral Ventricle

The trigone of the lateral ventricle is located deep in the brain, including important white matter fibers, and there are limited approaches to this area. The surgical approaches to the trigone reported so far include the paramedian high parietal lobe approach, the trans-middle-temporal transcortical or transsulcal approach, the interhemispheric transcallosal approach, the interhemispheric precuneus approach, and the distal Sylvian fissure approach [28]. The key concept in the approach to the trigone is to minimize damage to important superficial brain structures as well as deep white matter fibers. Endoscopic cylinder surgery is effective for trigone lesions because it allows for a minimal corridor approach. The authors mainly utilize a transsulcal approach through the high parietal or inferior temporal sulcus in endoscopic cylinder surgery.

The patient is positioned prone in the high parietal approach whereas supine lateral in the inferior temporal approach. The head is elevated according to the cylinder insertion angle and fixed with a head clamp. The choroid plexus is a good landmark during resection for trigone tumors. Especially in meningioma resections, securing the choroid plexus early in the removal procedure is the key to success since the choroid plexus arteriovenous system is generally the tumor feeder or drainer. The advantage of the inferior temporal approach is that the choroid plexus can be easily identified at the very early stage of surgery, but its disadvantages are the possibility of causing a disruption of the optic radiation and the difficulty of approaching the top of the trigone. On the other hand, the advantage of the high parietal approach is that the entire trigone can be easily observed, but its disadvantages include the possibility of postoperative parietal lobe disturbances, difficulty in identifying the choroid plexus early in the procedure, and the possibility that tumor decompression may be required. Based on these advantages and disadvantages, the approaching route should be determined according to the nature and location of the tumor. One option is to perform both approaches simultaneously, taking advantage of the minimal corridor of the endoscopic cylinder surgery (Figs. 7.4 and 7.5).

7.6.4 Third Ventricle

The third ventricle is situated at the center of the cranium and serves as a vital CSF pathway within the brain. It communicates anteriorly with the lateral ventricles through the bilateral foramen of Monro and posteriorly with the fourth ventricle through the cerebral aqueduct. The lateral walls are demarcated by the hypothalamus in the infero-anterior region and the thalamus in the superior-posterior region, while the floor consists of the tuber cinereum, mamillary body, and midbrain. The anterior wall is formed by the optic chiasm, lamina terminalis, and anterior commissure, whereas the posterior wall comprises the posterior commissure, habenula commissure, and pineal gland. Due to its location, the third ventricle is closely

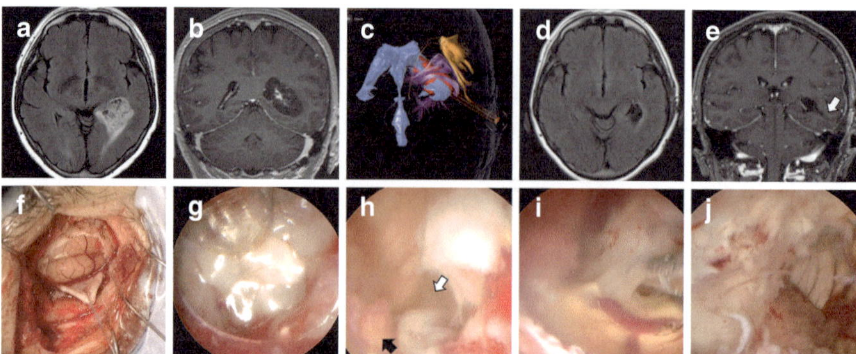

Fig. 7.4 A 60-year-old female presented with gradually worsening headaches. (**a**) MR FLAIR axial image reveals a high-intensity mass in the atrium of the left lateral ventricle. (**b**) The tumor shows less enhancement in gadolinium-enhanced MR coronal images. (**c**) Preoperative planning was performed using iPlan®, with the tumor shown in red and the ventricles in light blue. The superior longitudinal fascicles and the optic radiations were depicted in orange and purple lines, respectively, to avoid these vital subcortical fibers during cylinder insertion. (**d**) Postoperative MR FLAIR axial image displays the gross total removal of the tumor. (**e**) Postoperative gadolinium-enhanced MR coronal image demonstrates the gross total removal of the tumor with a minimal surgical trajectory scar. (**f**) A 5-cm skin incision and 3-cm craniotomy were made, exposing the middle and inferior temporal gyrus. (**g**) Internal decompression was performed by applying monopolar electrocautery to the aspiration tube to soften the tumor. (**h**) After tumor debulking, the body of the lateral ventricle (white arrow) and choroid plexus (black arrow) were observed under wet-field conditions. (**i**) A residual tumor was dissected from the ependyma. (**j**) Complete hemostasis and total removal were confirmed under wet-field conditions

surrounded by crucial brain structures, necessitating utmost caution during surgical interventions to preserve the integrity of the surrounding tissues.

The foramen of Monro is formed by the fornix in the anterior and medial aspects, and the internal cerebral vein is concealed by the choroid plexus in the posterior aspect. To minimize any strain on the foramen of Monro during surgery, the angle of cylinder insertion must be meticulously assessed, taking into account the precise location of the lesion. Preoperative MRI sagittal and coronal images can aid in estimating the optimal approach route from the lesion to the foramen of Monro. For instance, if the lesion is in the anterior half of the third ventricle, a slightly posterior approach may be favored, while for lesions in the posterior half, an anterior approach might be more appropriate (Fig. 7.6).

During surgery, the patient is positioned supine, and the head is fixed with a head clamp. The head is elevated and inclined according to the cylinder angle, particularly for anterior third ventricular lesions. The authors typically employ a transsulcal approach through the superior frontal sulcus.

After tumor resection, it is crucial to ensure a clear CSF pathway from the foramen of Monro to the cerebral aqueduct. However, if tumor removal is not feasible in the posterior part of the third ventricle, it is essential to perform a third ventriculostomy to achieve adequate spinal fluid drainage to the basilar cistern (Figs. 7.7 and 7.8).

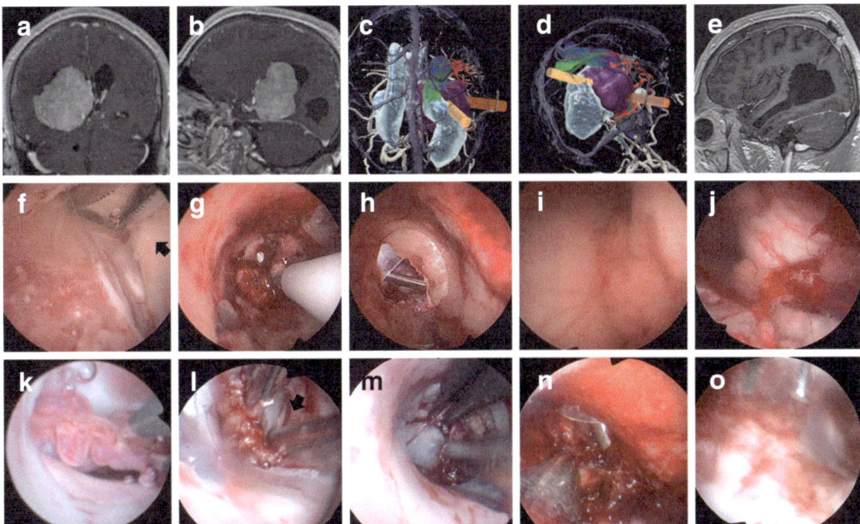

Fig. 7.5 A 46-year-old male presented with consciousness disturbance. (**a, b**) Gadolinium-enhanced MR coronal and sagittal images demonstrate a homogeneously enhancing mass in the atrium of the right lateral ventricle. (**c, d**) Preoperative planning was performed, with the tumor shown in purple and the ventricles in light blue. Double cylinder surgery was planned, inserted from the high parietal and inferior temporal routes. (**e**) Postoperative MR image shows the gross total removal of the tumor. Intraoperative findings from the high parietal route (**f–j**) and inferior temporal route (**k–o**). (**f**) The tumor was dissected from the thalamus (black arrow). (**g**) Tumor debulking was performed with an ultrasound aspirator. (**h**) After tumor debulking, the cylinder inserted from the inferior temporal route was observed. (**i, j**) After the removal of the tumor, total removal and complete hemostasis were confirmed under wet-field conditions. (**k**) Immediately after the insertion of the cylinder, the feeding artery from the choroid plexus was observed and coagulated. (**l**) Tumor dissection from the thalamus. (**m**) Tumor dissection of the posterior edge of the tumor. (**n**) After tumor debulking, the cylinder inserted from the high parietal route was observed. (**o**) Confirming total removal and complete hemostasis under wet-field conditions

7.6.5 Fourth Ventricle

The main tumors that occur in the fourth ventricle include medulloblastoma, ependymoma, and choroid plexus papilloma [34, 35]. The anterior aspect of the fourth ventricle is formed by the brainstem, while the posterior aspect is formed by the cerebellum. The trans-cerebello-medullary fissure approach has been developed and is now considered the standard microscopic surgical approach for fourth ventricle lesions [34, 36]. Additionally, endoscopic approaches have been explored to access the fourth ventricle, with two methods being reported: the trans-aqueductal approach through the lateral and third ventricles and the trans-Magendie-foraminal approach with the rigid endoscope [21, 37, 38]. In this section, we will introduce the endoscopic cylinder surgery with the trans-Magendie-foraminal approach.

During the procedure, the patient is placed in a prone position, and the head is raised, flexed, and slightly rotated to the right and then fixed with a head clamp [21].

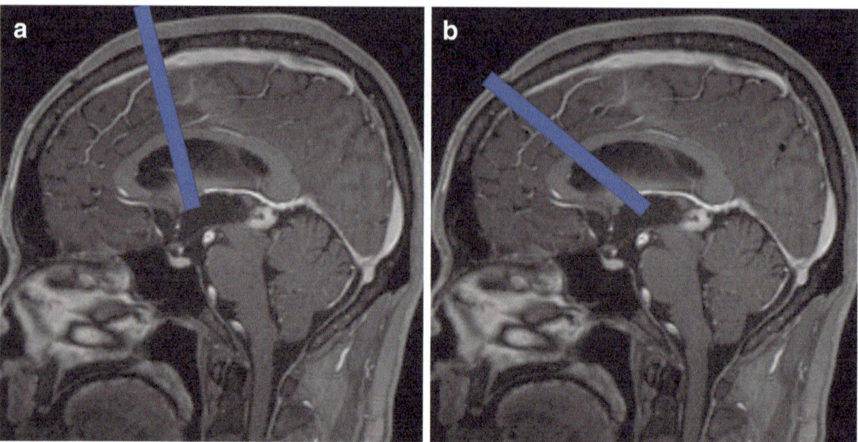

Fig. 7.6 Approaching the route for third ventricular lesions. If the tumor is located in the anterior third ventricle, accessing from the posterior side, similar to endoscopic third ventriculostomy, is suitable (**a**). However, if the tumor is located in the posterior third ventricle, a more anterior approach is recommended (**b**)

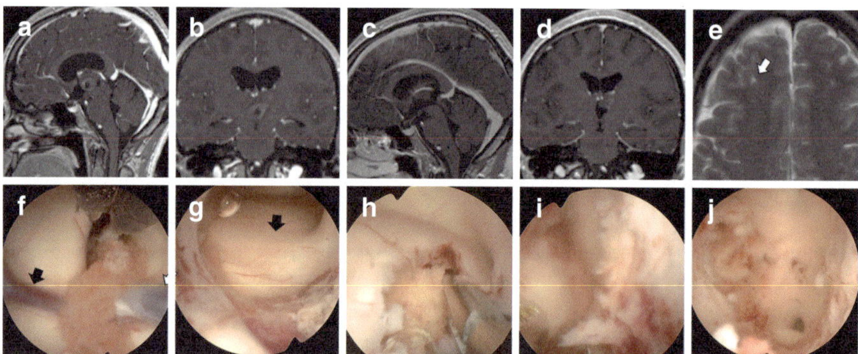

Fig. 7.7 A 26-year-old female presented with a headache. (**a, b**) Gadolinium-enhanced MR sagittal and coronal images demonstrate a mass lesion in the middle third ventricle. (**c, d**) Postoperative gadolinium-enhanced MR sagittal and coronal images show the subtotal removal of the tumor. (**e**) The postoperative MR T2-weighted image indicates a minimal trajectory scar (white arrow). (**f**) After insertion of the cylinder into the right lateral ventricle, the anterior septal vein (white arrow) and the thalamostriate vein (black arrow) were observed. (**g**) The cylinder was advanced into the third ventricle. The tumor was covered by the ependyma of the massa intermedia (black arrow). (**h, i**) Dissecting the tumor from the ependyma. (**j**) Confirming the patency of the cerebral aqueduct and achieving hemostasis under wet-field conditions

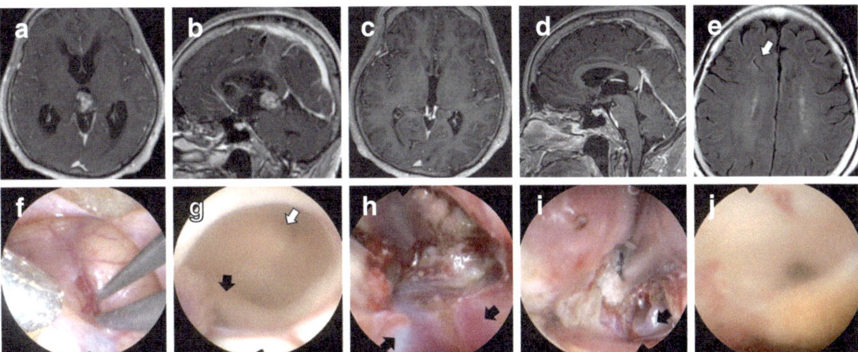

Fig. 7.8 A 67-year-old female presented with a gradually worsening headache and double vision. (**a, b**) Gadolinium-enhanced MR axial and sagittal images demonstrate a mass lesion in the posterior third ventricle. (**c, d**) Postoperative gadolinium-enhanced MR axial and sagittal images show the total removal of the tumor. (**e**) The postoperative MR FLAIR image indicates a minimal trajectory scar (white arrow). (**f**) Dissecting the superior frontal sulcus for the transsulcal insertion of the cylinder. (**g**) Endoscopic observation from the foramen of Monro. The massa intermedia (black arrow) and the mammillary body (white arrow) were observed. (**h**) The tumor was dissected from the bilateral internal cerebral veins (black arrow). (**i**) The tumor was dissected from the basal vein of Rosenthal (black arrow). (**j**) Confirming the cerebrospinal fluid pathway to the cerebral aqueduct

A small craniotomy of approximately 3 cm is performed at the base of the foramen magnum, and the dura mater is incised to expose the thick arachnoid membrane. After the incision of the thick arachnoid membrane, the foramen of Magendie becomes visible. At this moment, a straight anterior-posterior incision of the arachnoid makes it easy to perform the arachnoid plasty during closure. There is typically no adhesion in the bilateral cerebellar tonsils near the foramen of Magendie, allowing the smooth insertion of the cylinder into the fourth ventricle along the inferior surface of the vermis. The angle of the cylinder insertion should align with the posterior plane of the brainstem to prevent any contact or injury to the brainstem. Due to the difficulty of accessing the lateral direction, this technique should be limited to lesions located in the center of the fourth ventricle, which are less than 3 cm in diameter (Fig. 7.9).

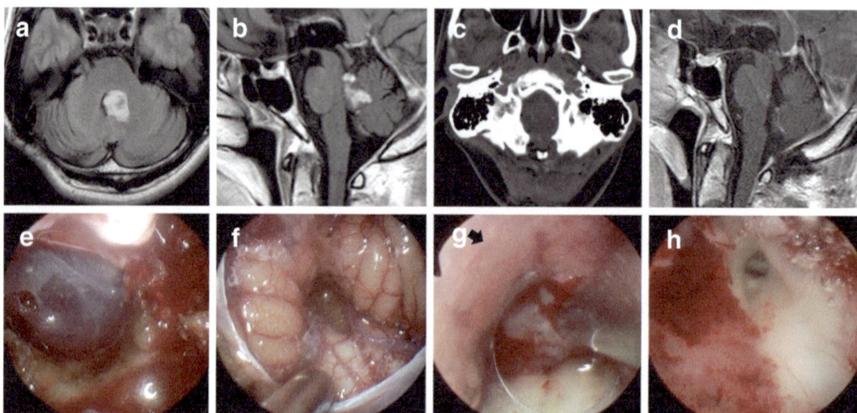

Fig. 7.9 A 70-year-old female presented with a gradually worsening headache. (**a**) The MR FLAIR axial image shows a mass lesion inside the fourth ventricle. (**b**) The gadolinium-enhanced MR sagittal image demonstrates a heterogeneously enhancing mass. (**c**) Postoperative CT shows a small craniotomy of the occipital bone. (**d**) The postoperative gadolinium-enhanced MR sagittal image demonstrates the total removal of the tumor. (**e**) After a 3-cm craniotomy, the thick arachnoid membrane was observed. (**f**) After insertion of the arachnoid, the foramen of Magendie was observed. There was no obvious adhesion between the bilateral tonsils. (**g**) The cylinder was inserted into the fourth ventricle, along with the vermis. The choroid plexus was observed through the transparent cylinder wall. (**h**) After the removal of the tumor, the cerebral aqueduct was observed

7.7 Conclusion

Endoscopic cylinder surgery represents a versatile and minimally invasive approach applicable to all ventricular systems. The endoscope can provide a clear field of view even underwater, enabling surgery while maintaining the shape of the ventricles. On the other hand, the narrow surgical field can be a cause of interference between the instruments. Surgical training is required to perform smooth surgical maneuvers in endoscopic cylinder surgery. Participating in hands-on training courses and gaining a comprehensive understanding of the procedure is highly recommended before performing this surgery.

References

1. Ostrom QT, Gittleman H, Truitt G, Boscia A, Kruchko C, Barnholtz-Sloan JS. CBTRUS statistical report: primary brain and other central nervous system tumors diagnosed in the United States in 2011-2015. Neuro-Oncology. 2018;20:iv1–iv86.
2. Monroy-Sosa A, Chakravarthi SS, de la Garza-Salazar JG, Garcia AM, Kassam AB. Principles of neuro-oncology: brain & skull base. Springer International Publishing; 2020. p. 1–982.

3. Zagzoog N, Reddy KK. Modern brain retractors and surgical brain injury: a review. World Neurosurg. 2020;142:93–103.
4. Mansour S, Echeverry N, Shapiro S, Snelling B. The use of BrainPath tubular retractors in the Management of Deep Brain Lesions: a review of current studies. World Neurosurg. 2020;134:155–63.
5. Kelly PJ, Goerss SJ, Kall BA. The stereotaxic retractor in computer-assisted stereotaxic microsurgery. Technical note. J Neurosurg. 1988;69:301–6.
6. Chen YN, Omay SB, Shetty SR, Liang B, Almeida JP, Ruiz-Treviño AS, Lavi E, Schwartz TII. Transtubular excisional biopsy as a rescue for a non-diagnostic stereotactic needle biopsy—case report and literature review. Acta Neurochir. 2017;159:1589–95.
7. Crevier L, Kassam A, Almenawer SA, Murty N, Reddy K. Minimal access to deep intracranial lesions using a serial dilatation technique. Neurosurg Rev. 2012;36:321–30.
8. Takeuchi K, Ohka F, Nagata Y, et al. Endoscopic trans-mini-cylinder biopsy for Intraparenchymal brain lesions. World Neurosurg. 2022;167:e1147–53.
9. Shapiro SZ, Sabacinski KA, Mansour SA, Echeverry NB, Shah SS, Stein AA, Snelling BM. Use of Vycor tubular retractors in the Management of Deep Brain Lesions: a review of current studies. World Neurosurg. 2020;133:283–90.
10. Eichberg DG, Buttrick S, Brusko GD, Ivan M, Starke RM, Komotar RJ. Use of tubular retractor for resection of deep-seated cerebral tumors and colloid cysts: single surgeon experience and review of the literature. World Neurosurg. 2018;112:e50–60.
11. Eichberg DG, Di L, Shah AH, Luther EM, Jackson C, Marenco-Hillembrand L, Chaichana KL, Ivan ME, Starke RM, Komotar RJ. Minimally invasive resection of intracranial lesions using tubular retractors: a large, multi-surgeon, multi-institutional series. J Neuro-Oncol. 2020;149:35–44.
12. Cohen-Gadol AA. Minitubular transcortical microsurgical approach for gross total resection of third ventricular colloid cysts: technique and assessment. World Neurosurg. 2013;79:207.e7–10.
13. Scranton RA, Fung SH, Britz GW. Transulcal parafascicular minimally invasive approach to deep and subcortical cavernomas: technical note. J Neurosurg. 2016;125:1360–6.
14. Echeverry N, Mansour S, MacKinnon G, Jaraki J, Shapiro S, Snelling B. Intracranial tubular retractor systems: a comparison and review of the literature of the BrainPath, Vycor, and METRx tubular retractors in the Management of Deep Brain Lesions. World Neurosurg. 2020;143:134–46.
15. Kutlay M, Kural C, Solmaz I, Tehli O, Temiz C, Daneyemez M, Izci Y. Fully endoscopic resection of intra-axial brain lesions using neuronavigated pediatric anoscope. Turk Neurosurg. 2016;26:491–9.
16. Kassam AB, Engh JA, Mintz AH, Prevedello DM. Completely endoscopic resection of intra-parenchymal brain tumors. J Neurosurg. 2009;110:116–23.
17. Assina R, Rubino S, Sarris CE, Gandhi CD, Prestigiacomo CJ. The history of brain retractors throughout the development of neurological surgery. Neurosurg Focus. 2014;36:E8.
18. Hong CS, Prevedello DM, Elder JB. Comparison of endoscope-versus microscope-assisted resection of deep-seated intracranial lesions using a minimally invasive port retractor system. J Neurosurg. 2016;124:799–810.
19. McLaughlin N, Prevedello DM, Engh J, Kelly DF, Kassam AB. Endoneurosurgical resection of intraventricular and intraparenchymal lesions using the port technique. World Neurosurg. 2013;79:S18.e1–8.
20. Nishihara T, Teraoka A, Morita A, Ueki K, Takai K, Kirino T. A transparent sheath for endoscopic surgery and its application in surgical evacuation of spontaneous intracerebral hematomas. Technical note. J Neurosurg. 2000;92:1053–5.
21. Nagata Y, Takeuchi K, Yamamoto T, Mizuno A, Wakabayashi T. Fully endoscopic Transcylinder trans-Magendie Foraminal approach for fourth ventricular Cavernoma: a technical case report. World Neurosurg. 2020;142:104–7.

22. Ishikawa T, Takeuchi K, Yamamoto T, Nagata Y, Natsume A. Importance of hydrostatic pressure and irrigation for hemostasis in neuroendoscopic surgery. Neurol Med Chir (Tokyo). 2021;61:117–23.
23. Fujii M, Maesawa S, Motomura K, Futamura M, Hayashi Y, Koba I, Wakabayashi T. Intraoperative subcortical mapping of a language-associated deep frontal tract connecting the superior frontal gyrus to Broca's area in the dominant hemisphere of patients with glioma. J Neurosurg. 2015;122:1390–6.
24. Lerner A, Mogensen MA, Kim PE, Shiroishi MS, Hwang DH, Law M. Clinical applications of diffusion tensor imaging. World Neurosurg. 2013;82:96–109.
25. Potgieser ARE, Wagemakers M, van Hulzen ALJ, de Jong BM, Hoving EW, Groen RJM. The role of diffusion tensor imaging in brain tumor surgery: a review of the literature. Clin Neurol Neurosurg. 2014;124:51–8.
26. Takeuchi K, Nagata Y, Tanahashi K, Araki Y, Mizuno A, Sasaki H, Harada H, Ito K, Saito R. Efficacy and safety of the endoscopic "wet-field" technique for removal of supratentorial cavernous malformations. Acta Neurochir. 2022;164:2587–94.
27. Dănăilă L. Primary tumors of the lateral ventricles of the brain. Chirurgia (Bucur). 2013;108:616–30.
28. Gazi Yaşargil M, Abdulrauf SI. Surgery of intraventricular tumors. Neurosurgery. 2008;62:1029–41.
29. Shucart WA, Stein BM. Transcallosal approach to the anterior ventricular system. Neurosurgery. 1978;3:339–43.
30. Anderson RCE, Ghatan S, Feldstein NA. Surgical approaches to tumors of the lateral ventricle. Neurosurg Clin N Am. 2003;14:509–25.
31. Komiyama M. Functional venous anatomy of the brain for neurosurgeons. Jpn J Neurosurg. 2017;26:488–95.
32. Zhang X, Zhang S, Chen Q, Ding W, Campbell BCV, Lou M. Ipsilateral prominent thalamostriate vein on susceptibility-weighted imaging predicts poor outcome after intravenous thrombolysis in acute ischemic stroke. Am J Neuroradiol. 2017;38:875–81.
33. Zhang XF, Li JC, Wen XD, Ren CG, Cai M, Chen C. Susceptibility-weighted imaging of the anatomic variation of thalamostriate vein and its tributaries. PLoS One. 2015;10:1–11.
34. Ghali MGZ. Telovelar surgical approach. Neurosurg Rev. 2021;44:61–76.
35. Ferguson SD, Levine NB, Suki D, Tsung AJ, Lang FF, Sawaya R, Weinberg JS, McCutcheon IE. The surgical treatment of tumors of the fourth ventricle: a single-institution experience. J Neurosurg. 2018;128:339–51.
36. Matsushima T, Rhoton AL, Lenkey C. Microsurgery of the fourth ventricle: part 1. Neurosurgery. 1982;11:631–67.
37. Hiroshima S, Saga T, Saito M, Tamura Y, Ogawa H, Anei R, Kamada K. Treatment of fourth ventricle arachnoid cyst via anterior hone of lateral ventricle using flexible endoscope. World Neurosurg. 2019;124:224–7.
38. Sharma BS, Sawarkar DP, Verma SK. Endoscopic Management of Fourth Ventricle Neurocysticercosis: description of the new technique in a case series of 5 cases and review of the literature. World Neurosurg. 2019;122:e647–54.

Chapter 8
Purely Endoscopic Treatment for Arachnoid Cysts

Joachim Oertel and Karen Radtke

8.1 Introduction

Arachnoid cysts are lesions consisting of an arachnoid membrane filled with a liquid similar to cerebrospinal fluid [1]. They are commonly described to make up about 1% of all intracranial mass lesions [2]. In a retrospective analysis by Al-Holou et al. of more than 48,000 patients who underwent magnetic resonance (MR) imaging of the brain, arachnoid cysts were found in 1.4%, with a significant male predominance [3]. About half of all arachnoid cysts were found in the posterior fossa, most commonly retrocerebellar and in the cerebellopontine angle. One third of all arachnoid cysts were located in the middle fossa. Arachnoid cysts in direct relation to the brainstem were extremely rare. Other rare locations were the anterior fossa or the interhemispheric gap.

Arachnoid cysts are described as mostly congenital lesions; rare cases have reported cysts as a result of intracranial hemorrhage, infections, or trauma [1, 4, 5]. However, even later in life, the spontaneous development of arachnoid cysts has been described without any obvious underlying cause [6, 7]. In these, a slit valve mechanism for the entrapment of the CSF is postulated [6, 7].

Most commonly, arachnoid cysts are asymptomatic and are thus an incidental finding in brain imaging [1]. Symptoms associated with arachnoid cysts occur in about 5% of patients [8]. Thus, the indication for surgical treatment should be critically evaluated for each patient.

J. Oertel (✉) · K. Radtke
Klinik für Neurochirurgie, Universitätklinikum des Saarlandes und Fakultät für Medizin, Universität des Saarlandes, Homburg, Saar, Germany
e-mail: Joachim.Oertel@uks.eu; Karen.Radtke@uks.eu

W. A. Azab (ed.), *Endoscope-controlled Transcranial Surgery*, Advances and Technical Standards in Neurosurgery 52,
https://doi.org/10.1007/978-3-031-61925-0_8

8.2 Clinical Presentation and Diagnostics

8.2.1 Symptoms

As described above, most arachnoid cysts are incidental findings in brain imaging. Typical symptoms described in the literature are headaches, the formation of hydrocephalus, seizures, vertigo, focal deficits due to cranial nerve impairment or cognitive deficits up to developmental retardation, as well as gait disturbance or ataxia [3, 8–12]. In children, the development of macrocephaly might be observed [9, 10]. The incidence of symptoms is reported to depend on the localization of the cysts, with suprasellar and cerebellopontine angle cysts as well as cysts in the ambient or quadrigeminal cistern causing symptoms more often than cysts in the middle fossa [3]. Suprasellar cysts can result in obstructive hydrocephalus by the compression of the third ventricle or the occlusion of the foramina of Monro or aqueduct [13]. Other symptoms might be hypothalamic or pituitary dysfunction or vision impairment due to mass effect on the optic chiasm [14]. Posterior fossa arachnoid cysts might also impair CSF flow by the obstruction of the fourth ventricle, aqueduct, or foramina of Luschka or Magendie [13]. Increased intracranial pressure (ICP) might also result in vision impairment and headaches. There is generally a slight risk of traumatic or nontraumatic arachnoid cyst rupture, which might result in subdural effusion or even an acute increase in intracranial pressure [15, 16], possibly warranting emergency treatment.

8.2.2 Radiographic Findings

The primary diagnostic tool for arachnoid cysts is radiographic imaging. In CT scans, arachnoid cysts appear as well-circumscribed lesions isodense to CSF, possibly resulting in the displacement of adjacent intracranial structures by exerting a mass effect. In MR imaging, arachnoid cysts also present as circumscribed lesions isointense to CSF. The arachnoid membrane might be visualized [17]. In FLAIR sequences and diffusion-weighted sequences (DWI), arachnoid cysts are equivalent to CSF [18]. Those sequences can be used to differentiate between arachnoid cysts and epidermoid cysts [8]. Arachnoid cysts show no contrast enhancement, which might help differentiate them from tumor-associated cysts. Computed tomography cisternography (CTC) [19] is frequently used to assess arachnoid cysts' communication with basal cisterns and/or ventricles. Magnetic resonance cisternography (MRC) [20] was long used as a gold standard for the evaluation of cyst communication. However, it has to be pointed out that the license for intrathecal application of gadolinium was suspended by the European Medical Association (EMA) for all EU member states in 2017.

8.3 Surgical Technique

8.3.1 Indications for Surgery

Surgical indication has to be evaluated individually in each patient. Small, asymptomatic cysts do not warrant surgical treatment. There is a general consensus that symptomatic arachnoid cysts should be treated surgically [4], especially patients with hydrocephalus, focal deficits, or seizures refractory to antiepileptics. In patients with less severe symptoms, such as chronic headaches or dizziness, surgery should be evaluated even more critically [8]. Choi et al. conducted a study in children with arachnoid cysts, showing that especially children with hydrocephalus and huge or enlarging cysts improved postoperatively. In contrast, headache or dizziness did not improve in more than 50% of cases [21]. As described previously, ruptured cysts might warrant emergency treatment due to an acute increase in intracranial pressure due to the hemorrhage caused by the cyst rupture.

To evaluate the need for surgery and anticipated postoperative benefit, CSF flow between the arachnoid cyst and the normal CSF space should be evaluated. The aim of surgery in arachnoid cysts is to restore CSF communication and thus relieve pressure inside the cyst, resolving local mass effect and chronically elevated intracranial pressure. If CTC or MRC shows the arachnoid cyst to already communicate with the subarachnoid space or ventricular system, the patient is not expected to benefit from surgery; thus, surgical treatment is generally not recommended.

8.3.2 Purely Endoscopic Treatment

In general, there are three options to treat arachnoid cysts surgically: resection, fenestration, or shunting. Each case should be evaluated individually; decision-making should respect the size and localization of the cyst regarding its proximity to the subarachnoid or ventricular space and adjacent neurovascular structures, as well as the safety and feasibility of resection and the experience of the surgeon.

This chapter focuses on the purely endoscopic treatment of arachnoid cysts, and thus, endoscopic cyst fenestration shall be described. For more detailed information, please refer to earlier publications of the authors [6, 7, 12].

After a thorough evaluation of the surgical indication, the optimal approach is planned. Ideally, the approach is mapped out in MRI images with the help of a neuronavigation system allowing a three-dimensional visualization of the trajectory. The positioning of the patient depends on the localization of the cyst and the planned trajectory. In general, arachnoid cyst surgery is performed under general anesthesia. The patient's head is positioned in a Mayfield skull clamp. In infants and children under 2 years of age, a horseshoe headrest might be used if additional bandages are applied for skull fixation. Typically, a single straight trajectory from the skin incision through the burr hole to the cyst and the CSF space is used. This trajectory should allow for restoring the communication of the cyst with the adjacent CSF space. The head should be rotated to have the burr hole at the highest point to have accurate neuronavigational guidance as long as possible. The burr hole position at the highest point prevents massive intraoperative CSF loss, significant brain shift, and postoperative pneumocephalus. After patient positioning, the neuronavigation system and intraoperative electrophysiological monitoring are installed. With the help of neuronavigation, the position of the burr hole is marked on the patient's head along the planned trajectory. A skin incision of 3–4 cm in length is made directly above the planned burr hole. After the exposure of the calvaria, a trepan is used to open up the skull. Bleeding from the bone and dura is stopped using bone wax and bipolar coagulation. The dura is opened in a cruciate fashion with the dural opening having the exact same size as the outer diameter of the endoscope to prevent blood leakage into the field of view. Vision is of utmost importance in all endoscopic cases, with obstructed view due to hemorrhage being one of the most frequent causes of conversion to microsurgery. Continuous irrigation with the ringer's solution helps in visualization.

The exact surgical steps depend on the localization of the cyst and the chosen surgical procedure and will be laid out below.

8.3.3 *Endoscopic Cystocisternostomy*

Endoscopic fenestration of the cyst into the basal cisterns is usually performed if a straight trajectory between a reasonably placed burr hole, the cyst, and the subarachnoid space can be planned. This is most commonly performed in middle fossa (Sylvian fissure) arachnoid cysts or in posterior fossa arachnoid cysts. Again, after the planning of the trajectory, the optimal place of the burr hole is marked on the patient's head. After trephination and dural opening, the work sheath is inserted with the help of neuronavigation to find the right angle. The work sheath is then inserted into the arachnoid cyst. The arachnoid membrane should not be separated from the dura to avoid cyst collapse. Then the cyst and adjacent neurovascular structures are inspected. Different angled endoscopes facilitate the inspection of the complete perimeter; an angulation of the endoscope itself should be strictly prevented. In middle fossa arachnoid cysts, typically the ipsilateral internal carotid artery and the ipsilateral optic and oculomotor nerves can be seen and thus avoided when opening the arachnoid membrane. Ideally, the opening is made between the ICA and optic nerve, where no perforating arteries should be in the way. Alternatively, an opening between the oculomotor nerve and the ICA and/or between the oculomotor nerve and the tentorial edge is possible. An opening between the ICA and oculomotor nerve poses the risk of harming the anterior choroidal artery, which traverses directly in between. However, it frequently can be identified through the arachnoid cyst wall and thus be avoided. Usually, the opening is performed by

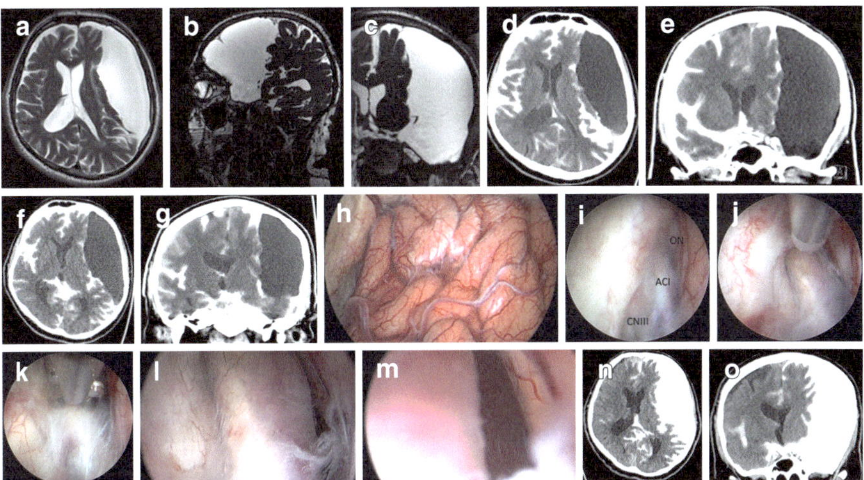

Fig. 8.1 Case 1 shows a 71-year-old male presented with vertigo and unsteady gait. MR tomography showed a very large left-sided frontotemporal space-occupying (Sylvian) arachnoid cyst with a midline shift to the right in axial (**a**), sagittal (**b**), and coronal T2-weighted images (**c**). CT cisternography was performed, which showed no communication of the cyst in axial slices (**d**) and coronal reconstruction (**e**) 1 h post contrast and no communication in axial slices (**f**) and coronal reconstruction (**g**) 2 h post contrast. Surgery was indicated. A cystocisternostomy into the basal cisterns was performed. Endoscopic images show the compression of the frontal and lateral lobes (**h**) and the anatomy at the opticocarotid window (**i**) with the optic nerve (ON), internal carotid artery (ACI), and oculomotor nerve (CNIII). Fenestration was performed with bipolar coagulation and membrane removal by grasping forceps at the ACI between the ACI and optic nerve and between the ACI and oculomotor nerve (**j–l**). At the final inspection of the fenestration, free CSF flow to the basal cisterns could be confirmed (**m**). Postoperatively, the patient still reported vertigo. Thus, another CT cisternography was performed, now showing immediate filling of the body of the cyst, confirming successful cyst fenestration in axial slice (**n**) and coronal reconstruction (**o**)

bipolar coagulation, followed by the enlargement of the stoma with grasping forceps or a balloon catheter. The authors recommend the placement of one large opening or multiple small openings to allow a near-physiological CSF flow and reduce the risk of reobstruction. After fenestration, the surgeon should be able to visualize the basal cisterns. If surgical success is verified, the cyst is thoroughly irrigated to flush out any remaining air; then the work sheath is carefully removed and watertight dural closure applied (Fig. 8.1).

8.3.4 Endoscopic Cystoventriculostomy

Endoscopic cystoventriculostomy is typically performed in patients with paraxial cysts when there is no connection of the cyst to the basal cisterns possible. These cases are rare, and their origin is unknown. However, these cases are very good candidates for a connection of the cysts to the ventricular system. The ideal approach for this surgical technique is a straight trajectory from the planned burr hole through the cyst into the ventricle. Since intraoperatively only the brain cortex can be frequently identified within the cyst, thorough preoperative planning of the ideal trajectory with a neuronavigation system is seen as absolutely mandatory by the authors. As described above, after trephination and dural opening, the work sheath is inserted into the cyst. The cyst is then thoroughly inspected, again using differently angled endoscopes. As mentioned, paraxial cysts typically lack anatomical landmarks. With the help of neuronavigation, the smallest distance between the cyst and ventricle is identified, and—if feasible (no eloquent structures!)—a fenestration through the brain parenchyma in the same style as described above is performed. Again, free CSF flow through the fenestration should be observed, and the endoscope should be advanced into the ventricle to confirm successful fenestration by visualizing intraventricular structures such as the choroid plexus or the foramen of Monro. A stent might be placed to ensure the patency of the fenestration. The endoscope is then carefully removed and dural plasty applied (Fig. 8.2).

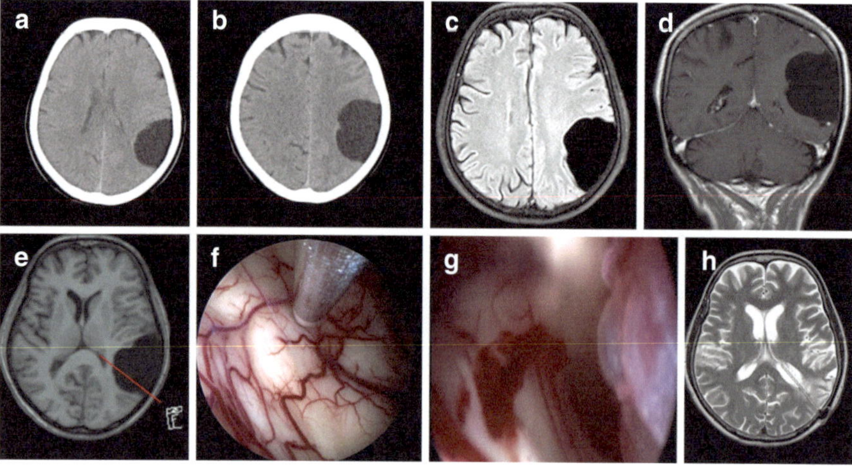

Fig. 8.2 Case 2 shows a 73-year-old woman with a paraxial cyst in the left parieto-occipital lobe (Fig. 8.2). She clinically presented with a seizure with initially right-sided hemiparesis and global aphasia, apraxia, and dysgraphia. The hemiparesis improved spontaneously; the other symptoms persisted. The cyst was first diagnosed 6 years prior by computer tomography (**a**); however, a distinct increase in size was shown on new CT (**b**) and new MR imaging (**c, d**). A straight trajectory from the burr hole through the body of the cyst through the brain parenchyma to the posterior lateral ventricle was planned (red line, **e**). Endoscopic cystoventriculostomy with stenting from the arachnoid cyst into the left lateral ventricle was performed. The perforation was done by blunt perforation; please note that absolutely no landmarks within the cyst are available (**f**). After perforation, the lateral ventricle is inspected by a 30° telescope (**g**). There were no intraoperative complications. Postoperative imaging shows the stent between the cyst and the lateral ventricle and the almost complete resolution of the arachnoid cyst (**h**). Neurological deficits improved directly after surgery. Three years postoperatively, the patient showed no neurological symptoms

8.3.5 *Ventriculocystostomy*

Ventriculocystostomy, the fenestration of a cyst into the ventricular system, is usually performed for cysts inside the ventricular system or quadrigeminal cysts. In these cases, usually a frontal approach is used by the authors. Frequently a trigonal approach is advocated by other neuroendoscopists. However, the authors of this chapter prefer the anterior approach for superior handling options because of the large ventricular space. A frontal approach allows easy navigation through the ventricular system and opening of the cyst with enough space to guide the endoscope. In trigonal approaches, the cyst is immediately in front of the endoscope tip and can be easily entered, but there is less space for maneuvering the endoscope inside the ventricle. In suboccipital approaches, the distance between the skull and cyst is short, which makes entering the cyst usually simple.

As for every endoscopic treatment of arachnoid cysts, the ideal trajectory has to be planned meticulously. Neuronavigation systems should be used to plan the ideal placement of the burr hole to determine the feasible pathway through the brain and to identify the ideal stoma position. Especially in suboccipital approaches and the posterior part of the lateral and third ventricles, a lot of thought should go into trajectory planning to avoid the deep cerebral veins.

In frontal approaches, the patient is placed in a supine position, head fixed in a Mayfield skull clamp. The burr hole is placed according to the preoperatively planned trajectory, usually around Kocher's point. In occipital approaches, either semi-sitting positioning or prone positioning is feasible. After burr hole application, the dura is opened, and the work sheath with trocar is advanced into the lateral ventricle. The ventricular system is thoroughly inspected; the anatomical structures and the cyst are identified. The stoma is created with either bipolar and/or laser coagulation and—if needed—enlarged using either a balloon catheter or grasping forceps. The stoma should be thoroughly inspected and the cyst then flushed with irrigation fluid. The endoscope can be advanced into the body of the cyst to ensure sufficient opening. A final inspection should be done while retracting the endoscope to rule out bleeding inside the ventricular system. Watertight suturing of the dura, closing of the burr hole, and suturing of the wound finalize the surgery.

In some cases, cysts obstruct physiological CSF flow through the foramen of Monro or the aqueduct, causing hydrocephalus. Then additional third ventriculocisternostomy might be indicated, allowing CSF flow from the third ventricle into the basal cisterns. Ideally, the approach is then planned to allow cystostomy as well as ventriculostomy. The endoscopic third ventriculostomy (ETV) should be performed before the cystostomy if possible because bleeding from the cyst might obstruct vision and make the ETV procedure unsafe afterward. ETV is deemed successful if the floor of the third ventricle and the Liliequist membrane are perforated, and the basilar artery in the interpeduncular cistern can be seen through the stoma.

For a suboccipital approach, either semi-sitting positioning or prone positioning is feasible. The head is also fixed in a Mayfield skull clamp. The burr hole is placed paramedian to avoid the superior sagittal sinus and suboccipitally, the median suboccipital sinus—if present. The work sheath is advanced to the area of interest, which might be supracerebellar, intraventricular, or at the foramen magnum. The vein of Galen and other deep cerebral brain must be avoided as the occlusion of these veins might have a fatal outcome due to venous congestive infarction.

The cyst is then perforated with either a laser or bipolar coagulation, the stoma then enlarged using a balloon catheter or grasping forceps, and the cyst wall resected. Thereafter, the endoscope is advanced into the cyst itself, and another stoma is done at the anterior wall of the cyst into the ventricular system. Neuronavigation helps ensure the ideal placement of the stoma. The stoma itself is then inspected; the endoscope might be advanced into the ventricular systems to ensure sufficient opening. Again, the endoscope is retracted carefully, the dura and bone are closed, and the wound is sutured (Fig. 8.3).

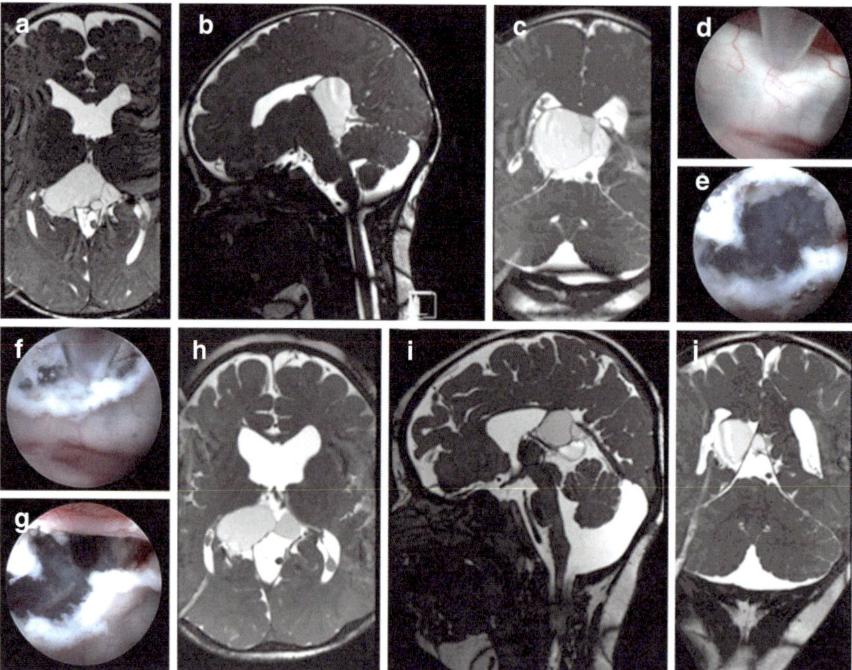

Fig. 8.3 Case 3 shows a 4-month-old girl with Aicardi syndrome. MR tomography showed multiple arachnoid cysts around the quadrigeminal plate on T2 images in the axial plane (**a**), sagittal plane (**b**), and coronal plane (**c**) among other cerebral anomalies. The girl was initially asymptomatic but later presented with seizures and developmental delay. Additionally, MR tomography showed an increase in cyst size; thus, surgery was indicated. A right frontal burr hole was performed; the endoscope was advanced into the lateral ventricle. A small layer of ependyma covered the cyst and was opened up with bipolar coagulation (**d**) until the cyst wall was seen (**e**). A ventriculocystostomy was performed on the upper cyst wall, leading to an immediate collapse of the cyst (**f**, **g**). Postoperatively, a decrease in cyst size was seen on T2 MR images in the axial plane (**h**), sagittal plane (**i**), and coronal plane (**j**)

8.3.6 Ventriculocystocisternostomy

Ventriculocystocisternostomy combines ventriculocystostomy with cystocisternography. It is usually performed in suprasellar cysts that lead to hydrocephalus by obstructing the physiological CSF pathway. The combined technique removes pressure from the midbrain and additionally restores CSF circulation.

Again, the optimal trajectory is planned in MRI imaging with the help of a neuronavigation system. The ideal trajectory connects both the inferior and superior cyst walls and their borders into the ventricular system and basal cisterns and also the burr hole while avoiding vascular structures and eloquent brain areas. After the supine positioning of the patient and fixation of the head in a Mayfield skull clamp and trephination, the dura is opened and the work sheath advanced under neuronavigational guidance. The lateral ventricle is punctured and thoroughly inspected. The endoscope is then advanced into the third ventricle. Usually, the superior portion of the cyst wall extends far up into the third ventricle and can be seen through the foramen of Monro from the lateral ventricle. The stoma should then be opened widely and parts of the membrane resected to prevent reocclusion. The endoscope is then advanced into the body of the cyst. A second stoma is performed in the inferior portion of the cyst wall into the interpeduncular cistern. Similar to ETV, injury to the basilar artery must be avoided due to its likely fatal outcome. In the end, free CSF flow through both stomata must be observable, and the basilar artery inside the interpeduncular cistern should be exposed. Oftentimes, the inferior cyst membrane is localized deeper than the third ventricle floor; thus, a stoma might have to be performed laterally to minimize the risk of perforating the trunk of the basilar artery. The endoscope is then retracted, and the dura, bone, and wound are closed in the usual manner (Fig. 8.4).

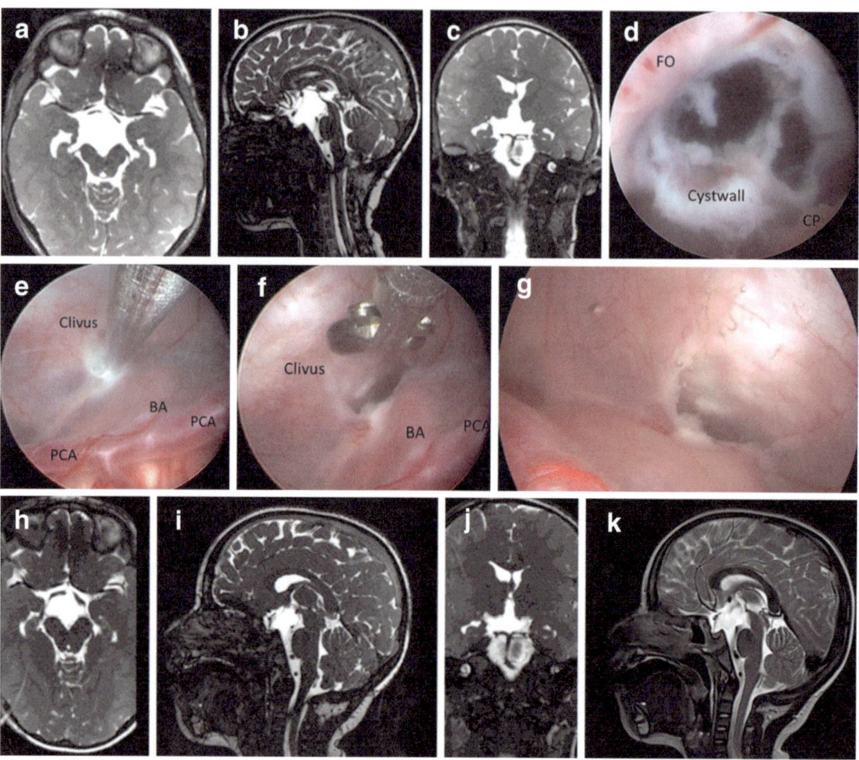

Fig. 8.4 Case 4 shows a child referred to our clinic at 2 years of age due to an arachnoid cyst, which had been diagnosed before birth. At the age of 2, pediatricians confirmed developmental delay. He had undergone MR tomography yearly, which showed no cyst growth but compression of the optic chiasm and third ventricle. Preoperative T2-weighted MR images are shown in axial (**a**), sagittal (**b**), and coronal projection (**c**). Surgery was performed at the age of 3. After thorough planning, an endoscope was advanced through the lateral ventricle. The foramen of Monro was identified. The cyst reached up to the foramen of Monro. There, the upper cyst wall was fenestrated using bipolar coagulation (**d**). Please note the fornix (FO) and the choroid plexus (CP) of the lateral ventricle as landmarks at the foramen of Monro. Then the endoscope was advanced into the body of the cyst, and a second perforation was performed at the floor of the third ventricle. (**e** and **f**) Show the blunt bipolar coagulation of the cyst wall, followed by the resection of the cyst wall with grasping forceps paramedian to the basilar artery (BA). For orientation, the posterior cerebral arteries (PCA) and the clivus are marked. A large ventriculocystocisternostomy resulted (**g**). Postoperative imaging shows a decrease in cyst size T2-weighted axial (**h**), sagittal (**i**), and coronal (**j**) MR images. Figure k shows in the T2-weighted sagittal MR image the vivid flow void sign at the floor of the third ventricle. There were no postoperative complications

8.4 Complications

8.4.1 Intraoperative Complications

One of the most common intraoperative complications of endoscopic cyst fenestration is bleeding [12, 22]. Mild hemorrhages can be treated by continuous irrigation with body temperature Ringer's solution. Even heavier bleeding might be controlled by irrigation alone. At least, irrigation can restore vision to allow the visualization and coagulation of the bleeding vessel. Other options to stop bleeding in intraventricular endoscopic procedures are the so-called small-chamber technique [23] and dry-field technique [24]. The authors recommend the dry-field technique in cases with heavy bleeding that cannot be controlled with irrigation alone. Here, all CSF is aspirated to allow better visualization of the bleeding vessel. A switch to microsurgery, which would allow bimanual manipulation at the cost of a more traumatic approach, is rarely necessary.

8.4.2 Postoperative Complications

The most common postoperative complications are infections, CSF leaks [25, 26], and the formation of subdural hematoma or hygroma [25, 26]. Infection should be avoided by applying single-shot antibiotics intraoperatively. The risk for CSF leaks decreases if the cyst is successfully fenestrated and CSF flow restored as pressure on the dural closure and skin is minimized. Other postoperative complications include hormonal disturbances or electrolyte imbalances and double vision due to cranial nerve palsy or irritation of the cerebellum [12].

8.5 Outcome

8.5.1 Postoperative Radiologic Findings

The authors recommend follow-up CT scans one day after the procedure to rule out immediate postoperative complications. If the patient deteriorates clinically, emergency CT scans are obtained immediately. Ideally, a collapse of the cyst and a decrease in ventricle size are seen in hydrocephalus patients. Brain structures should be decompressed sufficiently.

In the authors' center, MRI studies are conducted 3 months and 6–9 months postoperatively. Changes in cyst size are noted, and ventricle size is evaluated. If the success of the surgery remains questionable, CT or MR cisternography might be performed to assess the openness of the stoma.

In general, reports on neuroradiological outcomes vastly differ. A complete disappearance of the cyst is rare [27]. Reduction of cyst size is reported in about 50–70% of cases [9, 12, 25–27].

8.5.2 Clinical Improvement

Acute symptoms due to sudden elevated ICP such as vomiting and dizziness should resolve immediately postoperatively [10]. Symptoms such as headaches [9–12, 26–28], neurological deficits [9, 10, 27], and seizure frequence [9, 10, 26–28] are also reported to have a favorable outcome with improvement rates up to 100%. Chronic symptoms, such as macrocrania, might take longer to resolve. Still, it is reported that children usually show a return to normal head circumference after surgery [9, 10, 26–28]. The authors recommend that clinical assessment should be done in concordance with the recommendations for follow-up imaging. In children, particular attention has to be paid to head circumference and the stages of development. Patients and parents have to be educated on the symptoms of sudden elevation in ICP and have to be instructed to present to the hospital if those symptoms occur. Due to the possibility of the recurrence of arachnoid cysts [12], long-term follow-ups should be the standard for arachnoid cyst patients.

8.6 Conclusion

The authors recommend endoscopic fenestration as the first-line treatment for symptomatic, noncommunicating intracranial arachnoid cysts. To ensure operative success, consequent preoperative workup, good patient selection, and thorough planning of the ideal trajectory and approach are of utmost importance. Intraoperatively, it is crucial to be knowledgeable of neurovascular anatomy and be experienced in handling an endoscope in a small corridor to avoid and manage complications. If these precautions are followed, the endoscopic treatment of arachnoid cysts is a safe and feasible procedure for both patients and surgeons.

References

1. Öcal E. Understanding intracranial arachnoid cysts: a review of etiology, pathogenesis, and epidemiology. Childs Nerv Syst. 2023;39:73–8.
2. Vega-Sosa A, de Obieta-Cruz E, Hernández-Rojas MA. Intracranial arachnoid cyst. Cir Cir. 2010;78:551–6.
3. Al-Holou WN, et al. Prevalence and natural history of arachnoid cysts in adults. J Neurosurg. 2013;118:222–31.

4. Hall S, et al. Natural History of Intracranial Arachnoid Cysts. World Neurosurg. 2019;126:e1315–20.
5. Choi J-U, Kim D-S. Pathogenesis of Arachnoid Cyst: Congenital or Traumatic? Pediatr Neurosurg. 1998;29:260–6.
6. Oertel JMK, Baldauf J, Schroeder HWS, Gaab MR. Endoscopic cystoventriculostomy for treatment of paraxial arachnoid cysts: Clinical article. JNS. 2009;110:792–9.
7. Oertel J, Rediker J. Endoscopic techniques in Arachnoid Cyst Surgery. Chapter 11. In: Wester K, editor. Arachnoid cysts. clinical and surgical management. Elsevier Academic Press, London; 2018. p. 142–65.
8. Ahmed AK, Cohen AR. Intracranial arachnoid cysts. Childs Nerv Syst. 2023;39(10):2771–8. https://doi.org/10.1007/s00381-023-06066-0.
9. El-Ghandour NMF. Endoscopic treatment of middle cranial fossa arachnoid cysts in children: Clinical article. PED. 2012;9:231–8.
10. Schulz M, et al. Endoscopic and Microsurgical Treatment of Sylvian Fissure Arachnoid Cysts—Clinical and Radiological Outcome. World Neurosurg. 2015;84:327–36.
11. Gui S, et al. Assessment of endoscopic treatment for middle cranial fossa arachnoid cysts. Childs Nerv Syst. 2011;27:1121–8.
12. Oertel J, et al. Endoscopic Treatment of Intracranial Arachnoid Cysts: A Retrospective Analysis of a 25-Year Experience. Operative Surg. 2021;20:32–44.
13. Martínez-Lage JF, Pérez-Espejo MA, Almagro M-J, López-Guerrero AL. Hydrocephalus and arachnoid cysts. Childs Nerv Syst. 2011;27:1643–52.
14. Özek MM, Urgun K. Neuroendoscopic Management of Suprasellar Arachnoid Cysts. World Neurosurg. 2013;79:S19.e13-S19.e18.
15. Albuquerque FC, Giannotta SL. Arachnoid Cyst Rupture Producing Subdural Hygroma and Intracranial Hypertension: Case Reports. Neurosurgery. 1997;41:951–6.
16. Gelabert-González M, Fernández-Villa J, Cutrín-Prieto J, Garcìa Allut A, Martínez-Rumbo R. Arachnoid cyst rupture with subdural hygroma: report of three cases and literature review. Childs Nerv Syst. 2002;18:609–13.
17. Harsh GR, Edwards MSB, Wilson CB. Intracranial arachnoid cysts in children. J Neurosurg. 1986;64:835–42.
18. Adrien J, et al. Petrous and sphenoid arachnoid cysts: Diagnosis and management. Head Neck. 2015;37:823–8.
19. Wang X, Chen J, You C, Jiang S. CT cisternography in intracranial symptomatic arachnoid cysts: Classification and treatment. J Neurol Sci. 2012;318:125–30.
20. Tali ET, Ercan N, Kaymaz M, Pasaoglu A, Jinkins JR. Intrathecal gadolinium (gadopentetate dimeglumine) enhanced MR cisternography used to determine potential communication between the cerebrospinal fluid pathways and intracranial arachnoid cysts. Neuroradiology. 2004;46:744–54.
21. Choi JW, Lee JY, Phi JH, Kim S-K, Wang K-C. Stricter indications are recommended for fenestration surgery in intracranial arachnoid cysts of children. Childs Nerv Syst. 2015;31:77–86.
22. Prasjnar-Borak A, Oertel J, Antes S, Yilmaz U, Linsler S. Cerebral vasospasm after endoscopic fenestration of a temporal arachnoid cyst in a child - a are report and review of literature. Childs Nerv Syst. 2019;35:695–9.
23. Manwaring JC, El Damaty A, Baldauf J, Schroeder HWS. The Small-Chamber Irrigation Technique (SCIT): A Simple Maneuver for Managing Intraoperative Hemorrhage During Endoscopic Intraventricular Surgery. Operative Neurosurgery. 2014;10:375–9.
24. Oertel J, Linsler S, Csokonay A, Schroeder HWS, Senger S. Management of severe intraoperative hemorrhage during intraventricular neuroendoscopic procedures: the dry field technique. J Neurosurg. 2019;131:931–5.
25. Cinalli G, et al. Complications following endoscopic intracranial procedures in children. Childs Nerv Syst. 2007;23:633–44.
26. Di Rocco F, et al. Limits of endoscopic treatment of sylvian arachnoid cysts in children. Childs Nerv Syst. 2010;26:155–62.

27. Karabagli H, Etus V. Success of pure neuroendoscopic technique in the treatment of Sylvian arachnoid cysts in children. Childs Nerv Syst. 2012;28:445–52.
28. Spacca B, Kandasamy J, Mallucci CL, Genitori L. Endoscopic treatment of middle fossa arachnoid cysts: a series of 40 patients treated endoscopically in two centres. Childs Nerv Syst. 2010;26:163–72.

Chapter 9
Purely Endoscopic Evacuation of Intracranial Hematomas

Hisayuki Murai, Takuji Yamamoto, and Toru Nagasaka

9.1 Introduction

Cerebral hemorrhage is a frequent disease and one of the main causes for requiring nursing care. Even if cerebral hemorrhage occurs, the benefits would be immeasurable if not only the survival prognosis but also the functional prognosis could be improved. This chapter briefly reviews past research. We will discuss the usefulness and future prospects of hematoma removal surgery and introduce the standard surgical procedure currently performed in Japan.

9.2 What We Learned from Previous Research

In 1989, Auer et al. [1] found that although endoscopic deeply seated hematoma evacuation did not significantly improve the outcome, it was found to be useful for subcortical hemorrhage with a statistically significant difference. However, STICH (2005) [2] failed to demonstrate the usefulness of early surgery. In STICH II (2013) [3], the functional prognosis for subcortical hemorrhage tended to be better in the

H. Murai (✉)
Department of Neurosurgery, Saiseikai Narashino Hospital, Narashino, Japan
e-mail: murai@chiba-saiseikai.com

T. Yamamoto
Department of Neurosurgery, Juntendo University Shizuoka Hospital, Izunokuni, Japan
e-mail: tyamamoto@med-juntendo.jp

T. Nagasaka
Department of Pathology, Chub Rosai Hospital, Nagoya, Japan
e-mail: toru-ngy@umin.ac.jp, customerservice@tn-medical.net

© The Author(s), under exclusive license to Springer Nature Switzerland AG 2024
W. A. Azab (ed.), *Endoscope-controlled Transcranial Surgery*, Advances and Technical Standards in Neurosurgery 52,
https://doi.org/10.1007/978-3-031-61925-0_9

surgical treatment group, but it could not be said that it improved significantly. However, the survival rate improved in the surgical treatment group, and a considerable number of cases were transferred from the medical treatment group to surgical treatment, so it seems that the usefulness of surgery cannot be denied, and a secondary study was later conducted. Similarly, in some studies [4–6], there was a tendency for surgical treatment to be better, but the difference was not significant. It seemed that minimally invasive surgical treatment could improve the prognosis. In the MISTIE trial [7], a method of stereotactically inserting a drain and using tPA to lyse the hematoma was investigated, but its usefulness was not proven.

The results of the secondary analysis of MISTIE, STICH, and STICH II showed that the hematoma volume at the end of treatment affected the prognosis [8, 9], and surgical treatment tended to be more effective in moderate Glasgow Coma Scale (GCS) or large hematoma [10]. Regarding the timing of surgery, the early evacuation of intracerebral hemorrhage (ICH) with open surgery or a tissue plasminogen activator (tPA) does not provide better outcomes [9]. Hematoma stability may be beneficial before performing open surgery or thrombolysis. This means bleeding control might be difficult in both methods. But in endoscopic surgery, the bleeding point can be explored and coagulated. It was also suggested in the secondary analysis that the therapeutic window for hematoma evacuation might be somewhat longer [9].

9.3 Standard Endoscopic Hematoma Removal Method in Japan

Since Nishihara et al. [11] developed a transparent sheath in 2000, endoscopic hematoma removal has become a commonly performed procedure in Japan. According to a 2010 Japanese Society for Neuroendoscopy member survey, it is performed to the same extent as endoscopic third ventriculostomy. According to the primary report of a case registry study of experienced surgeons with over 100 cases (RICH-trend) [12], over 90% of surgeries were performed within 2 days after the onset of symptoms. The median time was 8 h after onset. Hematomas often become a little harder for 3–7 days after a stroke, and hematoma removal surgery tends to be avoided during this period. The hematoma may be also firmer in patients taking antithrombotic drugs such as warfarin, so measures such as preparing a thicker suction tube or physically crushing the hematoma with biopsy forceps are performed. There are a few papers with a high level of evidence regarding endoscopic hematoma removal, so surgeons are required to perform surgery in a less invasive manner and to carefully consider each case while taking account of their own skill level. For example, an inexperienced surgeon may choose to wait for several days until hemostasis has been achieved and the hematoma has softened.

9.4 Indications

Surgery for cerebellar hemorrhage (Fig. 9.1) seems to be the most effective because it shortens the surgical time and improves the prognosis [13, 14]. According to Kuramatsu et al. [15], surgery for cerebellar hemorrhage through suboccipital

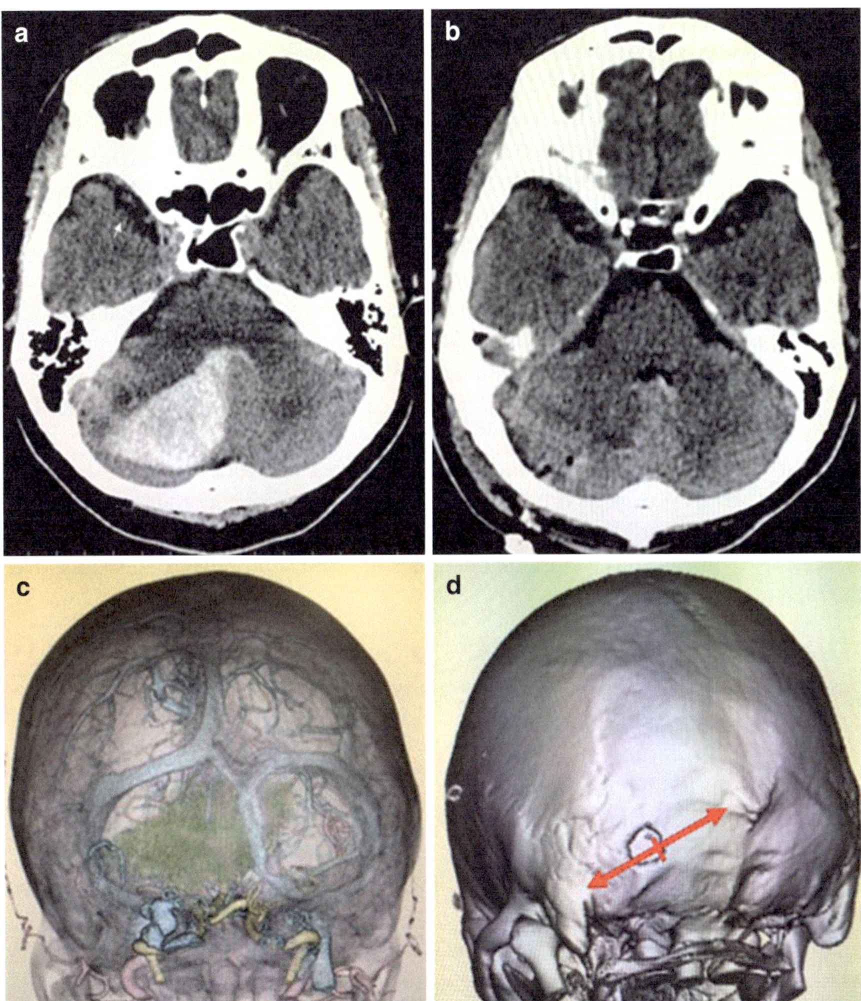

Fig. 9.1 Cerebellar hemorrhage. (**a**) preoperative CT, (**b**) postoperative CT. (**c**) To avoid sinus or venous injury, 3D CTA is recommended. Hematoma is indicated in green. (**d**) The standard burr hole site for endoscopic cerebellar hematoma evacuation is midpoint between the inion and mastoid

craniectomy had no significant effect on conservative treatment. However, according to Yamamoto et al. [13], there was no difference in the hematoma removal rate between craniectomy and endoscopy. The mean endoscopic surgical time is significantly shorter, approximately 70 min, and the need for shunts is significantly reduced. Second, intraventricular hemorrhage accompanied by hydrocephalus is a good indication. There have been reports that endoscopic hematoma removal has better outcomes than ventricular drain management alone [16, 17]. In the past, thalamic hemorrhage was often not an indication for surgery, but with endoscopy, it has become possible to enter the hematoma in the thalamus from the ventricle. Therefore, thalamic hemorrhage associated with acute hydrocephalus is also an indication for endoscopic surgery. Subcortical hemorrhage or putaminal hemorrhage exceeding 30 mL is also indicated. However, it is difficult to show improvement in functional prognosis for deep-seated cerebral hemorrhage. Recently, even in cases of deep-seated hematoma, there are some reports showing the superiority of the surgical group for moderate hematoma volume and moderate neurological symptoms. Yamamoto et al. [18] reported that endoscopic hematoma removal showed superior improvement over the internal medicine or craniotomy groups for hematoma volumes ranging from 30 mL to 60 mL and GCS scores of 9 to 12 points. Fujita et al. [19] reported that in early elderly patients (65 to 74 years old) with an ICH score of 3, both craniotomy and endoscopy showed superior improvement compared to medical treatment.

In Japan, unfortunately a multicenter randomized controlled trial has not been conducted. However, in facilities that have already introduced endoscopic hematoma removal, it is difficult to return to suboccipital craniectomy for cerebellar hemorrhage or to manage intraventricular hemorrhage with ventricular drains alone over the long period.

9.5 Instruments

The three essential and basic equipment are (1) a 0-degree rigid scope with an outer diameter of approximately 3 mm, (2) a transparent sheath, and (3) a suction coagulator (Fig. 9.2). There are some types of suction coagulators that can be used outside Japan, but in Japan, the ones made by Fujita medical instruments are often used and are available in several sizes.

Transparent sheaths (Fig. 9.3) include the acrylic Clear Sheath® manufactured by Machida and the plastic Neuroport® manufactured by Hakko sold by Olympus. There are two types of Clear Sheath® with an outer diameter of 6 mm and 8 mm, and Hakko's Neuroport® comes in two types with an outer diameter of 6 mm and 10 mm. Although a thin sheath is less invasive, the thickness must be selected according to the skill of the surgeon and the hardness of the hematoma.

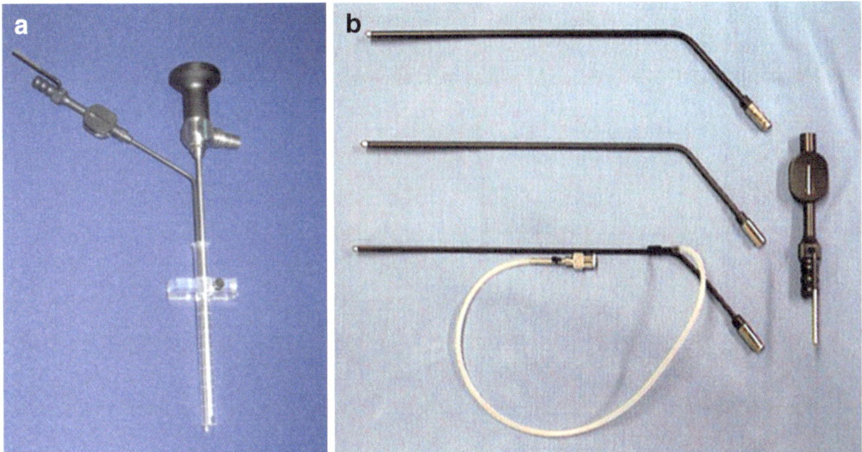

Fig. 9.2 Fundamental setup (**a**) and suction coagulators (**b**). There are three basic elements: a transparent sheath, a rigid scope, and a suction coagulator. Suction coagulators (Fujita Medical Instruments, Tokyo) come in various thicknesses

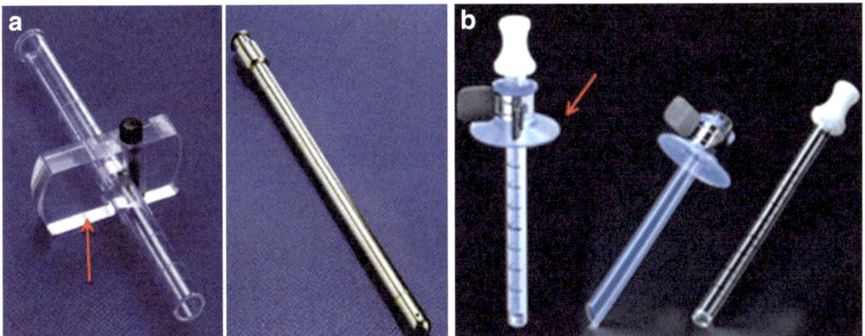

Fig. 9.3 Transparent guiding sheath. (**a**) MACHIDA Clear Sheath® is made of acryl glass. Two diameter sizes (OD 6 mm and 8 mm) are available. (**b**) Hakko/Olympus Neuroport® is made of plastic. Two diameter sizes (OD 6 mm and 10 mm) are available. Both have a stopper (arrow) to change the depth

9.6 Surgical Procedures

9.6.1 Entry Point and Tract

Consider the puncture site along the long axis of the hematoma as this allows for more efficient and less invasive hematoma removal. When the burr hole is located on the forehead, it is often moved to the hairline for cosmetic reasons. Puncture is performed under navigation or ultrasound guidance to be minimally invasive. Also, choose a tract that will not damage important nerve fibers. Instead of inserting a thick sheath from the beginning, always perform a test puncture with a thin puncture needle. Neuroport®'s stylet is also transparent, so you can puncture it while looking at the tip.

9.6.2 Internal Decompression

Once inside the hematoma cavity, aspirate and decompress the hematoma to some extent. If the hematoma is hard, do not try to force it out; instead, look for a soft spot. Generally, the edges of the hematoma are slightly softer.

9.6.3 Exploration of the Hematoma Cavity (Fig. 9.4, Modified from Nagasaka 2011 [20])

Once a certain amount of hematoma has been aspirated, the hematoma wall is explored while pulling up the sheath. The white matter that is the hematoma wall, the tip of the sheath, the suction tube, and the hematoma should be seen as much as possible on the monitor. Search and suction in a rotating motion within the hematoma cavity and proceed from shallow areas to deeper areas.

9.6.4 Hemostasis (Fig. 9.5, Modified from Nagasaka 2011 [20])

If fresh red blood is seen in some areas, this is a sign that the patient is still bleeding, and the bleeding point must be located and coagulated to stop the bleeding. White matter is soft, so if you press on the bleeding point, it will cause bleeding from deeper and cause damage to the white matter, so you must be careful. To coagulate the bleeding, lightly touch a suction coagulator to the bleeding point or apply light suction to the bleeding blood vessel and slowly pull it up while applying electricity to coagulate and stop the bleeding. A hard clot may be firmly attached to a bleeding blood vessel, in which case it is intentionally left in place.

9.6.5 Confirmation of Hemostasis

Irrigate and clean the hematoma cavity and confirm hemostasis. If it is difficult to confirm hemostasis, the hematoma cavity may be cleaned using a flexible scope.

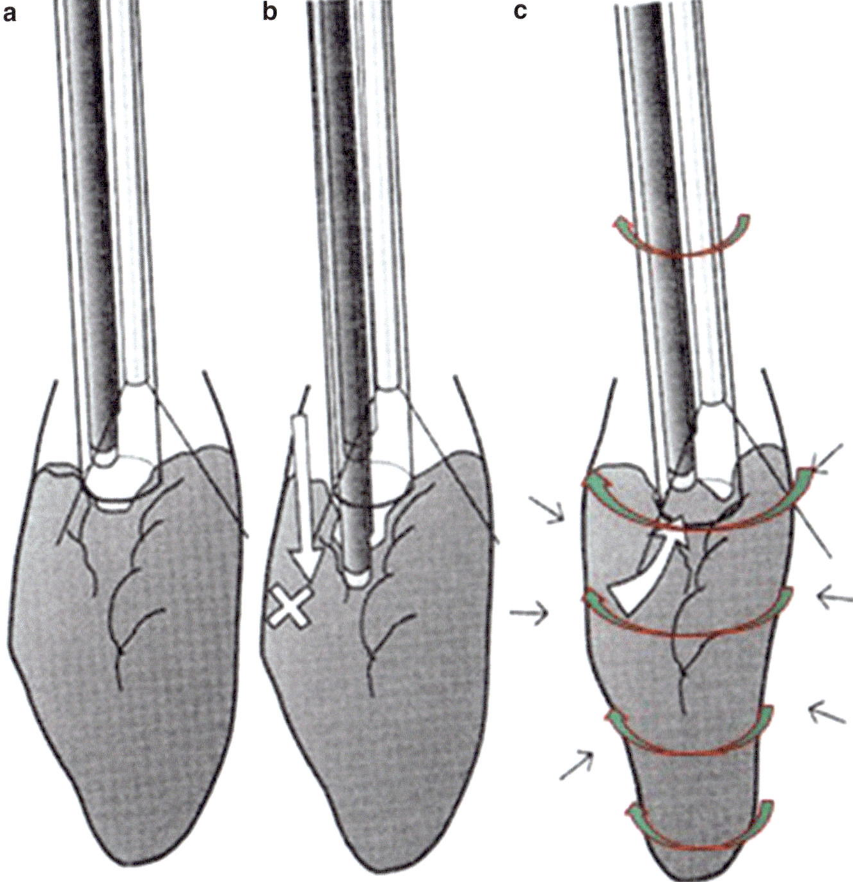

Fig. 9.4 Evacuation of hematoma (modified from Nagasaka 2011 [20]). The sucker tip should be placed inside or at the tip of the sheath (**a**). Sticking a sucker may injure the brain parenchyma and cause unexpected bleeding (**b**). Explore the hematoma cavity border and suck the hematoma from top to bottom (**c**). As the hematoma cavity becomes smaller, it becomes easy to move along the borders

9.6.6   Assistant's Role

Endoscopic hematoma removal is a two-person operation, and the assistant plays a major role. The assistant usually holds the sheath lightly so as not to impede the surgeon's movements, and when the surgeon pulls out the endoscope, the assistant holds the sheath firmly so that it does not fall out of the hematoma cavity. The assistant works with the surgeon to control the depth of the sheath by moving the stopper, but the stopper is often unnecessary with a skilled assistant. The assistant also cleans the inside of the sheath and hematoma cavity, the dirty rigid scope, etc., as appropriate.

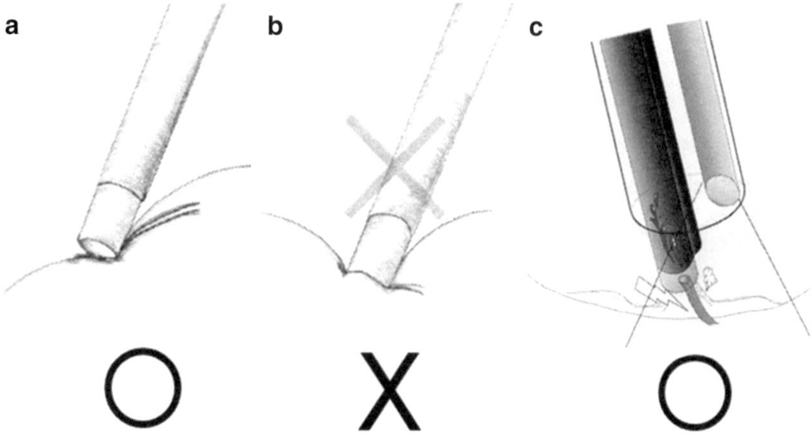

Fig. 9.5 Coagulation of bleeding point (modified from Nagasaka 2011 [20]). Pushing the bleeding point (**a**) makes it deeper and may damage the brain. Gently touch (**b**) or gently suck the bleeding vessel (**c**) and coagulate it

9.7 A Representative Case (Fig. 9.6)

A woman in her 50 s had a headache and vomiting, and a hematoma was found under the cortex of her right temporoparietal lobe. Since she had a history of angina pectoris several months ago and her heart function was not good, general anesthesia was considered dangerous and conservative treatment was started, but she was taking antithrombotic drugs, and the hematoma was growing. As the patient became drowsy and the vomiting became more frequent, hematoma removal was performed under local anesthesia. The burr was placed on the thinnest part of the cortex. Figure 9.6c is a representative image during surgery, with the white matter, hematoma, suction tube, and sheath tip on the monitor. The bleeding vessel was cauterized, and the surgery was completed in about an hour.

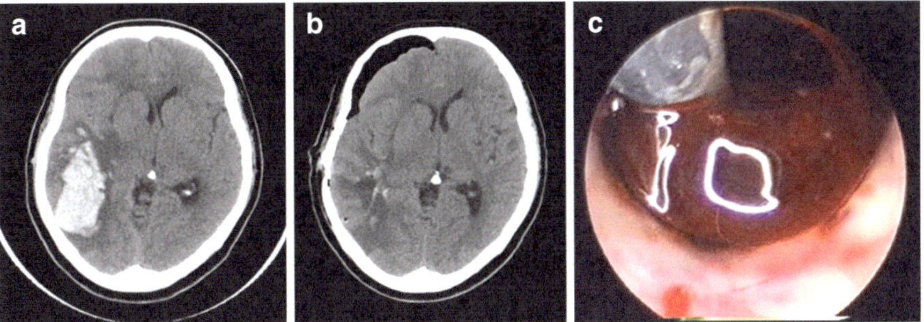

Fig. 9.6 A case of subcortical hematoma. (**a**) preoperative CT, (**b**) postoperative CT, (**c**) standard surgical view

9.8 Future Prospects

Recently, the results of the ENRICH study were reported [21, 22], including the effectiveness of minimally invasive surgery for lobar hematomas over medical treatment with a statistically significant difference. In cases of cerebral hemorrhage, if there is a region of the brain that can be recovered, the extent of hematoma removal conferred survival and functional benefits. Furthermore, the less invasive the surgery is, the more effective it can be expected to be. Hematoma removal using an endoscope seems to be highly effective and promising, but the current surgical techniques and equipment are still in the development stage. There is still much research to be done, and improvements in the surgery itself seem to be on the way. Operators should carefully decide on surgical indications, considering their own technique, the condition of each patient, and the available equipment. We hope that the Japanese surgical methods introduced in this chapter will contribute to improving surgical outcomes in each region.

Financial Support and Sponsorship Nil.

Conflicts of Interest There are no conflicts of interest.

References

1. Auer LM, Deinsberger W, Niederkorn K, et al. Endoscopic surgery versus medical treatment for spontaneous intracerebral hematoma: a randomized study. J Neurosurg. 1989;70:530–5.
2. Mendelow AD, Gregson BA, Fernandes HM, Murray GD, Teasdale GM, Hope DT, STICH Investigators, et al. Early surgery versus initial conservative treatment in patients with spontaneous supratentorial intracerebral haematomas in the International Surgical Trial in Intracerebral Haemorrhage (STICH): a randomised trial. Lancet. 2005;365:387–97.
3. Mendelow AD, Gregson BA, Rowan EN, Murray GD, Gholkar A, Mitchell PM, STICH II Investigators. Early surgery versus initial conservative treatment in patients with spontaneous supratentorial lobar intracerebral haematomas (STICH II): a randomised trial. Lancet. 2013;382:397–408.

4. Vespa P, Hanley D, Betz J, et al. ICES Investigators. ICES (Intraoperative Stereotactic Computed Tomography-Guided Endoscopic Surgery) for Brain Hemorrhage: A Multicenter Randomized Controlled Trial. Stroke. 2016;47(11):2749–55.

5. Kellner CP, Song R, Pan J, Nistal DA, et al. Long-term functional outcome following minimally invasive endoscopic intracerebral hemorrhage evacuation. J Neurointerv Surg. 2020;12(5):489–94.

6. Ali M, Zhang X, Ascanio LC, et al. Long-term functional independence after minimally invasive endoscopic intracerebral hemorrhage evacuation. J Neurosurg. 2022;138(1):154–64.

7. Hanley DF, Thompson RE, Rosenblum M, et al. MISTIE III Investigators. Efficacy and safety of minimally invasive surgery with thrombolysis in intracerebral haemorrhage evacuation (MISTIE III): a randomised, controlled, open-label, blinded endpoint phase 3 trial. Lancet. 2019;393(10175):1021–32.

8. de Havenon A, Joyce E, Yaghi S, et al. End-of-Treatment Intracerebral and Ventricular Hemorrhage Volume Predicts Outcome: A Secondary Analysis of MISTIE III. Stroke. 2020;51(2):652–4.

9. Polster SP, Carrión-Penagos J, Lyne SB, et al. Intracerebral Hemorrhage Volume Reduction and Timing of Intervention Versus Functional Benefit and Survival in the MISTIE III and STICH Trials. Neurosurgery. 2021;88(5):961–70.

10. Gregson BA, Mitchell P, Mendelow AD. Surgical Decision Making in Brain Hemorrhage New Analysis of the STICH, STICH II, and STITCH(Trauma) Randomized Trials. Stroke. 2019;50:1108–15.

11. Nishihara T, Teraoka A, Morita A, et al. A transparent sheath for endoscopic surgery and its application in surgical evacuation of spontaneous intracerebral hematomas. Technical note. J Neurosurg. 2000;92:1053–5.

12. Yamamoto T, Watabe T, Arakawa Y, et al. Registry of Intracerebral Hemorrhage treated by endoscopic hematoma evacuation: RICH-trend primary report. Presented at the Japanese Society for Neuroecndoscopy meeting, Nagoya, Japan; 2021.

13. Yamamoto T, Nakao Y, Mori K, et al. Endoscopic hematoma evacuation for hypertensive cerebellar hemorrhage. Minim Invasive Neurosurg. 2006;49:173–8.

14. Atsumi H, Baba T, Sunaga A, et al. Neuroendoscopic Evacuation for Spontaneous Cerebellar Hemorrhage Is a Safe and Secure Approach and May Become a Mainstream Technique. Neurol Med Chir (Tokyo). 2019;59(11):423–9.

15. Kuramatsu JB, Biffi A, Gerner ST, et al. Association of Surgical Hematoma Evacuation vs Conservative Treatment with Functional Outcome in Patients with Cerebellar Intracerebral Hemorrhage. JAMA. 2019;322(14):1392–403.

16. Chen CC, Liu CL, Tung YN, et al. Endoscopic surgery for intraventricular hemorrhage (IVH) caused by thalamic hemorrhage: comparisons of endoscopic surgery and external ventricular drainage (EVD) surgery. World Neurosurg. 2011;75(2):264–8.

17. Noiphithak R, Ratanavinitkul W, Yindeedej V, et al. Outcomes of Combined Endoscopic Surgery and Fibrinolytic Treatment Protocol for Intraventricular Hemorrhage: A Randomized Controlled Trial. World Neurosurg. 2023;172:e555–64. https://doi.org/10.1016/j.wneu.2023.01.080.

18. Yamamoto T, Esaki T, Nakao Y, et al. Endoscopic Hematoma Evacuation to Improve the Functional Outcome. Jpn J. 2011;Neurosurg(Tokyo)20:734–40.

19. Fujita N, Ueno H, Watanabe M, Nakao Y, Yamamoto T. Significance of endoscopic hematoma evacuation in elderly patients with spontaneous putaminal hemorrhage. Surg Neurol Int. 2021;12:121.

20. Nagasaka T. Neuroendoscopic surgery for intracerebral hemorrhage. Nagoya, Japan: TN-medical publishing; 2011.

21. Ratcliff JJ, Hall AJ, Porto E, et al. Early Minimally Invasive Removal of Intracerebral Hemorrhage (ENRICH): Study protocol for a multi-centered two-arm randomized adaptive trial. Front Neurol. 2023;14:1126958.

22. Hall A, et al. Very early minimally invasive removal of intracerebral hemorrhage: the ENIRCH trial. [Press Release]. Munich, Germany: Presented at the European Stroke Organisation Conference; 2023.

Chapter 10
Full Endoscopic Transcranial Resection of Meningiomas

Sebastian Senger, Karen Radtke, and Joachim Oertel

Abbreviations

CNS   Central nervous system
CT   Computer tomography
DSA   Digital subtraction angiography
FOV   Field of view
MRI   Magnetic resonance imaging
ROI   Region of interest

10.1   Introduction

Meningiomas are a group of mostly benign tumors stemming from arachnoid cap cells. They make up about one third of all primary brain tumors [1] and more than 50% of all nonmalignant brain tumors [2]. Due to their benign nature and usually slow growth rate, studies report incidental findings of meningiomas in almost 1–2% of healthy subjects who underwent cranial MRI, predominantly women [3, 4]. The commonly reported risk factors are ionization radiation, higher levels of reproductive hormones, and certain genetic aberrations [1]. About 35% of all meningiomas are located at the convexities or parasagittal, 10% are located at the falx cerebri, and another 10% in the cerebellopontine angle and around the sphenoid wing and sellar

S. Senger · K. Radtke · J. Oertel (✉)
Klinik für Neurochirurgie, Universitätsklinikum des Saarlandes und Fakultät für Medizin,
Universität des Saarlandes, Homburg Saar, Germany
e-mail: Sebastian.Senger@uks.eu; Karen.Radtke@uks.eu; Joachim.Oertel@uks.eu

© The Author(s), under exclusive license to Springer Nature Switzerland AG 2024
W. A. Azab (ed.), *Endoscope-controlled Transcranial Surgery*, Advances and Technical Standards in Neurosurgery 52,
https://doi.org/10.1007/978-3-031-61925-0_10

region each. Meningiomas of the olfactory groove and clivus make up about 5% of meningiomas each; even more rare locations include the cerebellar convexities or the foramen magnum [5]. Even though more than 80% of meningiomas are WHO grade 1 (2) and do not show invasion of the surrounding structures, they might warrant surgical resection due to the compression of the neighboring neurovascular structures, such as arteries of the skull base, cranial nerves, or the brain stem.

In general, meningioma surgery is challenging. On one hand, these lesions grow around delicate structures such as the cranial nerve and arteries and veins, which have to be preserved with surgical resection; on the other hand, meningiomas might cause significant brain edema, which makes surgical resection difficult because of the lack of space and the high risk of brain parenchyma damage.

Over the last 2–3 decades, the endoscope has become a valuable addition to the microscope in the resection of these tumors. Particularly, the endonasal route for skull base meningiomas resection has been intensively studied [6–8]. The transcranial approach, however, is still mainly performed under a microscopic view. Over the recent years, the endoscope has been more and more frequently introduced as an adjunct for inspection and assistance, while the main procedure remained microsurgical [9, 10]. But although the number of publications on this subject is notorious, only very few authors really addressed the advantages and pitfalls of the endoscopic-assisted technique [11]. The last change in visualization now comes from the introduction of various exoscopes into the market as an addition to or replacement for microscopes and endoscopes [12].

The endoscopic-controlled resection via a transcranial approach in contrast to the abovementioned techniques is a rather rarely performed procedure. Reasons for this might be that the surgeons still missed three-dimensional (3D) imaging with the most available endoscopes. Also, the high magnification and the endoscope tip in the immediate vicinity of the lesion might be of hindrance to large multilobulated lesions.

The authors of this chapter apply the endoscopic-controlled technique in a small subgroup of meningiomas. This chapter describes in detail the endoscopic-controlled technique of the authors for meningioma resection.

10.2 Indications/Contraindications

Meningioma surgery is always a serious task. Lesions that involve a high number of structures to be preserved and that require an approach from variable angles of view are not good candidates for an endoscopic-controlled approach.

Also, the size of the lesion and its vascularization, as well as its consistency, matter. The endoscope gives a very high magnification and perfect image resolution. However, the technique of the authors does not involve a 3D endoscope, so the technique is limited to a 2D view. In large lesions, very high magnification might be a hindrance to sufficient timely tumor resection. Furthermore, a highly vascularized meningioma with expected significant bleeding during resection is not a good candidate for endoscopic-controlled surgery. Finally, the degree of manipulation required influences the selection of the surgical technique. The more surgical time is needed for resection, the more likely the authors prefer a microsurgical approach.

The authors select an endoscopic-controlled approach for meningiomas that can be accessed in a straight approach with the application of a keyhole craniotomy.

10.3 Operative Technique

10.3.1 Preoperative Preparation

The authors use the endoscopic-controlled technique for small and medium-sized meningiomas that can be accessed through a straight approach via keyhole craniotomy. The major indications are lesions of the falx and of the anterior fossa, such as the olfactory rim, sellar floor, and sphenoid plane. Under general anesthesia and electrophysiological neuromonitoring, the patient is placed in a supine position, and the head is fixed in three-pin-sharp head fixation.

10.3.2 Keyhole Craniotomy to Falx Meningioma

In the endoscopic-controlled approach of falx meningioma, the head is anteflexed and not turned. No rotation is applied to facilitate a rather large surgical field in the anterior-posterior plane. This makes the positioning of the endoscope easier. Neuronavigation is referenced, and neuromonitoring, including motor-evoked potentials and sensory-evoked potentials, is applied. A keyhole burr hole is placed right on top of the sinus and a mini keyhole craniotomy is performed to the desired site. As a thumb rule, the craniotomy size is about 2×3 cm. The dura is opened toward the sagittal sinus, and holding sutures are applied. If needed, a retractor spatula is inserted, and endoscopy is introduced into the surgical field. The authors prefer to position the endoscope on the anterior or posterior edge of the surgical field and fix it to an endoscope-holding device. Subsequently, the tumor is visualized, and after debulking, the tumor is detached from its origin. Tumor origin at the falx is either coagulated or resected depending on the individual situation. After resection, hemostasis is obtained and the dura closed. The bone flap is inserted and fixed with titanium plates. Bone cement is applied to reconstruct a smooth plan, particularly in far anterior frontal craniotomy, to achieve a favorable cosmetic result.

10.3.2.1 Illustrative Case 1

A 45-year-old lady presented with a growing falcine lesion. The lesion was contrast enhancing in T1 MR images, which is highly suspicious for falcine meningioma. Fig. 10.1 shows the preoperative MR images. The ideal position for the bilateral skin incision and keyhole craniotomy is determined by neuronavigation. After burr hole placement, a small craniotomy is performed (Fig. 10.2a–d). The dura is opened toward the sagittal sinus, and holding sutures are applied (Fig. 10.3a, b). Then the tumor is exposed, a biopsy for the instant section is taken, and the tumor is debulked with an ultrasonic aspirator (Fig. 10.3c–e). Figure 10.3f shows the setup of the operating room with the screen, the applied endoscope connected to a holding device, and the surgical instruments in the surgical field. After complete resection, hemostasis is obtained (Fig. 10.3g). The tumor is excised after debulking in toto (Fig. 10.3h). Fig. 10.4a–d shows the postoperative CT, including the bone windows with a 16 mm craniotomy diameter.

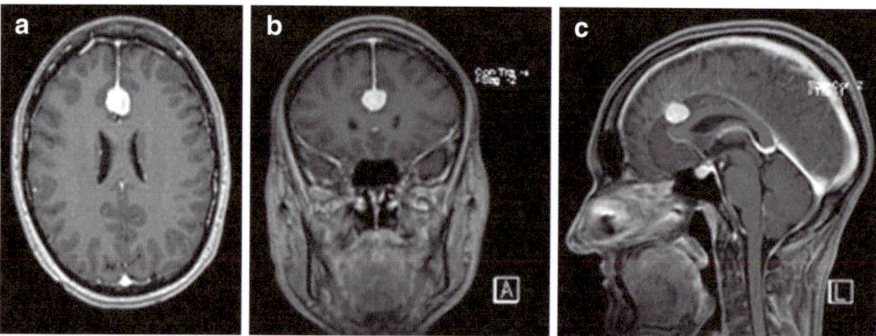

Fig. 10.1 (**a**) T1-weighted contrast-enhanced MR image in axial plane. (**b**) T1-weighted contrast-enhanced MR image in the coronal plane. (**c**) T1-weighted contrast-enhanced MR image in the sagittal plane. All three images show the medially located falcine meningioma of about 2.5 cm diameter

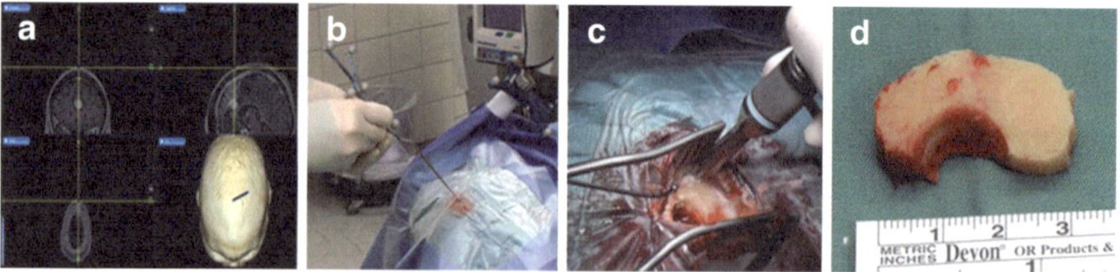

Fig. 10.2 (**a, b**) Referencing neuronavigation is very helpful in determining the ideal position for skin incision and craniotomy. (**c, d**) A small craniotomy is performed, resulting in a bone flap of about 2 × 3 cm

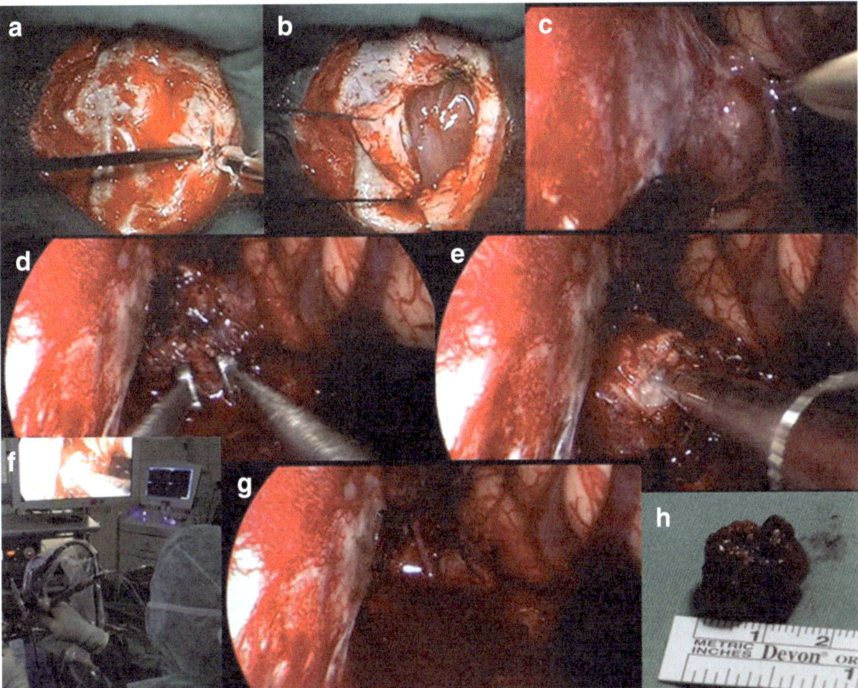

Fig. 10.3 (**a**, **b**) Dura opening toward the sagittal sinus. (**c**) Exposure of the tumor. (**d**) Sampling for the instantaneous section with neuropathology is performed. (**e**) The tumor is debulked with an ultrasonic aspirator. (**f**) Technical setup in the operating room with the screen, the applied endoscope connected to a holding device, and the surgical instruments in the surgical field. (**g**) After a complete resection, hemostasis is obtained. (**h**) A picture of the tumor after excision

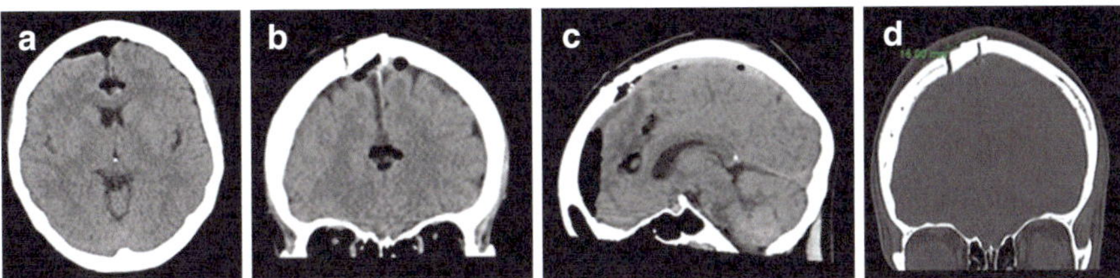

Fig. 10.4 (**a**) Axial slice of the postoperative computer tomography. (**b**, **c**) Coronal and sagittal reconstruction of the CT. (**d**) Coronal reconstruction of the computer tomography in bone window with a measurement of the craniotomy size

10.3.3 Supraorbital Keyhole Craniotomy

The supraorbital craniotomy has been frequently described. The skin incision is placed in the lateral half of the eyebrow, laterally from the supraorbital foramen with the supraorbital nerve. The orbicular muscle is dissected with a monopolar probe. The fascia of the temporal muscle is then incised directly at the orbital rim, and the temporal muscle is retracted. Exposure and mobilization of the temporal muscle should be restricted to a necessary minimum to prevent postoperative problems with chewing and to maintain a satisfactory cosmetic result. The craniotomy is then started with a burr hole posterior below the temporal line, and the craniotome is directed posteriorly than medially and finally anteriorly. Care should be taken to avoid opening the orbit. A bone flap with a width of about 2–3 cm and a height of about 2–3 cm results. After craniotomy, the anterior skull base is drilled extradurally. In lesions of the olfactory rim, the head is more turned contralaterally than in the lesion of the sella in which only a slight rotation of about 25–30° is applied. After craniotomy, the dura is opened toward the orbit and fixed with holding sutures. The endoscope is inserted, and CSF is drained by opening either the Sylvian fissure or the basal cisterns. If required, a spatula is inserted for brain retraction and fixed to a Leyla holding device. The tumor is exposed under endoscopic view and subsequently resected. In frontal skull base meningiomas, almost always these lesions are detached from the dura as a first step to devascularization. Finally, after the identification of all delicate structures that have to be preserved, the tumor is excised. After hemostasis, the dura is closed, the bone flap fixed with titanium screws, and the remaining craniotomy defect reconstructed with bone cement. The wound is closed layer by layer, and the skin is adapted with Steri-Strips wound bandage.

10.3.3.1 Illustrative Case 2

A 48-year-old lady presented with visual deterioration in the right eye. On MRI, a contrast-enhancing lesion of the sphenoid plane growing into the optic canal on the right was seen. Figure 10.5 shows the preoperative MR images. The patient was put in a prone position with the head slightly rotated to the left and slightly retroflexed posteriorly to facilitate brain retraction due to gravity (Fig. 10.6). After disinfection and draping, craniotomy is performed by placing the burr hole at the temporal bone, followed by craniotomy (Fig. 10.7a–d). Before the opening of the dura, the frontal skull base is flattened with a diamond burr (Fig. 10.8a). After the dural opening, the endoscope is inserted and the tumor at the sphenoid plane exposed and resected (Fig. 10.8b, c). Then the optic canal is drilled with a diamond burr, and the optic nerve is decompressed until no remnant compression is noted and no tumor is left

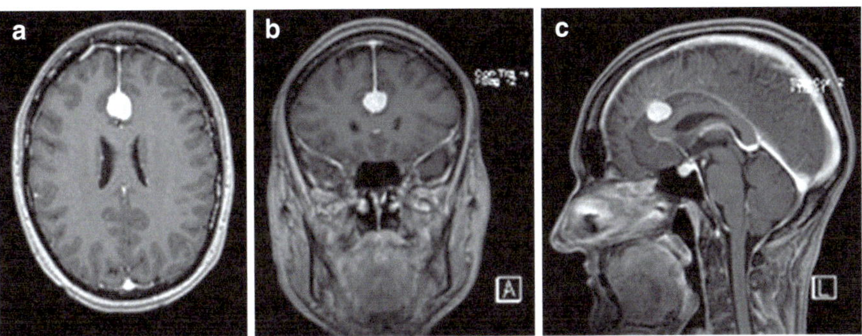

Figure. 10.5 (**a–c**) Meningioma of the sphenoid plane and right optic canal in T1-weighted contrast-enhanced MRI slices

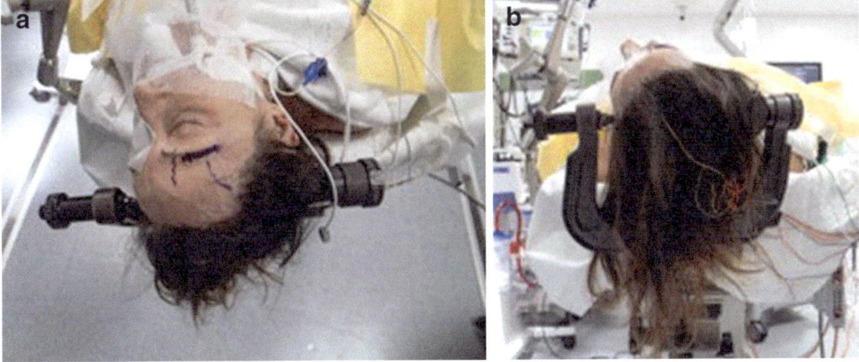

Fig. 10.6 (**a**) The head is slightly retroflexed to allow brain retraction by gravity. (**b**) Additionally, the head is rotated about 30° to the left

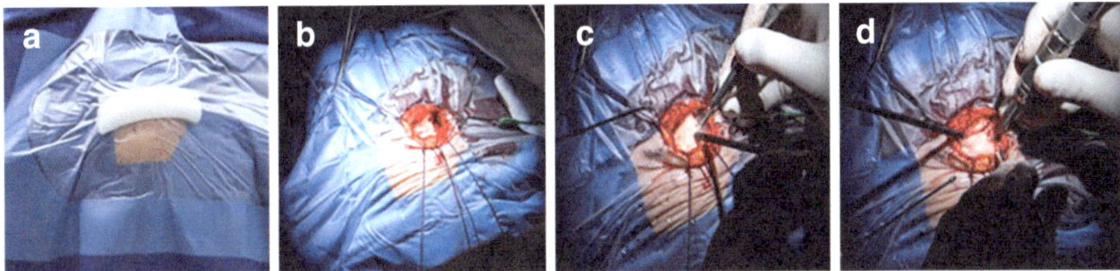

Fig. 10.7 (**a**) Surgical field after draping. (**b**) Dissection of the orbital muscle and temporal muscle with exposure of temporal bone. (**c**) Placement of burr hole. (**d**) Supraorbital craniotomy with craniotome

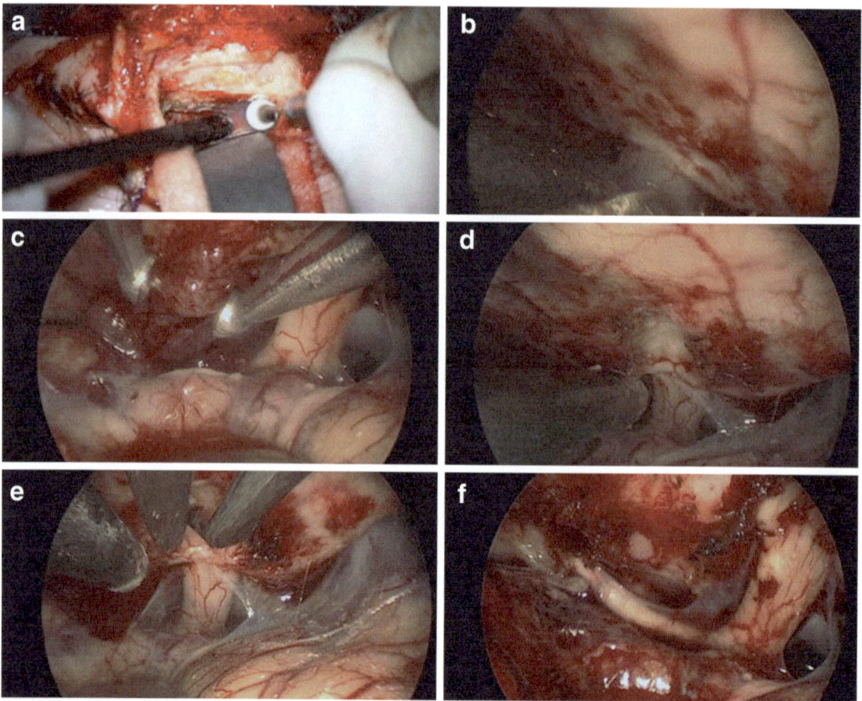

Fig. 10.8 (**a**) Extradural flattening of the frontal skull base with a diamond burr. (**b**, **c**) Insertion of the endoscope, identification of the tumor, and piecemeal resection. (**d**, **e**) Drilling of the optic canal and decompression of the optic nerve. (**f**) Final view at the surgical field with no remanent tumor and decompressed optic nerve

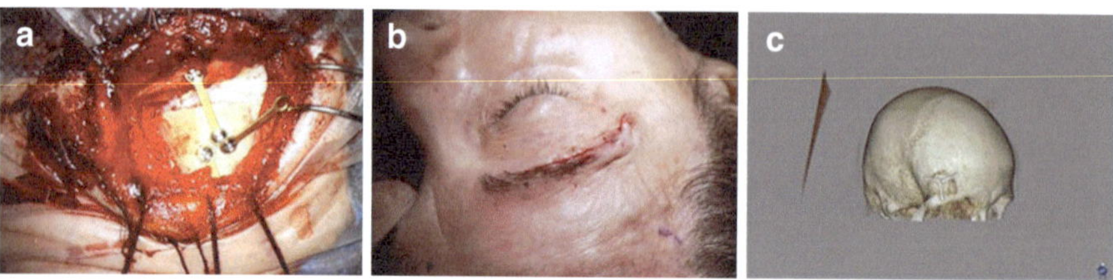

Fig. 10.9 (**a**) Fixation of the bone flap with titanium plates. (**b**) Favorable early postoperative cosmetic result. (**c**) Tight wound closure layer by layer with adaptation of the superficial skin by Steri-Strips. (**c**) 3D skull reconstruction to show the keyhole craniotomy

(Fig. 10.8d–f). The dura in a watertight fashion, and the bone flap is fixed with titanium plates (Fig. 10.9a). Cosmetically very favorable postoperative results are seen (Fig. 10.9b). On 3D reconstruction of postoperative computer tomography, the readers can appreciate the very small size of the craniotomy (Fig. 10.9c). On postoperative MRI, no remnant tumor can be detected (Fig. 10.10).

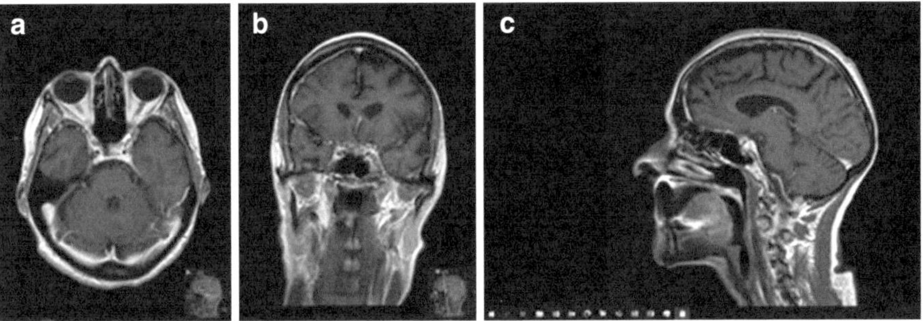

Fig. 10.10 Postoperative MRI in T1-weighted contrast-enhanced slices. (**a**) axial, (**b**) coronal, and (**c**) sagittal planes

10.4 Postoperative Management

The patient is extubated in the operating room and thereafter closely monitored in the neurointensive care unit. If the condition is stable and asymptomatic, the patient can be discharged to the ward. Immediate neuroimaging is optional if the patient remains neurologically stable, but usually a CT or MRI scan is performed during the in-hospital stay. No specific measures have to be undertaken for the endoscopic-controlled technique. Routine follow-up in all benign grade 1 meningiomas includes 3- and 6-month follow-up and follow-up on a yearly basis thereafter.

10.5 Complications

Complications of meningioma surgery can be divided into two groups: intraoperative and postoperative complications. Intraoperative complications are nerve and vessel injury as well as significant brain edema formation. Since with the endoscopic-controlled technique brain retraction is limited to a minimum and magnification of the surgical field is very high, the frequency of intraoperative complications should rather be lower than in microsurgical cases. Postoperative complications include postoperative hemorrhage, postoperative edema formation, and rarely vascular spasm. To the knowledge of the authors, no specific postoperative complication has been attributed to the endoscopic-controlled surgical technique.

10.6 Outcome and Prognosis

With a careful selection of the surgical candidate, the outcome of the endoscopic-controlled surgery in meningiomas should be very favorable. The overall prognosis is very good. However, the long-term prognosis depends on the biological behavior of the lesion rather than on the surgical technique applied.

10.7 Conclusion

The endoscopic-controlled surgical technique is a valuable alternative to a standard microsurgical approach for many indications. The endoscopic-controlled approach allows a very high magnification in combination with minimum keyhole craniotomies. In well-selected cases, this technique should be the procedure of choice. Nevertheless, the long-term prognosis depends rather on the biological nature of the meningioma; thus, the long-term prognosis cannot be influenced by the endoscopic-controlled technique.

References

1. Wiemels J, Wrensch M, Claus EB. Epidemiology and etiology of meningioma. J Neurooncol. 2010;99:307–14.
2. Ostrom QT, et al. CBTRUS Statistical Report: Primary Brain and Other Central Nervous System Tumors Diagnosed in the United States in 2015–2019. Neuro-Oncology. 2022;24:v1–v95.
3. Krampla W, et al. Frequency and risk factors for meningioma in clinically healthy 75-year-old patients: Results of the Transdanube Ageing Study (VITA). Cancer. 2004;100:1208–12.
4. Vernooij MW, et al. Incidental Findings on Brain MRI in the General Population. N Engl J Med. 2007;357:1821–8.
5. Hirayama R, et al. Voxel-based lesion mapping of meningioma: a comprehensive lesion location mapping of 260 lesions. J Neurosurg. 2018;128:1707–12.
6. Henderson F, et al. Endonasal transsphenoidal surgery for planum sphenoidale versus tuberculum sellae meningiomas. J Neurosurg. 2022;138:1338–46.
7. Schwartz TH, Morgenstern PF, Anand VK. Lessons learned in the evolution of endoscopic skull base surgery. J Neurosurg. 2019;130:337–46.
8. Mastantuoni C, et al. Midline skull base meningiomas: transcranial and endonasal perspectives. Cancers (Basel). 2022;10:2878.
9. Boissonneau S, et al. Transfalcine approach for the resection of a bilateral falx meningioma: Technical nuances and review of literature. Asian J Neurosurg. 2021;16:821–3.
10. Roser F, Rigante L. The endoscope-assisted contralateral paramedian approach to large falcine meningiomas. Acta Neurochirurgica (Wien). 2018;160:79–82.
11. Khan DZ, et al. The endoscope-assisted supraorbital "keyhole" approach for anterior skull base meningiomas: an updated meta-analysis. Acta Neurochirurgica (Wien). 2021;163:661–76.
12. Watanabe T, et al. Combined exoscopic and endoscopic two-step keyhole approach for intracranial meningiomas. Curr Oncol. 2022;29:5370–82.

Chapter 11
Fully Endoscopic Supraorbital Approach for Anterior Cranial Base Meningiomas

Waleed Abdelfattah Azab, Mustafa Najibullah, Zafdam Shabbir, Fatemah Alali, and Waleed Yousef

11.1 Introduction

Advances in endoscopic technology have significantly contributed to the development and refinement of minimally invasive brain surgery. As a matter of fact, minimally invasive approaches are associated with lower complication profile, comparable or even better outcomes, better cosmetic results, and faster recovery times in comparison to the conventional approaches [1–3]. Fully endoscopic or endoscope-controlled approaches are essentially keyhole approaches in which rigid endoscopes are the sole visualization tools used during the whole procedure.

Endoscopic assistance in cranial surgery emerged out of the need to operate via small openings and yet obtain appropriate visualization and control of the structures within the field—in other words, to perform a minimally invasive yet maximally effective surgery. At the early attempts of endoscope-assisted cranial surgery, it was noted that rigid endoscopes enabled overcoming the problem of suboptimal visualization when small exposures are used.

In 1974, Werner Prott, working then as an otosurgeon at the University of Würzburg, used a rigid endoscope to explore and operate within the cerebellopontine angle via a transpyramidal retrolabyrinthine approach through Trautmann's triangle. After a mastoidectomy, a bone flap with a diameter of 1 cm was made; then the endoscope was inserted through this narrow space between the sigmoid sinus, the superior petrosal sinus, the posterior semicircular canal, and the endolymphatic sac without damaging any functional structure of the inner ear or of the cerebellum [4]. In 1981, Falk Oppel and colleagues used a similar approach for sectioning the

W. A. Azab (✉) · M. Najibullah · Z. Shabbir · F. Alali · W. Yousef
Neurosurgery Department, Ibn Sina Hospital, Al-Sabah Medical Area, Kuwait City, Kuwait

© The Author(s), under exclusive license to Springer Nature Switzerland AG 2024
W. A. Azab (ed.), *Endoscope-controlled Transcranial Surgery*, Advances and Technical Standards in Neurosurgery 52,
https://doi.org/10.1007/978-3-031-61925-0_11

sensory root of trigeminal nerve, the glossopharyngeal nerve, and the cranial part of the vagus nerve to treat an intractable facial pain in a patient with recurrent upper jaw carcinoma [5].

Apuzzo and colleagues in 1977 described the use of Hopkins 70° and 120° side-viewing telescopes in a variety of approaches including intrasellar procedures by either the transsphenoidal or subfrontal routes to assist with visualization for complete gland ablation or total tumor excision. They also employed this endoscope-assisted strategy in aneurysm surgery while working in the vicinity of the circle of Willis, with particular emphasis on the assessment of adequacy and accuracy of clip placement, especially in lesions of the apex of the basilar artery [6].

Anterior skull base meningiomas encompass those meningiomas originating from the tuberculum sellae, the planum sphenoidale, or the olfactory groove. Olfactory groove meningiomas account for 8–13% of all intracranial meningiomas [7–9], while tuberculum sellae and planum sphenoidale meningiomas constitute around 10–15% of meningiomas and often present with visual disturbance due to compression of the optic nerves and chiasm [10, 11] (Fig. 11.1). Surgical excision is the main treatment modality for these tumors and should ideally aim at complete removal of the tumor as well as the dural tail and invaded bone [12], which is not easily achievable or even impossible in meningiomas involving the skull base. Surgical removal of tuberculum sellae and planum sphenoidale meningiomas is of special importance as it results in decompression of the optic nerves and chiasm and therefore prevents further visual deterioration and may reverse neural damage in some cases [13].

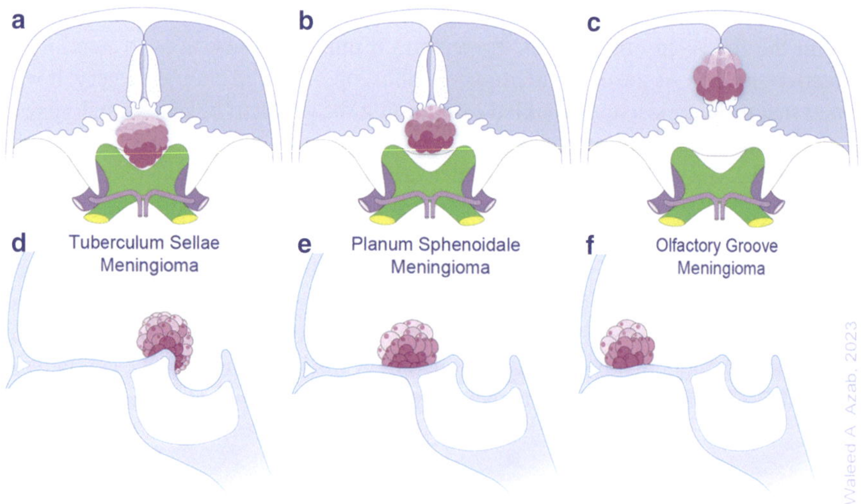

Fig. 11.1 Nomenclature of anterior skull base meningiomas according to anatomical origin in axial (**a–c**) and sagittal (**d–f**) planes. *(Modified from Azab W. et al. [23] under Creative Commons Attribution 4.0 International license* (https://creativecommons.org/licenses/by/4.0/))

For surgical excision of anterior skull base meningiomas, minimally invasive approaches in which rigid endoscopes are employed include the endoscopic endonasal approach [14–17] and the endoscope-assisted or endoscope-controlled supraorbital keyhole eyebrow approaches [1, 18–23]. Although the conventional microscopic supraorbital keyhole approach with or without endoscopic assistance is frequently utilized nowadays for treating these tumors, the fully endoscopic or endoscope-controlled version of the approach is not routinely practiced by neurosurgeons, with few series published so far.

In this chapter we describe the fully endoscopic or endoscope-controlled supraorbital keyhole approach for anterior cranial base meningiomas and focus mainly on its surgical technique and nuances.

11.2 The Supraorbital Keyhole Approach

Fedor Krause was the first to describe a supraorbital subfrontal exposure to excise an anterior skull base meningioma in 1908 [24]. In 1913, Charles Frazier used a supraorbital craniotomy with removal of the orbital rim and roof for resection of a "pituitary cyst" that he described as "seen projecting upward between optic tracts" and pointed out that the procedure offered "a splendid exposure of the region of the sella turcica" [25]. Elaborating on a variety of approaches for supratentorial pathologies that he devised, Donald Wilson was the first to use the term "keyhole surgery." He used small linear incisions and a 2-inch D'Errico trephine to create limited craniotomies that were still sufficient to operate through. In his technical note "Limited Exposure in Cerebral Surgery," published in 1971, he pointed out that such operating methodology avoided unnecessary exposure and potential damage of brain tissue and was also associated with better cosmetic results [26]. Axel Perneczky popularized the supraorbital keyhole approach through an eyebrow incision and demonstrated the importance of endoscopic assistance in this approach through many published large series of vascular and tumor cases [1, 3, 22, 27].

In comparison to the conventional approaches, the supraorbital keyhole approach minimizes brain retraction, tissue dissection, and length of the skin incision. Temporalis muscle dissection is also very limited so that temporalis muscle atrophy and the consequent mandibular pain and chewing problems are almost nonexistent. Moreover, the approach results in much better cosmetic results than the classic approaches [22, 23, 27, 28].

11.3 Rationale for the Fully Endoscopic Technique

The technical specifications and design of the currently available rigid endoscopes are associated with a group of unique features that define the endoscopic view and lay the basis for its superiority over the microscopic view during brain surgery

                                                                W. A. Azab et al.

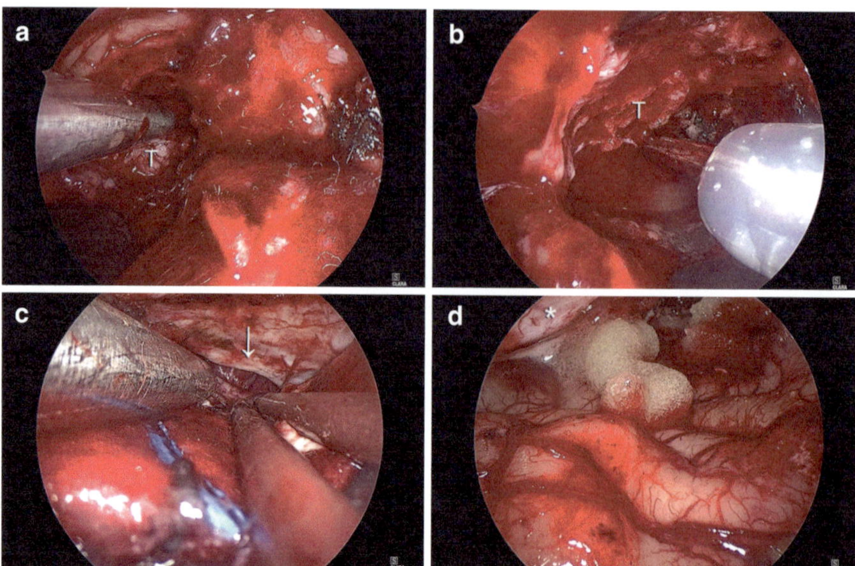

Fig. 11.2 The superiority of the endoscopic over the microscopic view exemplified by an endoscope-controlled supraorbital keyhole approach for resection of an olfactory meningioma. The larger depth of focus keeps the tumor (T) and other structures in focus during all stages of the procedure. The panoramic highly illuminated field of view is clearly seen with absence of shadows or haze. This is evident during initial debulking (**a**), resection of the basal attachment of the tumor using the CUSA (**b**), and performing hemostasis in a bimanual fashion at the very deep area near the crista galli (white arrow) (**c**). In (**d**), a final view of the inferior surface of the frontal lobe and the frontal base dura (asterisk) after tumor resection and hemostasis

(Fig. 11.2). When a rigid endoscope is inserted into the surgical field, a very highly illuminated area of interest is obtained because the light beam is completely brought inside the field without any loss of light energy at the edges of the craniotomy or cortical incision. Furthermore, the close proximity of the light source to the structures being viewed eliminates shadows within the field, adding to the extreme clarity of the endoscopic images. The superiority of the endoscopic view also results from the wide-angle view as well as the high color fidelity and image definition capabilities of today's state-of-the-art rigid endoscopes. In addition, rigid endoscopes are characterized by a greater depth of field. Therefore, the viewed objects remain in focus throughout a greater range of distances from the viewing lens. This means lesser need to adjust the focus of the endoscope during the procedure, and consequently a seamless operative workflow. The use of angled scopes also enables "looking around the corners" and thereby adds further to the efficacy and safety of the procedure as it brings concealed tumor remnants into view and obviates the need for retraction of neurovascular structures. On the contrary, the microscope in keyhole surgery requires frequent changing of the viewing angle to allow illumination and visualization of the area of interest deep in the surgical field, an inevitable consequence of the light source and the viewing lens being located outside the craniotomy. The loss of light energy at the edges of the small craniotomy and the dropped shadows on the structures within the field further contribute to the lesser quality of the microscopic view obtained during keyhole brain surgery [23].

The frequently raised concerns of endoscopic visualization include the lack of three-dimensionality, the need for familiarity with endoscopic devices, the need to develop eye-hand coordination, and the limitation of the operating range of movement of instruments [28]. These drawbacks are easily overcome by the surgeon's experience and are largely balanced by the superb image quality, increased radicality, and lower risk of complications that this form of surgery offers. In our opinion, rigid endoscopes are indispensable components of the array of surgical tools required to perform a keyhole brain surgery, and we firmly believe that they will eventually completely replace surgical microscopes for this type of surgery.

Specifically pertaining to excision of anterior cranial base meningiomas, the supraorbital keyhole approach with endoscopic assistance or control truly provides an excellent view to anterior skull base meningiomas. Optic nerve decompression is also possible under endoscopic view when angled scopes are used [29]. Recently, the purely endoscopic or endoscope-controlled supraorbital keyhole approach has been used with promising results [29, 30].

11.4 Pathological Anatomy of Anterior Skull Base Meningiomas

A thorough understanding of the pathological anatomy of anterior cranial base meningiomas is of crucial importance for surgical decision-making and execution of surgery. Tuberculum sellae meningiomas are in close anatomical proximity to the optic nerves, optic chiasm, internal carotid artery (ICA), anterior cerebral artery (ACA) complex, hypothalamus, pituitary stalk, and pituitary gland (Fig. 11.3). In comparison to planum sphenoidale meningiomas, true tuberculum sellae meningiomas are centered on the tuberculum sellae and grow in a posterosuperior direction displacing the optic nerves superolaterally [31] (Fig. 11.4a, b). Furthermore, tumor extension into one or both optic canals as well as vascular encasement can take place in many cases and adds to the technical difficulty of resecting these tumors (Fig. 11.4c, d). On the other hand, olfactory groove meningiomas are in close apposition to the olfactory nerves and tend to infiltrate the cribriform plate, invade the ethmoid and sphenoid sinuses, and engulf the anterior clinoid process as well as the vasculature in its vicinity [7, 9, 18, 23, 32].

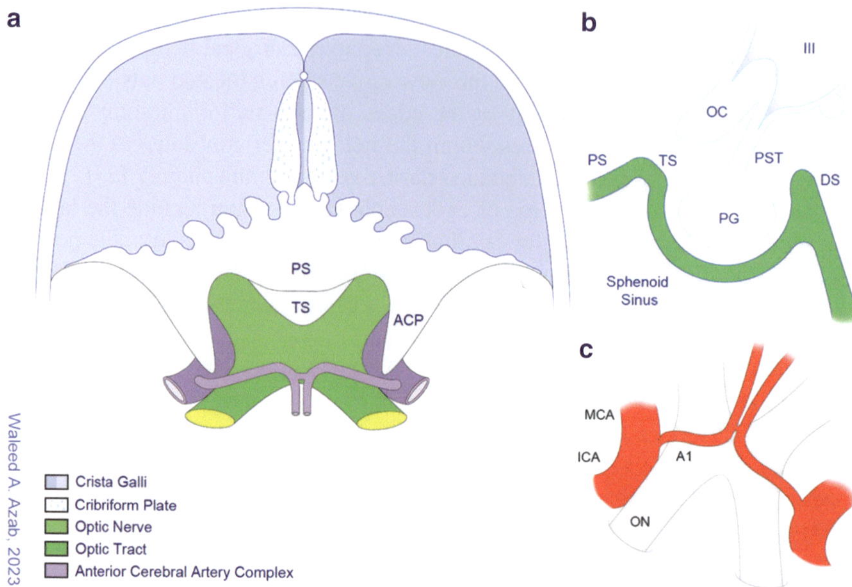

Fig. 11.3 Anatomical environment and structures related to anterior skull base meningiomas. Axial (**a**) and sagittal (**b**) views of the sellar region and structures in its vicinity that may specially be involved in tuberculum sellae and planum sphenoidale meningiomas. (**c**) View of the optic apparatus and the neighboring major vasculature. *A1* First segment of anterior cerebral artery, *ACP* Anterior clinoid process, *DS* Dorsum sellae, *ICA* Internal carotid artery, *MCA* Middle cerebral artery, *OC* Optic chiasm, *ON* Optic nerve, *PG* Pituitary gland, *PS* Planum sphenoidale, *PST* Pituitary stalk, *TS* Tuberculum sellae, *III* Third ventricle. (*Modified from Azab W. et al.* [23] *under Creative Commons Attribution 4.0 International license* (https://creativecommons.org/licenses/by/4.0/))

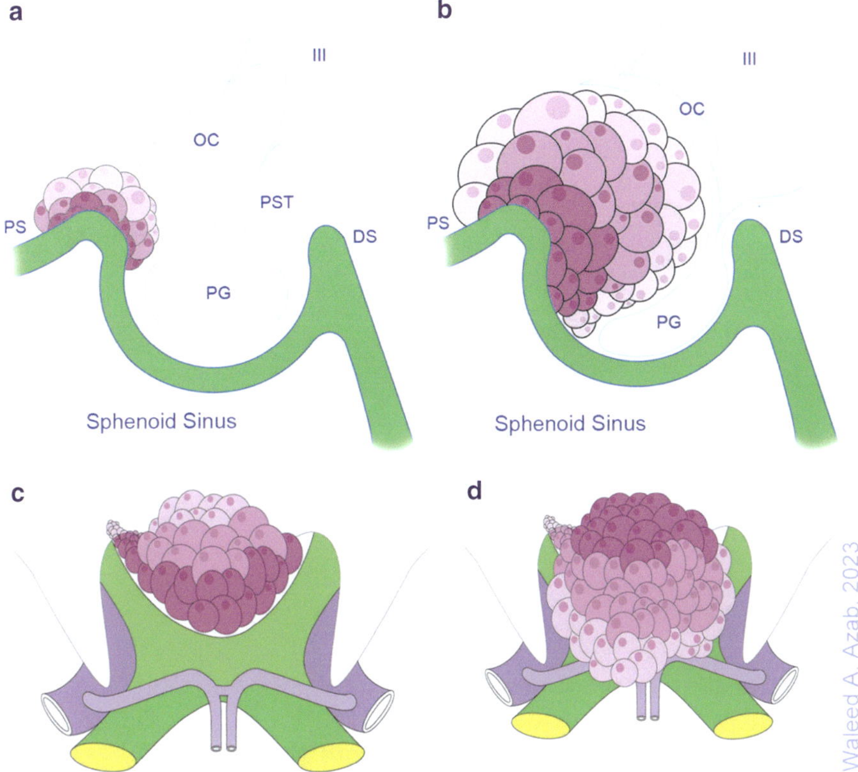

Fig. 11.4 Tuberculum sellae meningiomas can be small (**a**) or large (**b**) and are centered on the tuberculum sellae. They grow posterosuperiorly displacing the optic nerves superolaterally. Note the intrasellar extension and compression of the neighboring structures. They frequently extend into the optic canal (**c**) and may also encase blood vessels in the vicinity (**d**). *DS* Dorsum sellae, *OC* Optic chiasm, *PG* Pituitary gland, *PS* Planum sphenoidale, *PST* Pituitary stalk, *TS* Tuberculum sellae, *III* Third ventricle. (*Modified from Azab W.* et al. [23] *under Creative Commons Attribution 4.0 International license* (https://creativecommons.org/licenses/by/4.0/))

11.5 Surgical Technique

11.5.1 Operating Room Setup

The operating room setup is illustrated in Fig. 11.5 and is geared toward achieving an unobstructed line of view of the endoscope monitor by the surgical team and ergonomically appropriate working space around the patient's head. Neuronavigation is used as a routine.

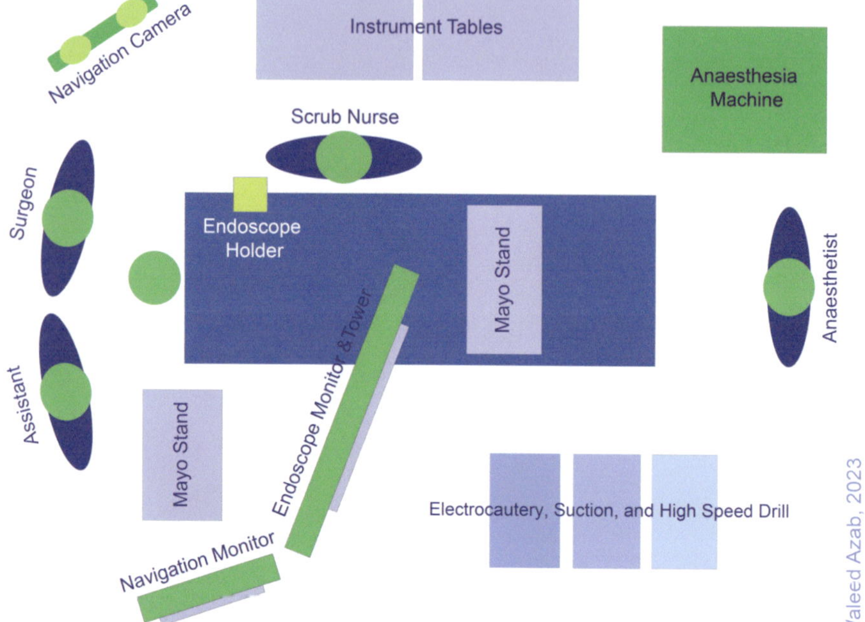

Fig. 11.5 The operating room setup for purely endoscopic supraorbital approach

11.5.2 Endoscopic Equipment Setup and Ergonomics

The rigid endoscope (0°, 30°, or 45°) is connected to a 4K endoscopic camera and inserted into the suction-irrigation sheath. The assembly is fixed to a holding mechanical arm (KARL STORZ, Germany) or to an intuitively movable manual support arm (ENDOFIX exo, AKTORmed, Germany). The endoscope holding arm is fixed to the side rail of operating table to the left of the operating surgeon, irrespective of whether a right- or left-sided approach is used. The endoscope tower and monitor are positioned on one side of the operating table so that a straight line of view by the operating surgeon is established (Fig. 11.6). At the initial phase of the procedure, the endoscope is fixed in an exoscopic position and is later inserted through the craniotomy as the next steps follow. At some points, the endoscope is held free hand by the assistant surgeon.

11.5.3 Positioning

The patient is positioned with the head elevated 20° above the level of the heart and fixed in three-pin head clamp. The patient's head is positioned using three movements of contralateral rotation, extension, and contralateral flexion (Fig. 11.7a). In

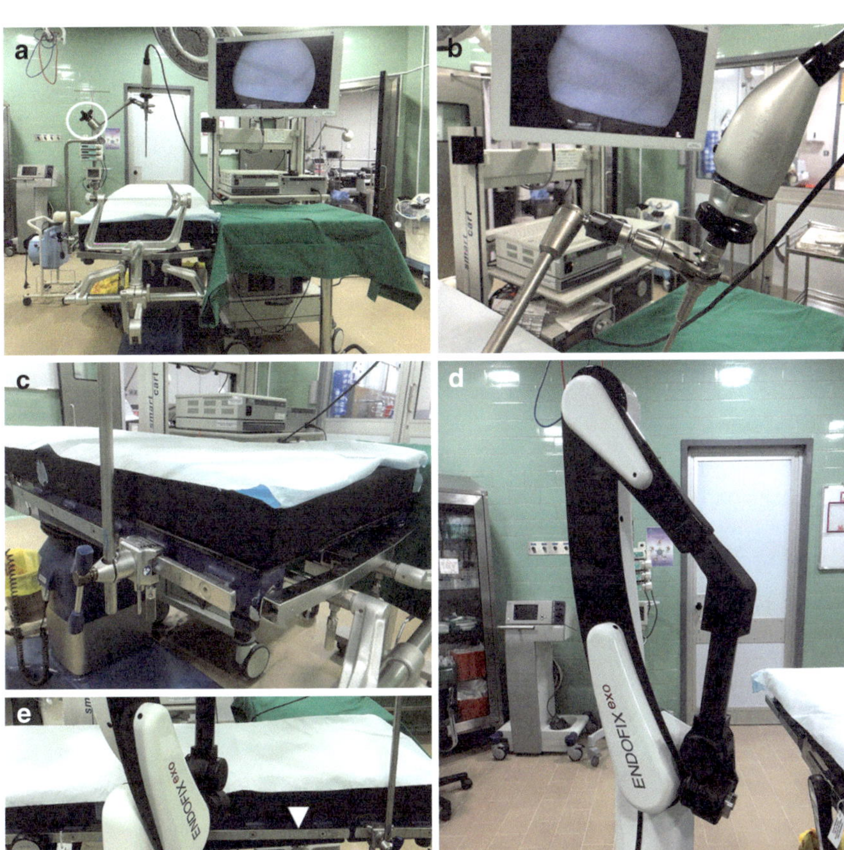

Fig. 11.6 (**a**) The rigid endoscope is connected to a 4K endoscopic camera and inserted into the suction-irrigation sheath. The assembly is fixed to a holding mechanical arm. The position of the scope can be adjusted (white circle) according to the required position. At the initial phase of the procedure, the endoscope is fixed in an exoscopic position. (**b**) A close-up view of the clamping jaw holding the endoscope and connecting it to the mechanical holding system. (**c**) The rotational socket clamps the mechanical holder to the side rail of the operating table at a point around 20 cm from its end. An intuitively movable manual support arm (ENDOFIX exo, AKTORmed, Germany) can be used instead of the mechanical holding arm (**d**) and is also fixed to the side rail of the operating table at a point around 50 cm from its end (arrowhead) (**e**)

contrast to the microscopic approach, full extension of the head should be avoided to prevent the endoscope shaft and camera of compromising the surgeon's working space. We insert a lumbar puncture needle after induction of general anesthesia and withdraw about 50 mL of CSF. This helps greatly to have a sufficiently slack frontal lobe after opening the dura. More CSF is released while the initial phase of the procedure goes on. These initial steps provide a sufficient space without the need to rely much on gravitational brain retraction offered by head extension.

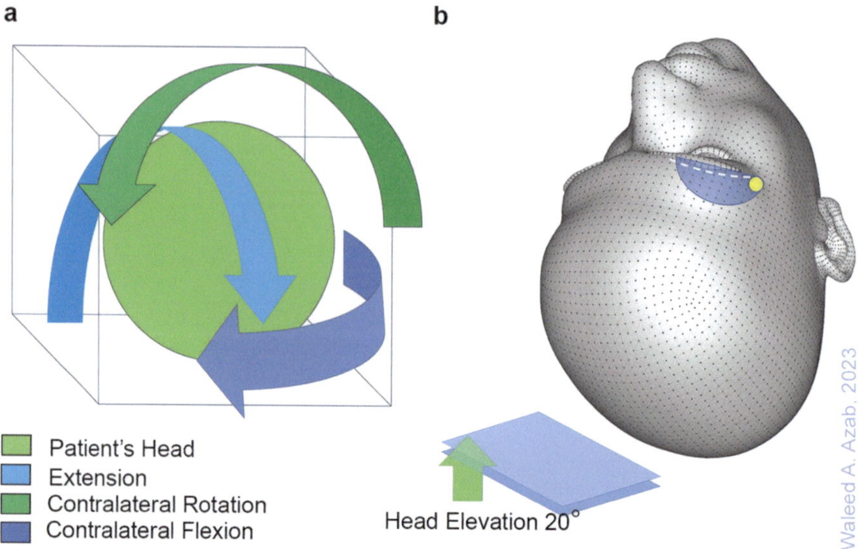

Fig. 11.7 Positioning and exposure for fully endoscopic supraorbital approach. The patient's head is positioned using three movements of contralateral rotation, extension, and contralateral flexion (**a**). In contrast to the microscopic approach, full extension of the head is to be avoided to prevent the endoscope shaft and camera of compromising the surgeon's working space. The eyebrow incision, burr hole, and craniotomy are demonstrated in (**b**)

11.5.4 Eyebrow Incision

The skin incision lies within or at the superior edge of the eyebrow and starts just lateral to the supraorbital notch, to avoid injury to the supraorbital nerve and consequent postoperative forehead numbness, and ends at the lateral end of the eyebrow over the zygomatic process (Fig. 11.7b). In some cases, the incision may be extended laterally for further 5–10 mm within a skin crease without significant cosmetic sequelae. At the superior temporal line, the temporalis fascia is incised using the monopolar coagulation for about 2 cm; then the frontalis fascia is cut from the temporal line in a semicircular fashion over the frontal bone with its base at the orbital rim. The temporalis muscle is subsequently dissected off the bone and retracted posteriorly for 1–2 cm [23]. Fish-hook retractors are used to retract the scalp. It is our practice not to retract the ocular edge of the incision. The use of fish-hooks is very important because of its low profile which helps achieving much less crowded field and allows more space for endoscope shaft and instrument manipulation.

11.5.5 Supraorbital Craniotomy

A single burr hole is made using a sharp pit attached to the high-speed drill in the temporal fossa lateral to the superior temporal line (Fig. 11.7b). The burr hole position is chosen at a point that is slightly higher than the classic MacCarty burr hole. A frontal direction of drilling prevents entering the orbit. A craniotome is then used to perform a 2–3.5 cm × 2–2.5 cm bone flap. Care should be taken to avoid opening the frontal air sinus at the medial border of the craniotomy.

11.5.6 Dural Opening and Intradural Steps

The dural flap is cut with its base at the orbital roof and is then reflected. Under endoscopic control, the subfrontal corridor is developed. The ipsilateral optic nerve and supraclinoid carotid artery are identified, and the arachnoid membranes of the optico-carotid and carotid-oculomotor cisterns are opened to allow CSF egress. CSF release adds to brain relaxation and greatly widens the surgical corridor.

The endoscope shaft is advanced and angulated and its focus is adjusted for a closer view according to the need. A handheld or Leyla retractor-mounted brain spatula is used to retract the frontal lobe and may be removed later. All the standard technical steps for meningioma removal are performed under endoscopic control and include devascularization at the dural attachment, dedressing with dissection of the arachnoid layer off the tumor surface, debulking using Cavitron Ultra-Sonic Aspirator (CUSA) or bipolar and suction, and developing the plane of cleavage around the tumor.

It is of note that tuberculum sellae meningiomas grow in a subchiasmatic location displacing the optic chiasm backward and the optic nerves laterally and superiorly creating a prechiasmatic working space and facilitating the resection of these tumors via a supraorbital eyebrow approach. In far anterior olfactory groove meningiomas, visualization of the attachment point of the tumor in the midline depression of the olfactory groove is possible with an angled endoscope and angled instruments [23].

Some important principles are very helpful during endoscope-controlled procedures. In general, angled low profile instruments are to be used, obviously because they occupy smaller area within the limited working space. Also, the suction-irrigation using a 50 mL syringe connected to the irrigation sheath and controlled by the assistant is very important for an uninterrupted seamless procedure, because it enables keeping the lens clean without the need to take the scope outside the surgical field. Also, the two-suction technique in which one suction gently pulls the tumor tissue while the other suction teases away the small vessels or the arachnoid attached to the tumor capsule is a very useful maneuver in tumors with a surrounding plane of cleavage. After confirmation of hemostasis, closure then proceeds in the standard fashion.

Many of the aforementioned steps and technical considerations are detailed in the following representative cases and their corresponding figures.

11.6 Representative Case 1

A 33-year-old female patient presented with history of headache and gradually progressive visual loss of the left eye. Her visual acuity was 20/40 on the right, and 20/200 on the left. Visual field examination revealed generalized depression of the left eye. Fundus examination revealed severe optic disc pallor on the left side and a normal fundus on the right side. Neurological examination was otherwise normal. MR imaging was consistent with a tuberculum sellae meningioma (Fig. 11.8). She underwent a purely endoscopic left supraorbital approach for excision of the tumor. Operative details of the procedure are demonstrated in Figs. 11.9 and 11.10. Postoperative MR imaging (Fig. 11.11) revealed gross total resection of the tumor. The patient did very well and regained vision of the left eye by 3 months postoperatively.

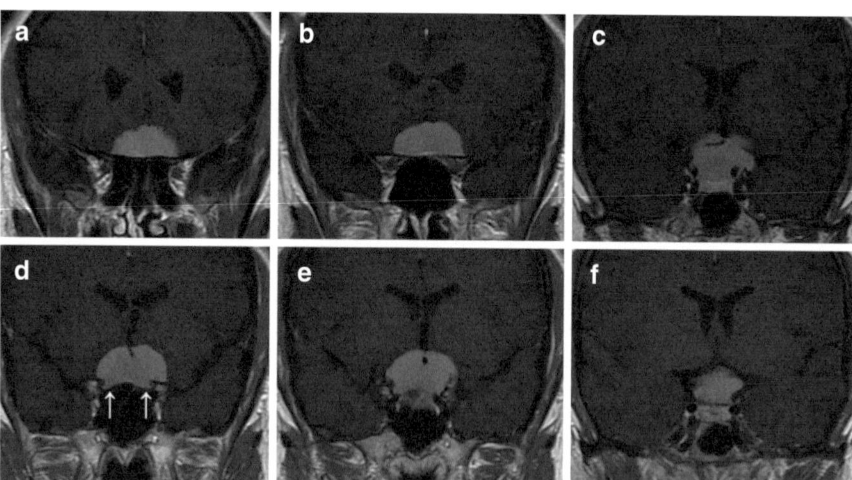

Fig. 11.8 Preoperative MRI of case 1 with tuberculum sellae meningioma. Serial coronal T1-weighted images with contrast (**a–f**). Encasement of ACA complex is seen in (**c–f**), and tumor extension into both optic canals (arrows) is seen in (**d**)

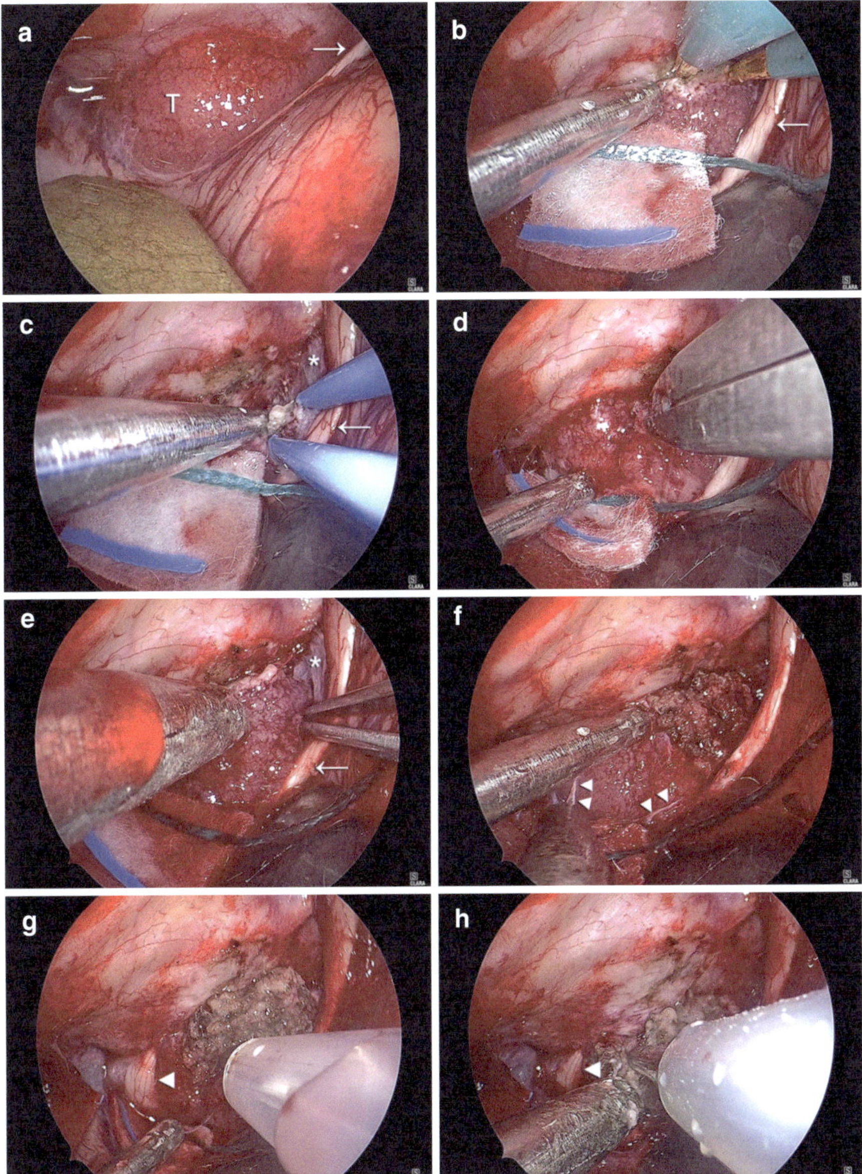

Fig. 11.9 Intraoperative views from case 1 with tuberculum sellae meningioma. (**a**) An initial view of the tumor after the left frontal lobe has been retracted. The olfactory nerve is seen (arrow). (**b**) The tumor basal attachment is bipolar coagulated for initial devascularization. The olfactory nerve is seen (arrow). (**c**) Further tumor coagulation and suction partially debulks the tumor. The arachnoid covering the tumor is exposed (asterisk). The olfactory nerve is seen (arrow). (**d**) Biopsy is taken using a pituitary forceps. (**e**) The arachnoid plane is further developed using a spreading movement of the shafts of a nontoothed forceps. (**f**) More tumor debulking and coagulation has been achieved, and the arachnoid membrane (double arrowheads) is further retracted off the tumor surface using one suction tube while another suction is used for countertraction of the tumor tissue. (**g**, **h**) CUSA is used for further tumor debulking and the left optic nerve (arrowhead) is now partially decompressed and exposed

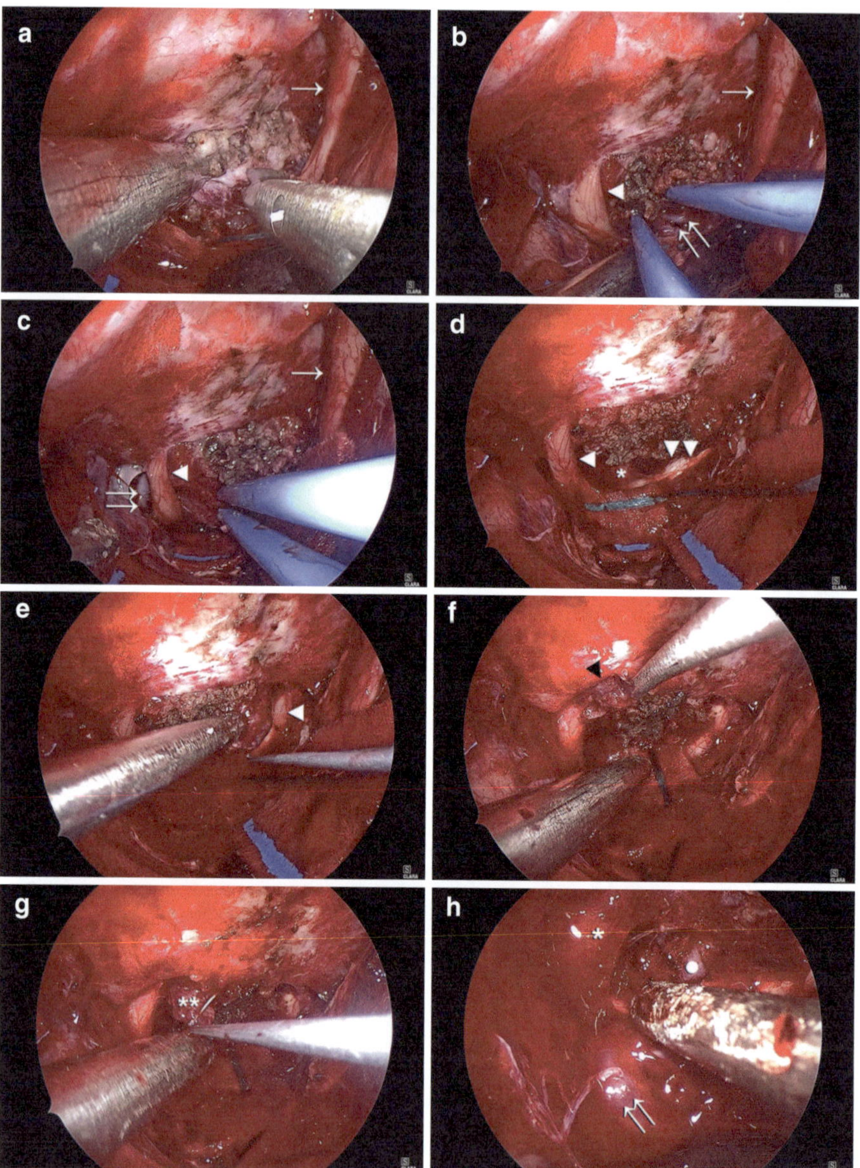

Fig. 11.10 Intraoperative views from case 1 with tuberculum sellae meningioma. (**a**) Tumor tissue is cut using a microscissors in a standard microsurgical fashion and debulked. (**b**) As tumor debulking progresses, the left optic nerve (arrowhead) is significantly decompressed, and the ACA complex (double arrows) is exposed. (**c**) The left supraclinoid ICA (double arrows) is seen lateral to the left optic nerve (arrowhead). (**d**) The right optic nerve (double arrowheads) and the pituitary stalk (asterisk) are now exposed in addition to the already exposed and decompressed left optic nerve (arrowhead). (**e**) A hook is used to remove the intracanalicular tumor compressing the right optic nerve (arrowhead). In (**f**), the left falciform ligament (black arrowhead) is cut using a sickle knife, and the intracanalicular tumor (double asterisk) is then removed using a hook to decompress the intracanalicular left optic nerve in (**g**). (**h**) View after tumor resection has been completed with the pituitary stalk (asterisk), right posterior communicating artery (white circle), and ACA complex (double arrows) being seen

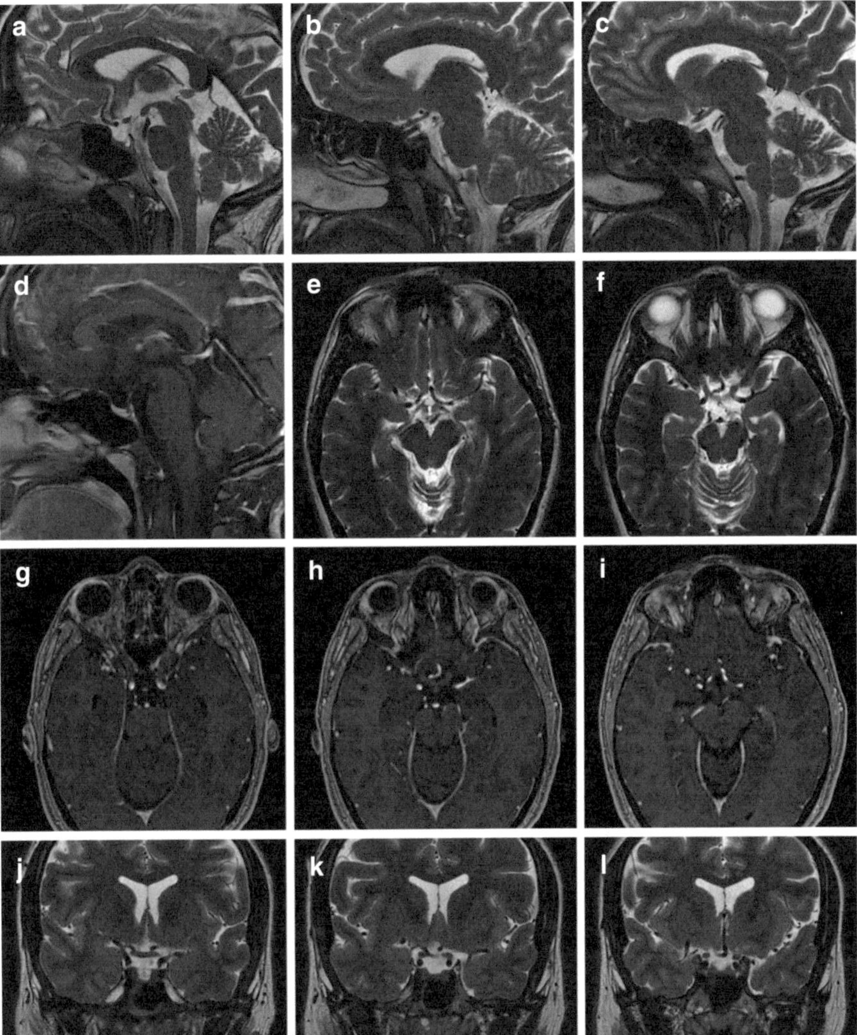

Fig. 11.11 Postoperative MRI of case 1 with tuberculum sellae meningioma revealed gross total resection. (**a–d**) Sagittal T2-weighted, (**e, f**) axial T2-weighted, (**g–i**) axial T1-weighted with contrast, and (**j–l**) coronal T2-weighted images

11.7 Representative Case 2

A 42-year-old female patient who was referred for evaluation of progressively severe daily headaches. Neurological examination was normal. The MRI findings (Fig. 11.12) were consistent with an olfactory groove meningioma. She underwent a purely endoscopic supraorbital approach for excision of the tumor. Operative

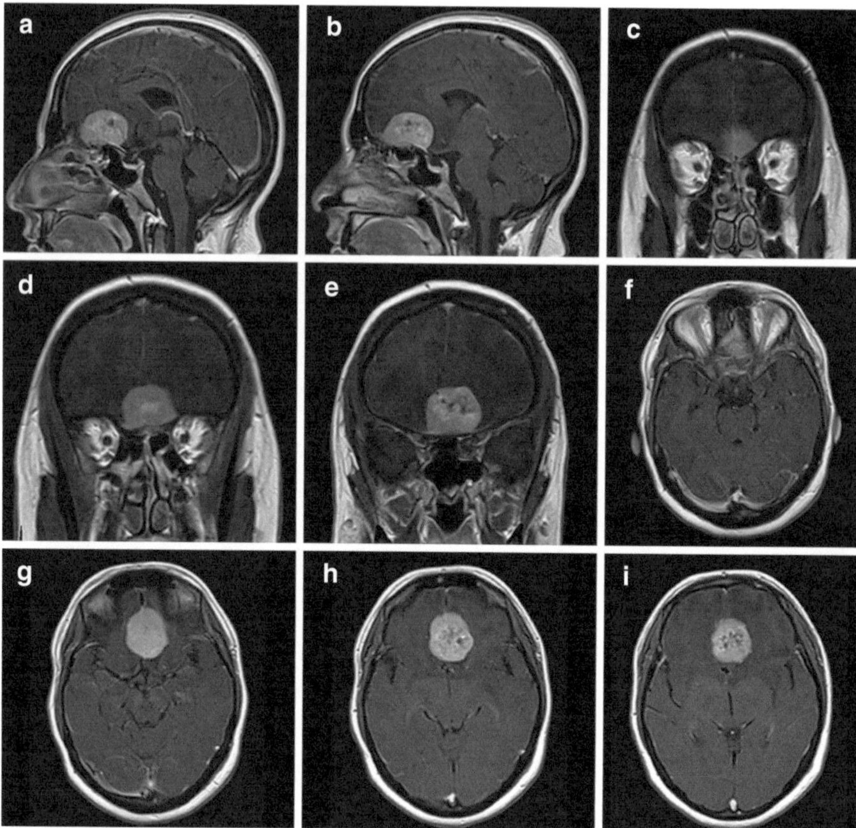

Fig. 11.12 Preoperative MRI of case 2 with olfactory groove meningioma. Serial sagittal (**a**, **b**), coronal (**c–e**), and axial (**f–i**) T1-weighted images with contrast

details of the procedure are demonstrated in Fig. 11.13. Postoperative MR imaging (Fig. 11.14) revealed near total resection of the tumor. The patient did very well and was discharged 6 days after surgery.

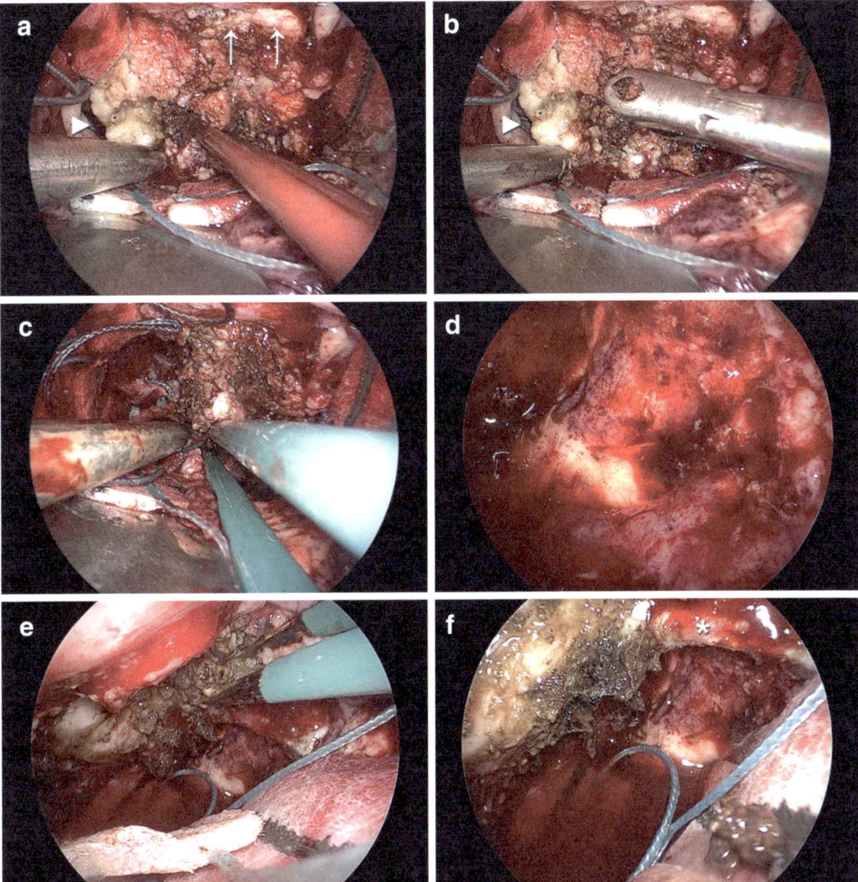

Fig. 11.13 Intraoperative views from case 2 with olfactory groove meningioma. (**a**) A view after initial debulking of the tumor has been achieved. Note the cottonoid patties inserted into the tumor's plane of cleavage (arrowhead). The basal attachment of the tumor (arrows) is seen. (**b**) Tumor piecemeal removal using a tumor forceps. (**c**) Bleeding control using bipolar as the tumor resection proceeds. A large part of the tumor has been removed at this stage. (**d**) The brain surface at the tumor bed is seen after most of the tumor has been resected. Bipolar of tumor tissue at the base of the tumor is performed using a 45° scope seen in (**e**) and a view of the completed resection of the tumor and the attachment of the falx cerebri (asterisk) (**f**)

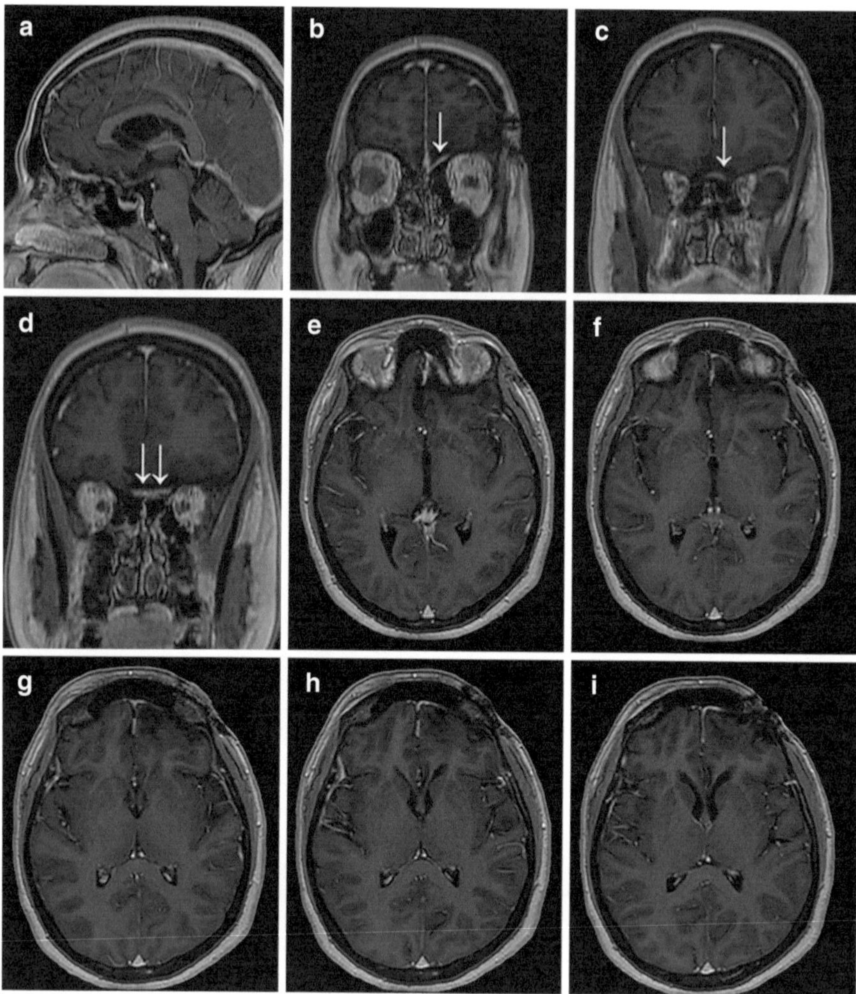

Fig. 11.14 Postoperative MRI of case 2 with olfactory groove meningioma. Serial sagittal (**a**), coronal (**b–d**), and axial (**e–i**) T1-weighted MR images with contrast revealed near total excision. An enhancing small area is seen at the tumor origin (arrows) and probably represents residual tumor

References

1. van Lindert E, Perneczky A, Fries G, Pierangeli E. The supraorbital keyhole approach to supratentorial aneurysms: concept and technique. Surg Neurol. 1998;49:481–90. https://doi.org/10.1016/S0090-3019(96)00539-3.
2. Ottenhausen M, Rumalla K, Alalade AF, Nair P, La Corte E. Decision-making algorithm for minimally invasive approaches to anterior skull base meningiomas. Neurosurg Focus. 2018;44(4):E7.

3. Perneczky A, Müller-Forell W, van Lindert E, Fries G. Keyhole concept in neurosurgery: with endoscope-assisted microsurgery and case studies. 1st ed. Stuttgart: Thieme Medical Publishers; 1999.
4. Prott W. Cisternoscopy—endoscopy of the cerebellopontine angle. Acta Neurochir. 1974;31:105–13.
5. Oppel F, Mulch G, Brock M. Endoscopic section of the sensory trigeminal root, the glossopharyngeal nerve, and the cranial part of the vagus for intractable facial pain caused by upper jaw carcinoma. Surg Neurol. 1981;16(2):92–5.
6. Apuzzo ML, Heifetz MD, Weiss MH, Kurze T. Neurosurgical endoscopy using the side-viewing telescope. J Neurosurg. 1977;46(3):398–400.
7. Liu J, Silva N, Sevak I, Eloy J. Transbasal versus endoscopic endonasal versus combined approaches for olfactory groove meningiomas: importance of approach selection. Neurosurg Focus. 2018;44(4):E8. https://doi.org/10.3171/2018.1.FOCUS17722.
8. Pallini R, Fernandez E, Lauretti L, Doglietto F, D'Alessandris QG, et al. Olfactory groove meningioma: report of 99 cases surgically treated at the Catholic University School of Medicine. Rome World Neurosurg. 2015;83:219–31.
9. Komotar R, Starke R, Raper D, Anand V, Schwartz T. Endoscopic endonasal versus open transcranial resection of anterior midline skull base meningiomas. World Neurosurg. 2012;77:713–24.
10. Kane AJ, Sughrue ME, Rutkowski MJ, Shangari G, Fang S, McDermott MW, et al. Anatomic location is a risk factor for atypical and malignant meningiomas. Cancer. 2011;117:1272–8.
11. Ruggeri A, Cappelletti M, Fazzolari B, Marotta N, Delfini R. Frontobasal midline meningiomas: is it right to shed doubt on the transcranial approaches? Updates and review of the literature. World Neurosurg. 2016;88:374–82.
12. Simpson D. The recurrence of intracranial meningiomas after surgical treatment. J Neurol Neurosurg Psychiatry. 1957;20:22–39.
13. Bander E, Singh H, Ogilvie C, Cusic R, Pisapia D, et al. Endoscopic endonasal versus transcranial approach to tuberculum sellae and planum sphenoidale meningiomas in a similar cohort of patients. J Neurosurg. 2018;128(1):40–8. https://doi.org/10.3171/2016.9.JNS16823.
14. Hayhurst C, Sughrue ME, Gore PA, Bonney PA, Burks JD, Teo C. Results with expanded endonasal resection of skull base meningiomas technical nuances and approach selection based on an early experience. Turk Neurosurg. 2016;26(5):662–70. https://doi.org/10.5137/1019-5149.JTN.16105-15.3.
15. Koutourousiou M, Fernandez-Miranda JC, Wang EW, Snyderman CH, Gardner PA. Endoscopic endonasal surgery for olfactory groove meningiomas: outcomes and limitations in 50 patients. Neurosurg Focus. 2014;37(4):E8.
16. Cavallo LM, de Divitiis O, Aydin S, Messina A, Esposito F, et al. Extended endoscopic endonasal transsphenoidal approach to the suprasellar area: anatomic considerations-part 1. Neurosurgery. 2007;61(3 Suppl):24–34.
17. de Divitiis E, Cavallo LM, Cappabianca P, Esposito F. Extended endoscopic endonasal transsphenoidal approach for the removal of suprasellar tumors: part 2. Neurosurgery. 2007;60(1):46–59.
18. Banu MA, Mehta A, Ottenhausen M, Fraser JF, Patel KS, et al. Endoscope-assisted endonasal versus supraorbital keyhole resection of olfactory groove meningiomas: comparison and combination of 2 minimally invasive approaches. J Neurosurg. 2016;124:605–20.
19. Gandhoke GS, Pease M, Smith KJ, Sekula RF Jr. Supraorbital versus endoscopic endonasal approaches for olfactory groove meningiomas: a cost-minimization study. World Neurosurg. 2017;105:126–36.
20. Telera S, Carapella CM, Caroli F, Crispo F, Cristalli G, et al. Supraorbital keyhole approach for removal of midline anterior cranial fossa meningiomas: a series of 20 consecutive cases. Neurosurg Rev. 2012;35:67–83.

21. Iacoangeli M, Nocchi N, Nasi D, Rienzo DI, A, Dobran M. Minimally invasive supraorbital key-hole approach for the treatment of anterior cranial fossa meningiomas. Neurol Med Chir (Tokyo). 2016;56(4):180–5.
22. Reisch R, Perneczky A. Ten-year experience with the supraorbital subfrontal approach through an eyebrow skin incision. Neurosurgery. 2005;57(4 Suppl):242–55.
23. Azab WA, Elmaghraby MA, Zaidan SN, Mostafa KH. Endoscope-assisted transcranial surgery for anterior skull base meningiomas. Mini-invasive Surg. 2020;4:88. https://doi.org/10.20517/2574-1225.2020.75.
24. Krause F, Haubold H. Surgery of the brain and spinal cord, based on personal experiences. Thorek M [Trans]. New York: Rebman Company; 1909–1912.
25. Frazier C. An approach to the hypophysis through the anterior cranial fossa. Ann Surg. 1913;57:145–50. https://doi.org/10.1097/00000658-191302000-00001.
26. Wilson DH. Limited exposure in cerebral surgery: technical note. J Neurosurg. 1971;34:102–6. https://doi.org/10.3171/jns.1971.34.1.0102.
27. Fries G, Perneczky A. Endoscope-assisted brain surgery—part 2—analysis of 380 procedures. Neurosurgery. 1998;42(2):226–32.
28. Linsler S, Fischer G, Skliarenko V, Stadie A, Oertel J. Endoscopic assisted supraorbital key-hole approach or endoscopic endonasal approach in cases of tuberculum sellae meningioma: which surgical route should be favored? World Neurosurg. 2017;104:601–11. https://doi.org/10.1016/j.wneu.2017.05.023.
29. Arnaout MM, Luzzi S, Galzio R, Aziz K. Supraorbital keyhole approach: pure endoscopic and endoscope-assisted perspective. Clin Neurol Neurosurg. 2020;189:105623. https://doi.org/10.1016/j.clineuro.2019.105623.
30. Berhouma M, Jacquesson T, Jouanneau E. The fully endoscopic supraorbital transeyebrow keyhole approach to the anterior and middle skull base. Acta Neurochir. 2011;153:1949–54. https://doi.org/10.1007/s00701-011-1089-z.
31. Magill M, Morshed R, Lucas C, Aghi M, Theodosopoulos P, et al. Tuberculum sellae meningiomas: grading scale to assess surgical outcomes using the transcranial versus transsphenoidal approach. Neurosurg Focus. 2018;44(4):E9. https://doi.org/10.3171/2018.1.FOCUS17753.
32. Guinto G. Olfactory groove meningiomaas. World Neurosurg. 2015;83:1046–7.

Chapter 12
Endoscopic Eyebrow Approach for Aneurysms

Gerrit Fischer and Joachim Oertel

Abbreviations

A1	Proximal segment of the anterior cerebral artery
ACA	Anterior cerebral artery
AChorA	Anterior choroidal artery
ACoA	Anterior communicating artery
An	Aneurysm
BA	Basilar artery
ICA	Internal carotid artery
M1	Proximal segment of the middle cerebral artery
MCA	Middle cerebral artery
P1	Proximal segment of posterior cerebral artery
PCoA	Posterior communicating artery
SCA	Superior cerebellar artery

12.1 Introduction

The appearance of endovascular techniques has significantly changed the treatment modalities of intracranial aneurysms. Since then, surgical treatment is not only competing with the potential course of aneurysm-related affections but with less

G. Fischer · J. Oertel (✉)
Department of Neurosurgery, Saarland University Hospital, Homburg, Saar, Germany

Faculty of Medicine, Saarland University, Homburg, Saar, Germany
e-mail: Gerrit.Fischer@uks.eu; Joachim.Oertel@uks.eu

© The Author(s), under exclusive license to Springer Nature Switzerland AG 2024
W. A. Azab (ed.), *Endoscope-controlled Transcranial Surgery*, Advances and Technical Standards in Neurosurgery 52,
https://doi.org/10.1007/978-3-031-61925-0_12

invasive endovascular treatment procedures. Nevertheless, surgery remains the most definitive treatment option for many intracranial aneurysms, particularly in complex or broad-based lesions [1–4]. Plus, considerable effort has been made to reduce surgical invasiveness while enabling an effective utilization of the surgical area since Axel Perneczky introduced the supraorbital eyebrow approach as a core part of his keyhole concept in neurosurgery [5, 6].

The purpose of surgical management is to completely occlude the aneurysm while preserving flow in the involved parent, branching, and perforating arteries and avoiding affection of surrounding neural structures. Based on microsurgical principles of dissection and exposure, the quality of clip placement is mainly maintained and assured by direct intraoperative inspection. However, microscopic visualization is limited by the straight line of view and even more so in a keyhole approach. The application of additional methods like intraoperative microvascular Doppler sonography and near-infrared indocyanine green videoangiography for direct intraoperative neurovascular assessment has been introduced to the neurosurgical armamentarium and seems to be used on a regular asis [7–11]. But those techniques are also limited to front view information. The additional application of high-quality rigid endoscopes provides excellent wide-angle and close-up visualization of areas hidden under microscopic view. The enhancement of the visual field before, during, and after microsurgical aneurysm occlusion seems to be a safe and effective method to increase the quality of treatment [12–20].

12.2 Indications/Contraindications

Aneurysm surgery is always a serious task even the most experienced neurovascular surgeons never take lightly. Using a supraorbital eyebrow approach does not facilitate this aspect at all. However, the advantage compared with the pterional approach is that the anterior part of the temporal lobe does not obscure the access to most of the supratentorial sections especially the pre-, retro-, and suprasellar area. The Sylvian fissure does not necessarily need to be dissected. In addition, the supraorbital approach allows early access to the medial part of the Sylvian fissure, which slants directly in the lateral half of the corridor and thus may easily be split from medial to lateral without manipulation of the temporal lobe. If performed properly, the supraorbital keyhole approach can provide excellent access to the following vascular sections: ACoA, ACA, ipsilateral and medial circumference of the contralateral ICA, ipsilateral MCA and contralateral M1–M2 segments, AChorA, PCoA, BA apex, both P1 segments and ipsilateral PCoA-PCA junction, as well as both proximal SCA. The approach is considerably limited in cases of large complex aneurysms and giant aneurysms and not recommendable in BA aneurysms located beneath the dorsum sellae. Careful consideration must also be taken in cases of severe SAH and expected brain edema.

12.3 Operative Technique

12.3.1 Preoperative Preparation

Every surgical aneurysm case is reviewed to tailor the least invasive optimum procedure based on preoperative condition of the patient, on aneurysm site and size, and on individual anatomical findings. Under general anesthesia and electrophysiological neuromonitoring, the patient is positioned in a supine position, and the head is fixed in a MAYFIELD holder. The head is then rotated about 10°–60° to the contralateral side. The degree of rotation is determined by the precise location of the lesion and the individual pathoanatomical findings. In approaches to ipsilateral MCA aneurysms, a 10°–20° rotation is recommended. In approaches to the carotid artery region, a 20°–40° head rotation may be required and in approaches to ACOM and contralateral MCA a 40°–60° rotation. In a next step, the head is retroflexed about 10°–15° to support gravity-related self-retraction of the frontal lobe. Then the head is lateroflexed about 5°–10° to the contralateral side also depending on the precise location of the lesion and the pathoanatomic situation of each patient. Thereby, an ergonomic working position for the surgeon can be established and access to high-riding BA tip aneurysms is facilitated. An example of the surgical positioning is shown in Fig. 12.1a. For the appropriate skin incision, the important anatomical landmarks such as the superior temporal line, zygomatic arch, lateral border of the frontal paranasal sinus, and position of the supraorbital foramen with the supraorbital nerve are marked with a sterile pen. Thereafter the borders of the craniotomy are marked, taking into consideration the position of the lesion and the landmarks drawn on the skin. A standard skin incision does not exist, as the individual anatomy of each patient must be respected (Fig. 12.1b).

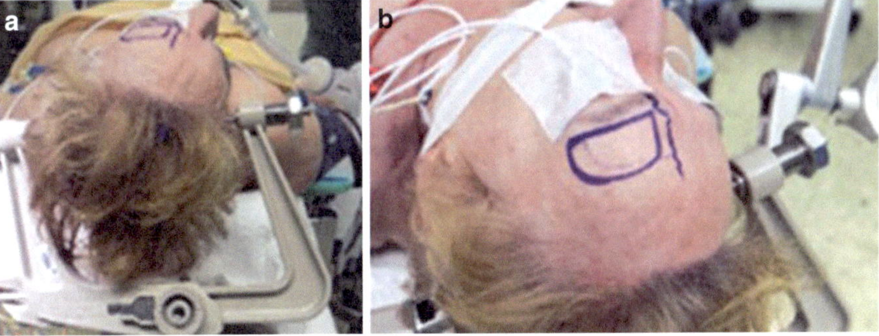

Fig. 12.1 (**a**) Positioning of the head. (**b**) An example for the skin incision based on the supraorbital nerve branch position and the position and configuration of the eyebrows

12.3.2 *Supraorbital Keyhole Craniotomy*

Usually, the skin incision is placed in the lateral half of the eyebrow, laterally from the supraorbital foramen and the neurovascular bundle. The orbicular muscle is split with a monopolar electrode knife above the orbital rim until the anterior temporal line. The fascia of the temporal muscle is then incised also with a monopolar electrode knife at a length of 15–30 mm directly at the lateral orbital rim. The temporal muscle is pushed backward and retracted posteriorly. Exposure and mobilization of the temporal muscle should be restricted to a necessary minimum to prevent postoperative problems with chewing and to maintain a satisfactory cosmetic result (Fig. 12.2a). The craniotomy is then started with a burr hole posterior to the temporal line (Fig. 12.2b). Postoperatively, the area behind the temporal line is covered by the temporal muscle, so that a burr hole in this place does usually not cause any cosmetic problems. The direction of drilling must be rather posteriorly than in a medial direction to avoid penetration of the orbit. Thereafter, considering the lateral border of the frontal paranasal sinus, a bone flap with a width of about 20–30 mm and a height of 15–20 mm is crated with a high-speed craniotome (Fig. 12.2c).

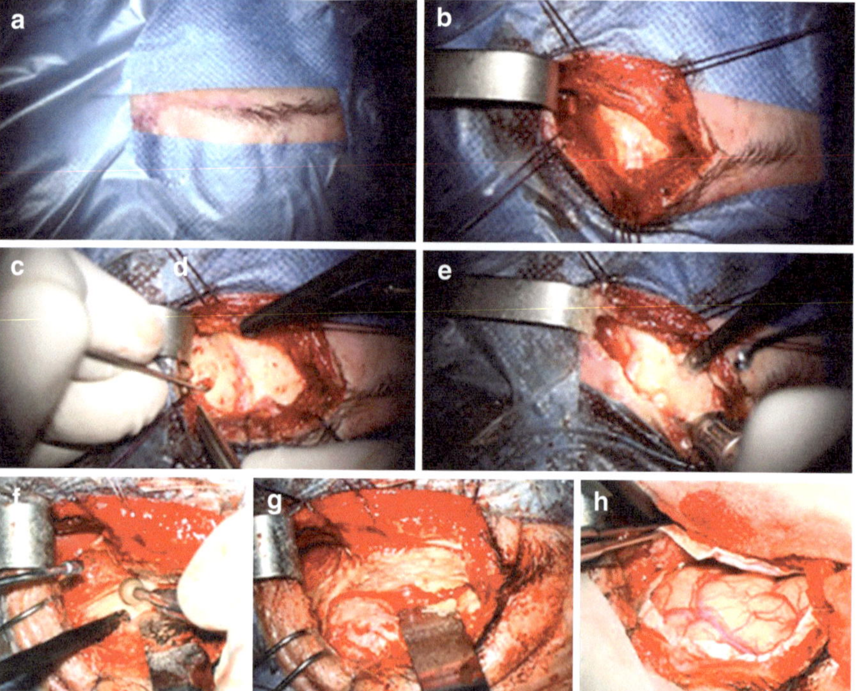

Fig. 12.2 (**a**) Position for skin incision after draping. (**b**) Incision of temporal muscle and application of retraction sutures. (**c**) Placement of burr hole at temporal bone. (**d**) Application of craniotomy. (**e**) Surgical field after removal of bone flap. (**f**) Extradural drilling to flatten the frontal skull base with a diamond burr. (**g**) Dural opening toward the frontal base (**h**)

An important step of the craniotomy after removal of the bone flap is the drilling of the inner edge of the bone above the orbital rim to obtain optimum alignment with the orbital roof. This can be performed with protection of the dura with either a sucker or a retractor blade (Fig. 12.2d). Small osseous extension of the orbital roof, which could shade the microscope light beam and restrict the optical field later during intradural dissection, should also be drilled off extradurally (Fig. 12.2e). In cases of MCA aneurysms located underneath the frontal basal level, the medial and lateral part of the sphenoid wing should be drilled away as well (Fig. 12.2f). The dura is opened in a slightly curved fashion with its base toward the orbital rim (Fig. 12.2g).

12.3.3 Description of the Procedure

Three different endoscopic applications can be defined for aneurysm surgery:

1. Inspection prior to clipping
2. Clipping under endoscopic view
3. Post-clipping evaluation

The initial aneurysm exposure is performed in standard microsurgical technique. The arachnoidal preparation contains a wide exposure of the basal cisterns (Fig. 12.3a, b).

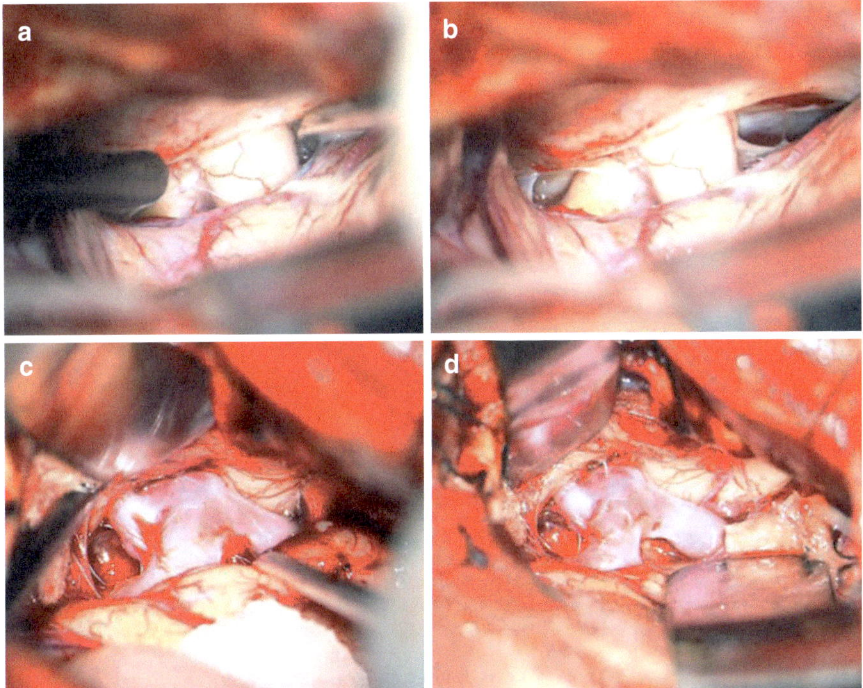

Fig. 12.3 (**a**, **b**) Exposure of left optic nerve and carotid artery. (**c**, **d**) Exposure of MCA aneurysm in the Sylvian fissure

In case of hemorrhage, the blood clots should be washed away thoroughly. The Sylvian fissure is opened from medial to lateral providing immediate control over the proximal M1 segment if necessary (Fig. 12.3c, d).

The endoscope is introduced freehand into the surgical field if additional topographic information is thought to be important. The relationship of the aneurysm to parent, branching, and perforating arteries as well as adjacent structures can be visualized in detail. The insertion of the endoscope must be carefully controlled under microscopic view. Particular attention should be paid to avoid any contact of the endoscope with aneurysm, vessels, and adjacent cranial nerves (Fig. 12.4a). Then, further dissection and aneurysm clipping are performed under the microscope (Fig. 12.4b, c). After clip placement, endoscopic insertion is performed to assess clip position, to confirm completeness of aneurysm obliteration, and to exclude parent, branching, or perforating vessel occlusion or constriction (Fig. 12.4d). If indicated, the clip is repositioned under microscopic view. To complement the visual information on the anatomical situations after clip application, flow assessment in the aneurysm sack and the involved parent, branching, and perforating arteries is performed using micro-Doppler and indocyanine green videoangiography (Fig. 12.4e).

In cases where clip application under direct endoscopic view is desirable, the endoscope should be fixed into the surgical field with an appropriate holding device.

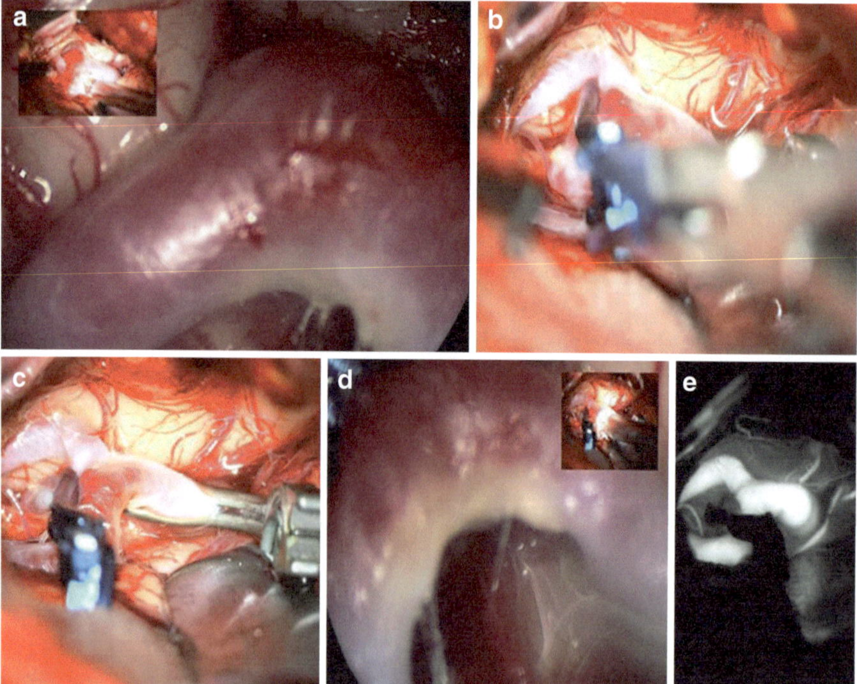

Fig. 12.4 (**a**) Endoscopic inspection of MCA bifurcation. (**b**) Microsurgical clip application. (**c**) Inspection of clipping results under microscopic view. (**d**) Endoscopic inspection behind the MCA main vessel to exclude clipping of perforators or compromise of branching MCA arteries. (**e**) Post-clipping ICG angiography under microscopic or endoscopic view

Care should be taken that the endoscope shaft and camera system do not obstruct the microscopic view and restrict microsurgical maneuvers in case of aneurysm rupture. So immediate switch to the microscope should be possible at all times.

Figure 12.5 details the endoscopic controlled clipping of a right MCA aneurysm. First the aneurysm and all arteries including parent and branching vessels were exposed (Fig. 12.5a). Then the aneurysm is mobilized and the posterior wall is freed of any adhesions (Fig. 12.5b). The aneurysm neck is separated from the anterior branch of the MCA trifurcation (Fig. 12.5c). A clip with a perfect firm fit in the clip applier is inserted (Fig. 12.5d). The anterior branch is pushed anteriorly with the clip (Fig. 12.5e). The clip is ideally positioned and slowly closed at the neck of the aneurysm (Fig. 12.5f, g). Microvascular Doppler sonography is applied to rule out remaining aneurysm perfusion (Fig. 12.5h) and compromise of branching and parent arteries (Fig. 12.5i). Finally endoscopic 2D ICG angiography was applied which showed complete aneurysm occlusion and no compromise of the branching and parent arteries (Fig. 12.5j).

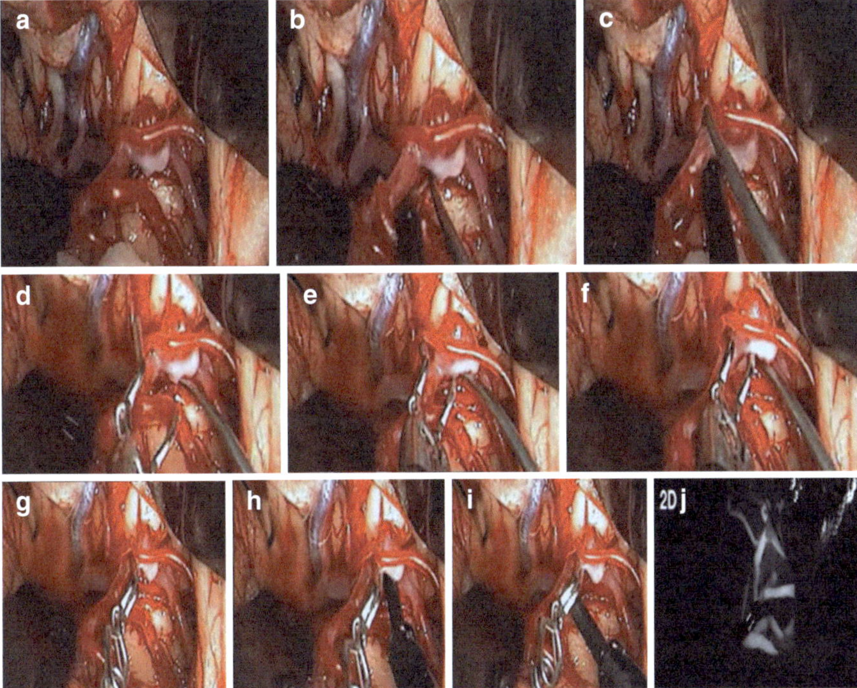

Fig. 12.5 (**a**) Exposure of aneurysm and all arteries including parent and branching vessels. (**b, c**) Removal of adhesions and dissection between anterior branching vessel and aneurysm neck. (**d, e**) Application of clip in a perfect firm fit in the clip applier in the ideal position. (**f, g**) Subsequent slow closure of the clip under continuous observation for vessel compromise. (**h, i**) Application of microvascular Doppler sonography to evaluate perfusion of vessels and aneurysm. (**j**) Endoscopic 2D ICG angiography shows complete aneurysm occlusion and no compromise of the branching and parent arteries

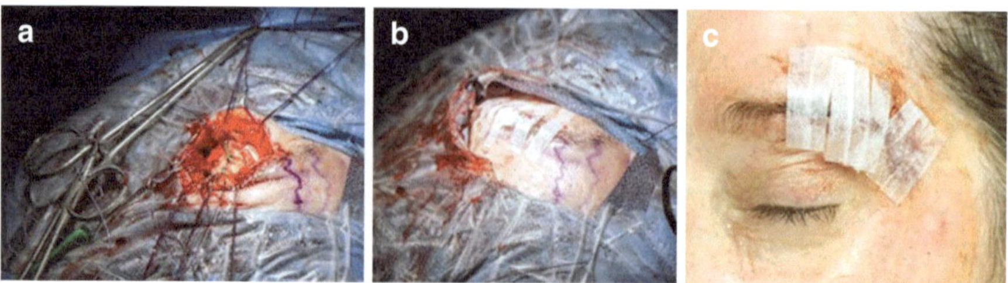

Fig. 12.6 (**a**) Fixation of the bone flap with titanium plates. (**b**) Tight wound closure layer by layer with adaptation of the superficial skin by Steri-Strips. (**c**) Significant reduction of approach trauma and superior cosmetic results by supraorbital key hole approach

12.3.3.1 Wound Closure

Closure of the wound does not differ from other microsurgical procedures. The intradural space is carefully refilled with Ringer solution at body temperature. The dura is closed watertight with running or interrupted sutures. A plate of gel foam is placed extradurally, and the bone flap is fixed with mini plates or other bone fixation techniques (Fig. 12.6a). The fascia and muscle layer are closed with interrupted sutures and the subcutaneous and skin layer with interrupted intracutaneous sutures and Steri-Strips (Fig. 12.6b, c).

12.4 Postoperative Management

The patient is extubated in the operating room and thereafter closely monitored in the neurointensive care unit. If the condition is stable and asymptomatic, the patient can be discharged to the ward. Immediate neuroimaging is optional if the patient remains neurologically stable, but usually a CT or MRI scan is performed. To evaluate the definitive clipping result, DSA is performed 3 days to 6 weeks postoperatively. Clinical follow-up is assessed every 2–3 months initially, then every 6–12 months, and later on every few years.

12.5 Illustrative Case

A 68-year-old lady presented with a history of headache and nausea, no other neurological deficits or preexisting illness. MRI and DSA revealed a broad-based aneurysm of the left MCA bifurcation (Fig. 12.7a–c). After various consultations, the patient opted for surgical treatment.

The aneurysm was clipped via a left supraorbital approach in the above-described manner. For details, please refer to Figs. 12.1, 12.2, 12.3, 12.4, 12.5, 12.6. The

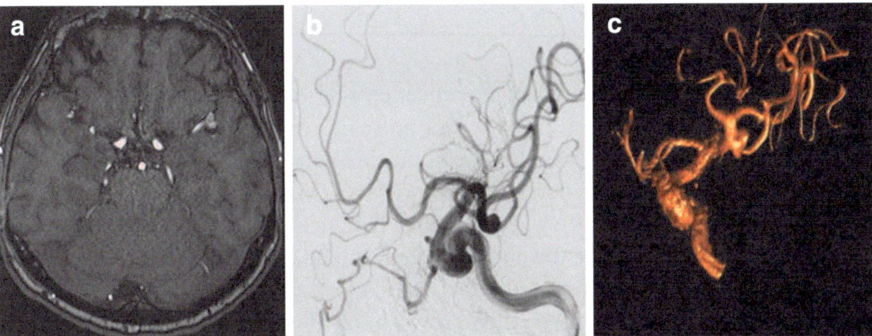

Fig. 12.7 (**a**) Preoperative MR image. (**b**, **c**) Preoperative digital subtraction angiography including 3D reconstruction

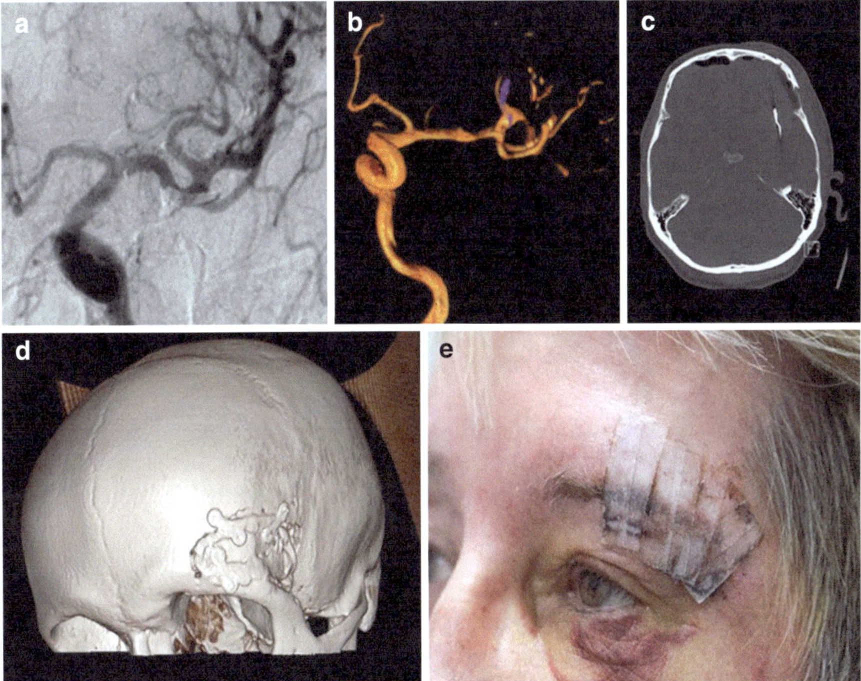

Fig. 12.8 (**a**, **b**) Postoperative digital subtraction angiography (**a**) including 3D reconstruction (**b**). (**c**) Postoperative CT in bone windows to show the craniotomy size. (**d**) 3D skull reconstruction to show the keyhole craniotomy. (**e**) Favorable early postoperative cosmetic result

postoperative course was uneventful; there was no new neurological deficit. Postoperative CT scan and DSA showed no intracranial complications and a perfect reconstruction of the MCA bifurcation without an aneurysm remnant (Fig. 12.8a–c). The patient could be discharged on the third postoperative day. Shortly after, she resumed her normal daily activities with a good cosmetical result (Fig. 12.8d, e).

12.6 Complications

Published experience with endoscopic procedures in aneurysm surgery is limited to several clinical retrospective articles, and no major complications in conjunction with the endoscope were presented. In certain cases, the contact with the endoscope with the aneurysm caused a premature rupture [16]. Contact with cranial nerves was reported to cause transient palsy [16, 19]. One case was described with a small local cortical contusion caused by the endoscope but remained clinically silent [19]. The experience of the authors covers about 500 aneurysm cases treated endoscopically. In these not a single complication of the application of the endoscope could be identified. However, like in all endoscopic procedures, while the advantages of the application of the endoscope are notorious, the main disadvantage is the immediate loss of an overview of the surgical field in case of aneurysm rupture. Thus, it remains recommended to always be prepared to treat the aneurysm in a microsurgical fashion although these situations might be rare and none of such cases have been experienced by the authors.

12.7 Outcome and Prognosis

The supraorbital eyebrow approach is about to find its way into neurovascular routine. It harbors a low rate of complications and provides highly favorable cosmetic results [7, 14, 18, 20]. The application of endoscopes was found to have a significant impact in the application of small keyhole approaches [16–20]. Concerning the author's experience, endoscopic inspection prior to clipping might reduce overexposure and overmobilization of the aneurysm. It was found that the rate of intraoperative rupture was decreased by endoscopic inspection prior to clipping [18]. Temporary clipping on a regular basis was not found necessary. In the post-clipping control, rearrangement of the applied clip or additional clipping due to incomplete aneurysm occlusion or neck remnants was found necessary in 19% of these cases. The consecutive clip rearrangements for incompletely clipped aneurysm led to a reduction of the complication rate down to 3.8% for incomplete aneurysm clipping [18] (instead of 18.9% in the overall aneurysm literature) [4]. Clip rearrangement due to unattended parent, branch, or perforator occlusion was performed in 6.1% of cases. Respectively, the complication rate for compromise of associated arteries was 2.3% [18] (instead of 4.6% in the overall aneurysm literature) [4]. Clipping under direct endoscopic control remains a rather rare event. In the author's opinion, purely endoscopic clipping operations should be limited to few carefully selected cases when an aneurysm rupture is highly unlikely. In case of intraoperative aneurysm rupture, an intracranial endoscope becomes immediately useless, and an external visualization device like a microscope or exoscope must be at hand immediately to solve the situation.

12.8 Conclusion

The supraorbital eyebrow approach is a safe and effective yet elegant approach in the treatment of most aneurysms of the anterior circulation. The additional enhancement of the visual field provided by the endoscope before, during, and after microsurgical aneurysm clipping might decrease the rate of intraoperative aneurysm ruptures and unexpected findings concerning completeness of aneurysm occlusion and compromise of involved parent, branching, and perforating vessels. It could be advisable to have the endoscope at hand at any operative aneurysm procedure since it may be a safe and effective application to increase the quality of aneurysm treatment.

References

1. David CA, Vishteh AG, Spetzler RF, et al. Late angiographic follow-up review of surgically treated aneurysms. J Neurosurg. 1999;91:396–401.
2. Fogelholm R, Hernesniemi J, Vapalahti M. Impact of early surgery on outcome after aneurysmal subarachnoid hemorrhage. A population-based study. Stroke. 1993;24:1649–54.
3. Hernesniemi J, Vapalahti M, Niskanen M, et al. One-year outcome in early aneurysm surgery: a 14 years experience. Acta Neurochir. 1993;122:1–10.
4. Macdonald RL, Wallace MC, Kestle JR. Role of angiography following aneurysm surgery. J Neurosurg. 1993;79:826–32.
5. van Lindert E, Perneczky A, Fries G, Pierangeli. The supraorbital keyhole approach to supratentorial aneurysms: concept and technique E. Surg Neurol. 1998;49(5):481–9.
6. Fischer G, Stadie A, Reisch R, Hopf NJ, Fries G, Böcher-Schwarz H, van Lindert E, Ungersböck K, Knosp E, Oertel J, Perneczky A. The keyhole concept in aneurysm surgery: results of the past 20 years. Neurosurgery. 2011;68(1 Suppl Operative):45–51.
7. Fischer G, Stadie A, Oertel JM. Near-infrared indocyanine green videoangiography versus microvascular Doppler sonography in aneurysm surgery. Acta Neurochir. 2010;152:1519–25.
8. Raabe A, Beck J, Gerlach R, Zimmermann M, Seifert V. Near-infrared indocyanine green video angiography: a new method for intraoperative assessment of vascular flow. Neurosurgery. 2003;52:132–9; discussion 139.
9. Amin-Hanjani S, Meglio G, Gatto R, Bauer A, Charbel FT. The utility of intraoperative blood flow measurement during aneurysm surgery using an ultrasonic perivascular flow probe. Neurosurgery. 2006;58:ONS-305–12; discussion ONS-312.
10. Dashti R, Laakso A, Niemela M, Porras M, Hernesniemi J. Microscope-integrated near-infrared indocyanine green videoangiography during surgery of intracranial aneurysms: the Helsinki experience. Surg Neurol. 2009;71:543–50; discussion 550.
11. Firsching R, Synowitz HJ, Hanebeck J. Practicability of intraoperative microvascular Doppler sonography in aneurysm surgery. Minim Invasive Neurosurg. 2000;43:144–8.
12. Fries G, Perneczky A. Endoscope-assisted brain surgery: part 2—analysis of 380 procedures. Neurosurgery. 1998;42:226–31; discussion 231–222.
13. Perneczky A, Fries G. Endoscope-assisted brain surgery: part 1—evolution, basic concept, and current technique. Neurosurgery. 1998;42:219–24; discussion 224–215.
14. Perneczky A, Boecher-Schwarz HG. Endoscope-assisted microsurgery for cerebral aneurysms. Neurol Med Chir (Tokyo). 1998;38(Suppl):33–4.
15. Hopf NJ, Perneczky A. Endoscopic neurosurgery and endoscope-assisted microneurosurgery for the treatment of intracranial cysts. Neurosurgery. 1998;43:1330–6; discussion 1336–1337.

16. Kalavakonda C, Sekhar LN, Ramachandran P, Hechl P. Endoscope-assisted microsurgery for intracranial aneurysms. Neurosurgery. 2002;51:1119–26; discussion 1126–1117.
17. Kato Y, Sano H, Nagahisa S, et al. Endoscope-assisted microsurgery for cerebral aneurysms. Minim Invasive Neurosurg. 2000;43:91–7.
18. Fischer G, Oertel J, Perneczky A. Endoscopy in aneurysm surgery. Neurosurgery. 2012;70(2 Suppl Operative):184–90.
19. Galzio RJ, Di Cola F, Dehcordi SR, Ricc A, De Paulis D. Endoscope-assisted microneurosurgery for intracranial aneurysms. Front Neurol. 2013;4:201–14.
20. Reisch R, Fischer G, Stadie A, Kockro R, Cesnulis E, Hopf N. The supraorbital endoscopic approach for aneurysms. World Neurosurg. 2014;82(6 Suppl):130–7.

Chapter 13
Endoscopic Supraorbital Translaminar Approach

Mehdi Khaleghi, Kyle C. Wu, and Daniel M. Prevedello

13.1 Introduction

Third ventricular tumors have long posed a significant challenge for neurosurgeons. The complex neurovascular anatomy surrounding these lesions demands meticulous planning and impeccable technique to ensure safe resection while minimizing potential risks [1–6].

Various surgical approaches have been developed to address the anatomic restrictions that might be encountered when facing critical structures surrounding the third ventricle such as the optic apparatus, hypothalamus, and the circle of Willis. The selection of an optimal surgical approach to this region requires a thorough assessment of tumor characteristics, location within the ventricle, degree, and direction of the tumor projection outside the ventricle, and its relationship with surrounding critical structures. Additionally, the surgeon's experience and familiarity with a selected approach and the patient's overall condition are considerations when choosing a surgical approach.

Traditionally, open microsurgical approaches, through the lateral ventricle (transfrontal or transcallosal-transforaminal) or lamina terminalis (anterior, anterolateral transcranial), have been utilized to access the third ventricle. However, these methods come with risks related to the relevant surrounding anatomy, necessitating the exploration of alternative techniques [2–4]. Traditional anterior transcranial approaches necessitate a large bicoronal skin incision with extensive soft tissue dissection and craniotomy, potentially leading to suboptimal cosmesis and

M. Khaleghi · K. C. Wu · D. M. Prevedello (✉)
Department of Neurosurgery, The James Cancer Hospital and Wexner Medical Center, The Ohio State University, Columbus, OH, USA
e-mail: mehdi.khaleghi@osumc.edu; kyle.wu@osumc.edu; daniel.prevedello@osumc.edu

© The Author(s), under exclusive license to Springer Nature Switzerland AG 2024
W. A. Azab (ed.), *Endoscope-controlled Transcranial Surgery*, Advances and Technical Standards in Neurosurgery 52,
https://doi.org/10.1007/978-3-031-61925-0_13

postoperative discomfort. Initially introduced by King [7], the trans-lamina terminalis approach through a pterional craniotomy was described to provide a secure pathway for addressing third ventricular tumors [7]. However, while anterolateral approaches via pterional or orbitozygomatic craniotomies are familiar to neurosurgeons, they come with limitations in tumors with significant extension in the rostrocaudal axis, risk of injury to the frontal branch of the facial nerve, and temporalis muscle atrophy. The transfrontal transforaminal approach has a restricted angle of attack for tumors with a significant lateral extension within the third ventricle, and the ipsilateral plane between the tumor and hypothalamus may be of difficult visualization. This approach may also increase the risks of postoperative seizures and permanent short-term memory loss due to cortical violation and forniceal injury, respectively. Although the interhemispheric transcallosal route to the foramen of Monro avoids cortical transgression, it poses risks of injury to the bridging veins that may drain eloquent areas as well as holds the potential for disconnection syndrome [1–4, 8, 9].

In the recent decade, the growing interest in minimally invasive skull base approaches has led to the evolution of the endoscopic endonasal transtuberculum/transplanum and minimally invasive microscopic supraorbital approaches to reach the lesions of the third ventricle and anterior cranial base [5, 6, 10–12]. The endoscopic endonasal approach (EEA) with transplanum/transtuberculum extension offers a minimally invasive technique with direct midline visualization through the third ventricular floor and enables early decompression of the optic apparatus, resulting in a favorable visual outcome. Despite its benefits, this approach entails a steep learning curve and a slightly higher risk of postoperative cerebrospinal fluid (CSF) leak than transcranial approaches, despite modern skull base repair techniques. Managing major arterial bleeding through the narrow endonasal corridor remains a challenge, given limitations in endoscopic electrocautery and clip application equipment. In cases of intraventricular or retrochiasmatic craniopharyngiomas (i.e., "prefixed optic chiasm"), the space between the optic chiasm and the superior aspect of the pituitary gland may not necessarily be expanded by the tumor, creating minimal working space. The endoscopic endonasal translaminar approach through the suprachiasmatic corridor could be a viable option. However, it risks compression injury of the optic chiasm and may provide a very narrow corridor and limited surgical freedom. The subtle risk of causing pituitary dysfunction and limitations in young children with a conchal-type sphenoid sinus are other drawbacks of an endonasal approach [5, 6, 13–15].

This chapter focuses on the endoscopic supraorbital translaminar approach (ESOTLA), which presents a promising evolution of traditional microsurgical techniques. By combining a minimally invasive keyhole approach with endoscopic visualization through the lamina terminalis, the ESOTLA offers a wider view and enhanced illumination around the blind corners of the third ventricle while minimizing the need for frontal lobe retraction. Notably, this approach overcomes the limited rostrocaudal access of its open microsurgical counterpart while addressing complex cases of retrochiasmatic craniopharyngioma that may be challenging to reach safely using conventional EEA [11, 16–18].

13.2 Differential Diagnosis and Evaluation

Accurate differentiation of lesions involving the third ventricle is imperative for effective management and surgical planning. The differential for benign lesions includes craniopharyngioma, pineocytoma, colloid cyst, meningioma, chordoid glioma, choroid plexus papilloma, and cavernous malformation. However, a comprehensive differential diagnosis should include malignant lesions such as metastasis, glioblastoma, ependymoma, and lymphoma [19].

Considering the clinical presentation, imaging characteristics, and complementary investigations like cerebrospinal fluid analysis or stereotactic biopsy may facilitate an accurate diagnosis before definitive treatment. Neuroimaging, particularly magnetic resonance imaging (MRI) with gadolinium, plays a crucial role in evaluating lesion location, size, characteristics, and relation to nearby neurovascular structures. Nonetheless, histopathologic examination remains the gold standard for achieving the diagnosis and developing the final treatment plan.

13.3 Advantages and Indication

The visualization provided by the ESOTLA offers a straightforward route to third ventricular lesions while allowing for an improved extent of resection in tumors with significant anterior or lateral extension. This approach provides a good visualization of the ventral cerebral peduncles, which can be accessed ideally via a contralateral ESOTLA. Utilizing an endoscopic route to reach the lamina terminalis has several advantages. It obviates frontal lobe retraction, reducing the risk of venous infarct, seizure, and postoperative basal frontal-associated neurocognitive deficits. It also minimizes soft tissue dissection leading to a significantly shorter operative time. In addition, this approach has the advantage of allowing for early and postoperative CSF diversion through fenestration of the lamina terminalis, which is especially relevant in cases with obstructive hydrocephalus and incomplete tumor resection. These technical advantages translate into enhanced surgical outcomes and shorter postoperative hospital stays in selected cases [11, 13, 16–18, 20].

In general, the ESOTLA is ideally suited for specific lesions within the third ventricle, such as purely intraventricular craniopharyngiomas, colloid cysts, chordoid glioma, and hypothalamic gliomas.

13.4 Contraindications

Although there are no specific contraindications of the ESOTLA, certain tumor characteristics may cause the surgeon to select a different approach. Large multi-compartment tumors with significant rostral extension to the lateral ventricle may require considerable traction of the optic chiasm and anterior cerebrovascular complex, posing a substantial challenge for circumferentially isolating the tumor solely through ESOTLA. In such instances, the transfrontal transforaminal approach may be combined with ESOTLA to address this limitation.

For craniopharyngiomas arising mainly from the pituitary stalk with significant extension into the suprasellar and interpeduncular cisterns, the ESOTLA provides limited access, and infrachiasmatic endoscopic or anterolateral approaches may offer a better extent of resection and overall outcome. As mentioned earlier, dealing with highly vascular tumors may also be challenging, given the limited endoscopic maneuverability to manage major arterial injuries. Furthermore, in patients with significant laterally extended frontal sinus, the increased risk of CSF leak may make this approach less favorable.

13.5 Case Description

A 44-year-old male presented with complaints of fatigue, poor sleep, and polyuria. A hormonal study revealed low testosterone and low urine specific gravity, indicative of diabetes insipidus. The patient was otherwise neurologically intact with full visual fields on ophthalmologic evaluation. Further investigation with contrasted brain MRI revealed a solid-cystic retrochiasmatic suprasellar mass measuring $29 \times 26 \times 24$ mm. The mass was found to arise from the superior part of the infundibulum, predominantly occupying the third ventricle. Notably, it considerably splayed the optic tracts and caused vasogenic edema in the optic chiasm and right hypothalamus. Additionally, the posteroinferior aspect of the tumor closely approached the cerebral peduncles and posterior cerebral arteries, while the anterior pole of the tumor abutted the right supraclinoid internal carotid artery (ICA) and A1 segment of the right anterior cerebral artery (ACA) (Fig. 13.1). However, no calcification was found in the head CT scan. The appearance of the mass was suggestive of craniopharyngioma. After discussing the likely diagnosis and the need for surgical intervention to achieve maximal safe resection, the patient elected to undergo surgery.

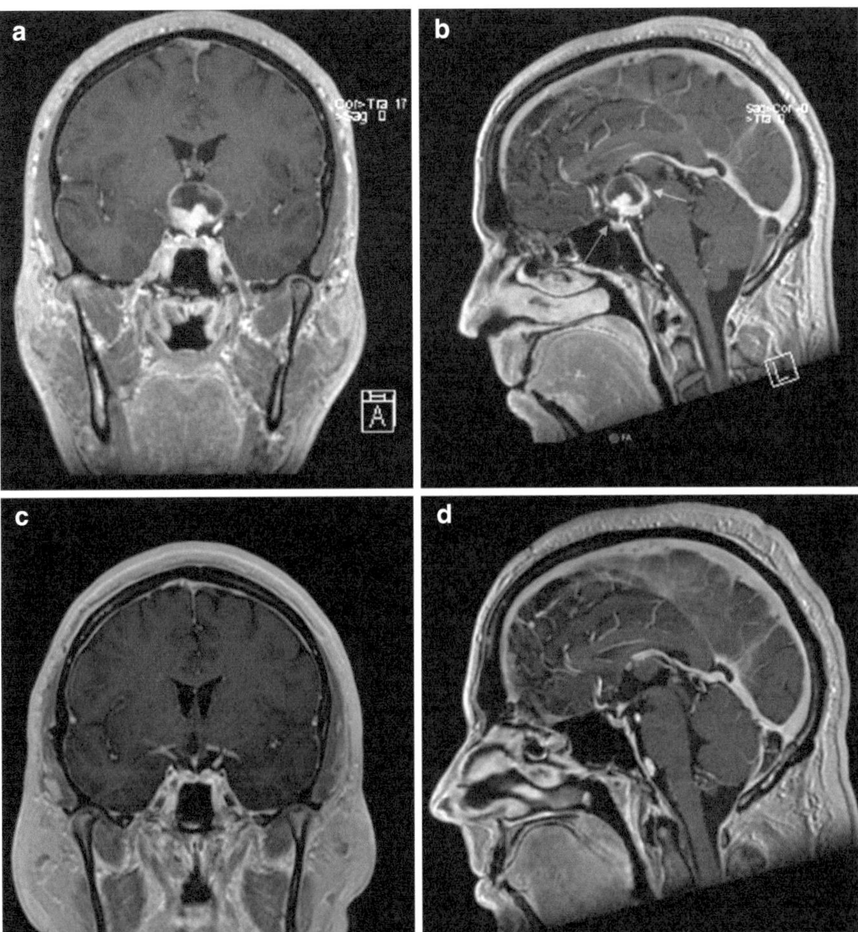

Fig. 13.1 Contrast-enhanced MRI of the patient. *Preoperative* (**a**) coronal and (**b**) sagittal views showing a retrochiasmatic heterogeneous enhancing cystic-solid suprasellar mass with prominent intraventricular extension and sellar sparing, consistent with craniopharyngioma. Note the narrow angle between the upper anterior border of the pituitary gland and the optic chiasm (blue *arrow*) and the proximity of the tumor to the cerebral peduncles (green arrow). 1-year *postoperative* (**c**) coronal and (**d**) sagittal views demonstrated no residual or recurrence following targeted therapy

13.6 Approach of Choice

In this case, the tumor was predominantly intraventricular without an intrasellar component. The fact that the tumor had no calcification increased the possibility of a "papillary" craniopharyngioma. Moreover, the inferior displacement of the optic apparatus and infundibulum created a narrow corridor between the pituitary gland and optic chiasm, rendering the transplanum/transtuberculum EEA less favorable, particularly on a patient with most of the pituitary gland function preserved. While the addition of an EEA to anterolateral approaches as a combined "above and below" approach may be effective in managing multi-compartmental intraventricular craniopharyngiomas, this tumor characteristic could be adequately addressed through a single-stage supraorbital corridor with the aid of the angled endoscope. The utilization of the endoscope allowed for excellent visualization of the entire floor of the third ventricle, including the cerebral peduncles and posterior aspect of the circle of Willis. It is important to note that the dominant retrochiasmatic portion of the tumor would be difficult to access via microsurgical translaminar approaches, necessitating aggressive chiasmatic retraction and potentially compromising visual function in an otherwise visually intact patient. Therefore, we decided to proceed with a one-stage ESOTLA, with the primary goal of a maximal safe resection of the tumor while preserving the optic apparatus and the hypothalamic function, followed by treating the tumor with BRAF inhibitors once papillary craniopharyngioma is confirmed.

13.7 Surgical Technique

Under general anesthesia, the patient was positioned supine with the head fixed in a three-pin head holder. Baseline somatosensory evoked potential (SSEP) monitoring was applied. The torso was slightly elevated, and the head was extended 15° to have the ipsilateral frontal lobe naturally fall away from the skull base, obviating the need for fixed frontal retraction. The head was turned 30° to the contralateral side to optimally reach the central portion of the lamina terminalis and other midline structures. To safeguard the eyes, Tegaderm dressings were applied following temporary tarsorrhaphy. After prepping and draping the surgical site, an incision was made over the superior third of the eyebrow at an angle parallel to hair follicles, starting a few millimeters lateral to the supraorbital notch and extending to the lateral end of the eyebrow. While protecting the orbicularis oculi muscle fibers, a subgaleal dissection was carried out, and the pericranium and temporalis fascia were exposed. Then the pericranium was elevated in a reverse U-shaped manner, based on the supraorbital rim, and retracted inferiorly. The temporalis muscle was detached bluntly and retracted posterolaterally without the use of electrocautery. A keyhole burr hole was placed posterior to the frontozygomatic suture, just inferior to the superior temporal line, and dissected away from the inferior frontal dura. Neuronavigation was used to identify the location of the frontal sinus, and a roughly 2 × 2 cm supraorbital craniotomy was performed above the orbital rim and lateral to the supraorbital notch, with care taken to avoid violating the frontal sinus. This craniotomy size provided sufficient space for endoscopic dissection of the para-chiasmatic cisterns and tumor removal within the third ventricle (Fig. 13.2). In the case of inadvertent entry into the frontal sinus, the opening is sealed with a periosteal flap and augmented with

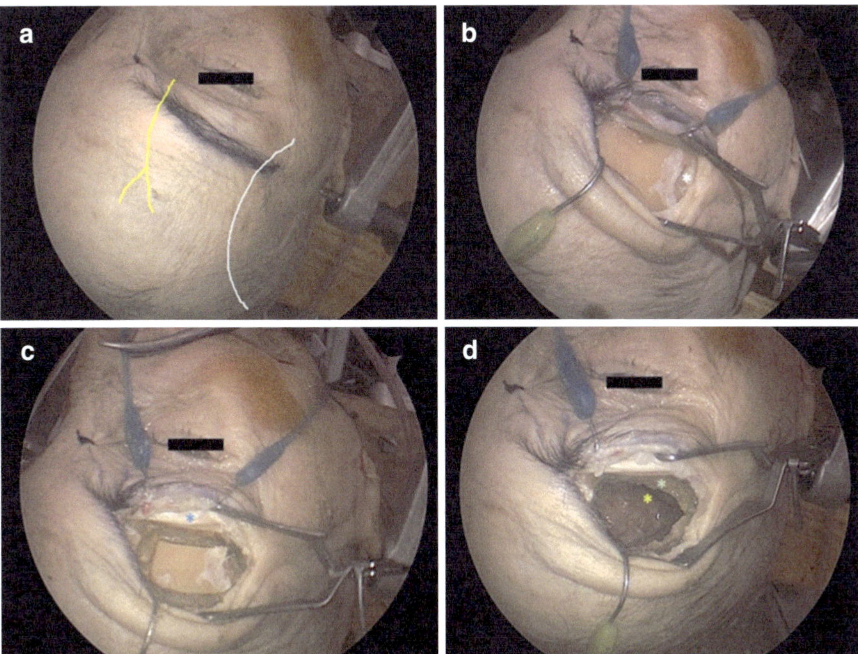

Fig. 13.2 Cadaveric dissection demonstrating stepwise supraorbital keyhole craniotomy. (**a**) Creating a trans-eyebrow incision between the supraorbital neurovascular bundle (yellow line) and superior temporal line (white line). (**b**) Retracting the pericranium inferiorly and detaching the temporalis muscle (white star). (**c**) Creating a craniotomy superior to the supraorbital ridge (blue star). (**d**) Flattening the orbital roof (green star) and dural opening to expose the inferolateral frontal lobe (yellow star)

Gelfoam to ensure gasket-seal closure. Preservation of the frontal sinus mucosa is preferred to maintain physiological drainage.

The dura was bluntly dissected from the orbital roof to flatten the anterior cranial base using a round diamond burr. This maneuver enables direct endoscopic visualization parallel to the anterior skull base without frontal lobe retraction. The endoscope (KARL STORZ Endoscopy-America, CA) with 0° and 45° rod lenses (18 cm in length, 4 mm in diameter) was then introduced into the field and held against the inferior edge of craniotomy as a rest point throughout the procedure. The dura was opened in a reverse C shape with an inferior base and retracted using a suture to gravity. Using a two-surgeon four-hand technique, the arachnoid dissection was performed under the ipsilateral frontal lobe in a lateral to medial direction to allow the frontal lobe to fall away from the skull base due to gravity. Once the ipsilateral sylvian cistern was centered in the field, the endoscope was moved from a lateral to medial trajectory along the lesser wing of the sphenoid to avoid injury to the ipsilateral olfactory nerve. Opening of the opticocarotid and chiasmatic cisterns allowed for further relaxation of the frontal lobe and better identification of the optic chiasm, ipsilateral optic nerve, and internal carotid artery (ICA). With a more medial

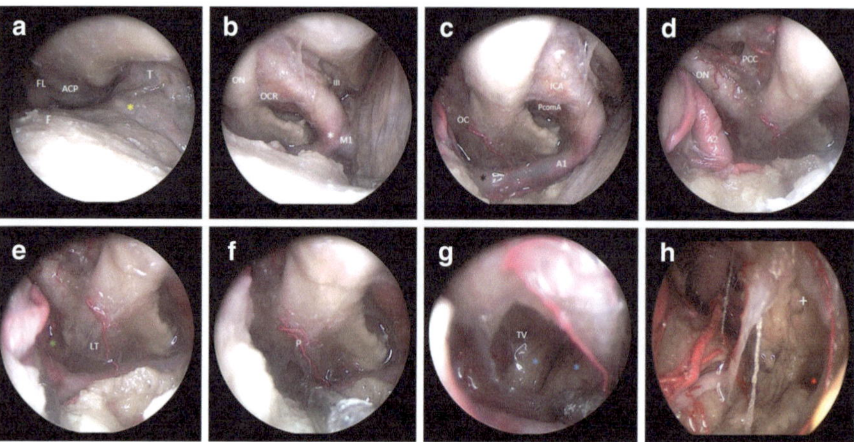

Fig. 13.3 Stepwise cadaveric dissection of the intradural anatomic landmarks during right-sided ESOTLA. (**a**) A lateral to medial subfrontal arachnoid dissection and early exposure of the sylvian cistern (yellow star). (**b**) Opening of the opticocarotid recess and exposure of the internal carotid artery bifurcation (white star). (**c**) Following the right A1 over the optic chiasm to expose the AcomA (black star). (**d**) Opening of the suprachiasmatic cistern and the left opticocarotid recess. (**e**) Identifying the left A1 (green star) and the lamina terminalis. (**f**) Sharp opening of the lamina terminalis. (**g**) Exposing of bilateral thalami (blue stars) within the third ventricle. (**h**) Identifying the retrochiasmatic space (white plus) and floor of the third ventricle (red star) using a 45° endoscope. *A1, A2* First and second segments of anterior cerebral artery, *ACP* Anterior clinoid process, *F* Frontal lobe, *FL* Falciform ligament, *ICA* Internal carotid artery, *LT* Lamina terminalis, *M1* First segment of the middle cerebral artery, *OC* Optic chiasm, *OCR* Opticocarotid recess, *ON* Optic nerve, *P* Perforator artery, *PCC* Prechiasmatic cistern, *PcomA* Posterior communicating artery, *T* Temporal lobe, *TV* Third ventricle, *III* Oculomotor nerve

trajectory, the contralateral opticocarotid cistern was exposed, enabling the identification of the contralateral ICA and optic nerve. Following the ipsilateral ICA toward its bifurcation and more distal, the ACA-anterior communicating artery (AcomA) complex was identified lying over the chiasm, typically within 3 mm of the anterior edge of the chiasm (Fig. 13.3). Meticulously preserving the perforators supplying the optic chiasm is crucial for optimal postoperative visual outcome.

Following the opening of the lamina terminalis cistern, the lamina terminalis was identified as a thin oblique membrane located posterior and superior to the optic chiasm and was significantly bulged by the tumor. The central avascular plane of the lamina terminalis was then identified and opened sharply. The limitation in identifying this avascular plane can be overcome by gently mobilizing the ACA-AcomA complex upward. After entering the third ventricle, the tumor capsule was opened, and the cystic portion of the tumor was evacuated. Internal debulking of the solid portion of the tumor was then performed using a combination of an ultrasonic aspirator (Sonopet, Stryker, Kalamazoo, MI) and a morcellation-aspiration device (NICO Myriad, NICO Corp., Indianapolis, IN). Once sufficient debulking was achieved, meticulous bimanual extracapsular sharp dissection was carried out to separate the tumor capsule from the hypothalamus, optic chiasm, and bilateral

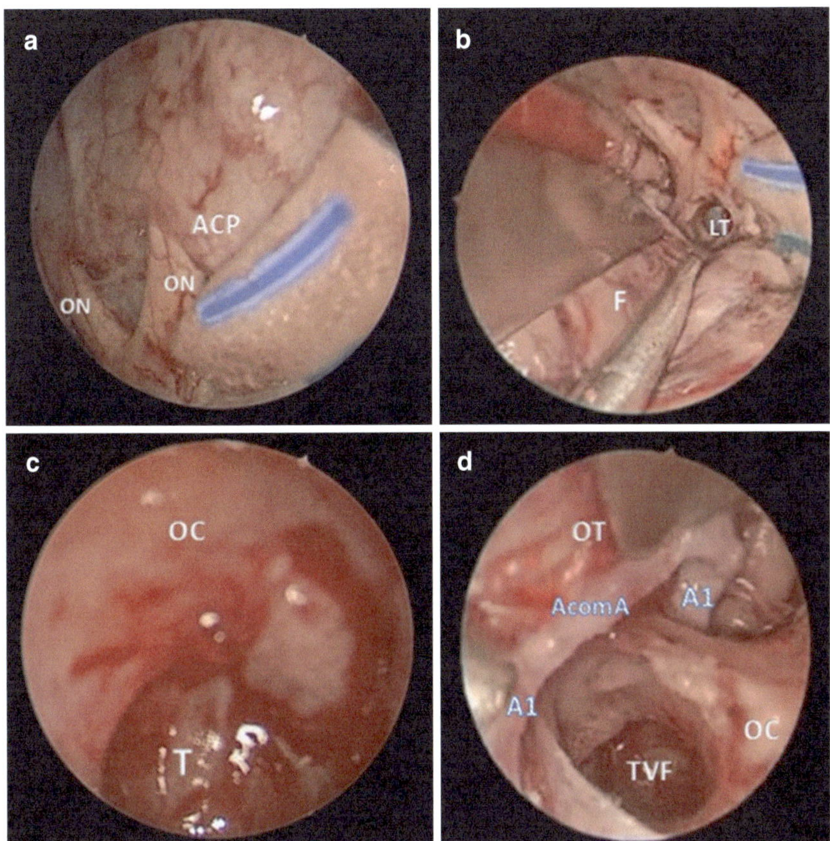

Fig. 13.4 Intraoperative views of the patient. Stepwise access to the third ventricle craniopharyngioma through the endoscopic supraorbital translaminar approach (ESOTLA). (**a**) Subfrontal dissection in a lateral to medial trajectory. (**b**) Opening of the lamina terminalis. (**c**) Internal debulking of the tumor. (**d**) Access to the floor of the third ventricle and retrochiasmatic portion of the tumor using a 45° endoscope. *A1* First segment of the anterior cerebral artery, *AcomA* Anterior communicating artery, *ACP* Anterior clinoid process, *F* Right frontal lobe, *LT* Lamina terminalis, *OC* Optic chiasm, *ON* Optic nerve, *OT* Optic tract, *T* Tumor, *TVF* Third ventricle floor

posterior cerebral arteries (PCAs). Then the tumor capsule was rolled centrally and resected in a piecemeal fashion, leaving a small shell of the tumor that was firmly attached to the floor of the third ventricle (Fig. 13.4).

Trying to achieve a gross total removal demanded significant traction on the hypothalamus and possible severe neurological deficits and was thus avoided based on the goals of the surgery. It is imperative to dissect the tumor capsule sharply and respect the arachnoid plane when isolating a craniopharyngioma to minimize this risk. Using the 45° endoscope and rotating it allowed visualization of the third ventricular floor from anterior to posterior, and the blind corners were assessed for areas of residual tumor.

13.8 Repair

Following meticulous hemostasis, dural closure was performed in a watertight fashion to minimize the risk of postoperative pseudomeningocele formation, ensuring optimal wound healing and reducing hospital stay. To obliterate any potential epidural dead space, the basal dura was tacked up inferiorly. The bone flap was then repositioned and fixed using a low-profile titanium plate and a burr hole cover, carefully considering the contour of the supraorbital ridge to address cosmetic concerns while ensuring stable fixation. The temporalis fascia was then secured to the bone flap to prevent muscle atrophy and preserve mastication. Lastly, the galea was closed using 4-0 Vicryl interrupted sutures followed by 6-0 subcuticular running stitches for the skin. Low-profile dressing and head wrap were applied for the next day to prevent soft tissue edema.

13.9 Postoperative Course

The patient tolerated the surgery well and woke up with an intact neurological examination and a full visual confrontation test. He resumed a regular diet and ambulated early after surgery. The patient was discharged 2 days postoperatively. Subsequent histological examination confirmed papillary craniopharyngioma with a positive BRAF V600E mutation. A week after the surgery, the incision was well healed with no signs of erythema or discharge, and the suture was removed. Postoperative MRI revealed a small residual tumor on the infundibulum leading to the initiation of adjuvant BRAF inhibitor therapy. Postoperative changes were noted at the 1-year surveillance MRI, and no evidence of residual or recurrence was found. The cosmetic outcome of the surgery was excellent, with no signs of visible scarring or alopecia at the surgical site. The patient has been followed for 4 years, and he is neurologically intact with partial hypopituitarism.

13.10 Complications

The ESOTLA, while an effective minimally invasive approach for addressing third ventricular lesions, is not without risk. However, no complications have been observed in the senior surgeon's (D.P.) experience. Frontal paresthesia from supraorbital nerve injury is rare when performing the skin incision lateral to the supraorbital notch. The risk of injury to the frontal branch of the facial nerve and resulting eyebrow asymmetry can be reduced by limiting the lateral extension of the incision and avoiding the use of cautery for temporalis muscle dissection. There is an alternative superior eyelid incision for this approach that is hidden by supratarsal crease and precludes the risk of eyebrow alopecia. However, it still harbors the risk of orbital septum violation.

Minimizing the need for frontal lobe retraction, the ESOTLA presents a potential advantage over microscopic techniques, resulting in a lower risk to memory, executive planning, and personality change. By carefully performing subfrontal arachnoid dissection in a lateral to medial trajectory, olfactory nerve injury can be avoided. Of significant concern are hypothalamic and optic apparatus injuries arising from significant traction or vascular compromise. These may be mitigated through the use of an angled endoscope and sharp extracapsular dissection. However, in cases where severe adhesions to the lateral wall or floor of the third ventricle are encountered, a strategic decision to leave the most redundant part of the tumor behind and proceed with adjuvant therapy may be more justifiable.

13.11 Commentary

The experience of the senior surgeon (D.P.) in dealing with lesions within the third ventricle demonstrates that the lamina terminalis and whole dimension of the third ventricle were easily accessed by ESOTLA in the hand of skilled endoscopic neurosurgeons, using a two-surgeon four-hand technique. There were no limitations to working freedom either behind the chiasm or on the third ventricular floor. While the small size of the supraorbital craniotomy might have posed a limited angle of attack in the open microscopic version of this approach compared to anterolateral approaches, this obstacle was effectively managed by employing angled lenses and strategic rotation within the surgical field.

13.12 Conclusion

The ESOTLA represents a promising and effective alternative corridor for addressing lesions within the third ventricle, resulting in excellent neurological and cosmetic outcomes. This chapter describes the technical aspects of this approach, offering insights into its application, advantages, and potential limitations. As we explore this novel technique, we hope to contribute to the growing body of knowledge in neurosurgery and further refine this approach to managing third ventricular lesions effectively and safely.

References

1. Krishna V, Blaker B, Kosnik L, Patel S, Vandergrift W. Trans-lamina terminalis approach to third ventricle using supraorbital craniotomy: technique description and literature review for outcome comparison with anterior, lateral and trans-sphenoidal corridors. Minim Invasive Neurosurg. 2011;54(5–6):236–42.
2. Shi XE, Wu B, Fan T, Zhou ZQ, Zhang YL. Craniopharyngioma: surgical experience of 309 cases in China. Clin Neurol Neurosurg. 2008;110(2):151–9.

3. Charalampaki P, Filippi R, Welschehold S, Conrad J, Perneczky A. Tumors of the lateral and third ventricle: removal under endoscope-assisted keyhole conditions. Neurosurgery. 2008;62(6 Suppl 3):1049–58.
4. Fahlbusch R, Honegger J, Paulus W, Huk W, Buchfelder M. Surgical treatment of craniopharyngiomas: experience with 168 patients. J Neurosurg. 1999;90(2):237–50.
5. Cavallo LM, Prevedello DM, Solari D, Gardner PA, Esposito F, Snyderman CH, et al. Extended endoscopic endonasal transsphenoidal approach for residual or recurrent craniopharyngiomas. J Neurosurg. 2009;111(3):578–89.
6. Kassam AB, Gardner PA, Snyderman CH, Carrau RL, Mintz AH, Prevedello DM. Expanded endonasal approach, a fully endoscopic transnasal approach for the resection of midline suprasellar craniopharyngiomas: a new classification based on the infundibulum. J Neurosurg. 2008;108(4):715–28.
7. King TT. Removal of intraventricular craniopharyngiomas through the lamina terminalis. Acta Neurochir. 1979;45(3–4):277–86.
8. Shucart WA, Stein BM. Transcallosal approach to the anterior ventricular system. Neurosurgery. 1978;3(3):339–43.
9. Beaumont TL, Limbrick DD, Patel B, Chicoine MR, Rich KM, Dacey RG. Surgical management of colloid cysts of the third ventricle: a single-institution comparison of endoscopic and microsurgical resection. J Neurosurg. 2022:1–9.
10. Ormond DR, Hadjipanayis CG. The supraorbital keyhole craniotomy through an eyebrow incision: its origins and evolution. Minim Invasive Surg. 2013;2013:296469.
11. Abdou MS, Cohen AR. Endoscopic surgery of the third ventricle: the subfrontal trans-lamina terminalis approach. Minim Invasive Neuros. 2000;43(4):208–11.
12. Cai M, Ye Z, Ling C, Zhang B, Hou B. Trans-eyebrow supraorbital keyhole approach in suprasellar and third ventricular craniopharyngioma surgery: the experience of 27 cases and a literature review. J Neuro-Oncol. 2019;141(2):363–71.
13. Gazzeri R, Nishiyama Y, Teo C. Endoscopic supraorbital eyebrow approach for the surgical treatment of extraaxialand intraaxial tumors. Neurosurg Focus. 2014;37(4):E20.
14. de Divitiis E, Cavallo LM, Cappabianca P, Esposito F. Extended endoscopic endonasal transsphenoidal approach for the removal of suprasellar tumors: part 2. Neurosurgery. 2007;60(1):46–58; discussion −9.
15. Cavallo LM, de Divitiis O, Aydin S, Messina A, Esposito F, Iaconetta G, et al. Extended endoscopic endonasal transsphenoidal approach to the suprasellar area: anatomic considerations—part 1. Neurosurgery. 2008;62(6 Suppl 3):1202–12.
16. Iacoangeli M, Colasanti R, Esposito D, Di Rienzo A, di Somma L, Dobran M, et al. Supraorbital subfrontal trans-laminar endoscope-assisted approach for tumors of the posterior third ventricle. Acta Neurochir. 2017;159(4):645–54.
17. Martinez-Perez R, Albonette-Felicio T, Hardesty DA, Shahein M, Carrau RL, Prevedello DM. The endoscopic supraorbital translaminar approach: a technical note. Acta Neurochir. 2021;163(3):635–41.
18. Spena G, Fasel J, Tribolet N, Radovanovic I. Subfrontal endoscopic fenestration of lamina terminalis: an anatomical study. Minim Invasive Neurosurg. 2008;51(6):319–23.
19. Ahmed SI, Javed G, Laghari AA, Bareeqa SB, Aziz K, Khan M, et al. Third ventricular tumors: a comprehensive literature review. Cureus. 2018;10(10):e3417.
20. Arnaout MM, Luzzi S, Galzio R, Aziz K. Supraorbital keyhole approach: pure endoscopic and endoscope-assisted perspective. Clin Neurol Neurosurg. 2020;189:105623.

Chapter 14
Transorbital Route to Intracranial Space

Alberto Di Somma, Marta Codes, Giulia Guizzardi, Alejandra Mosteiro, Roberto Tafuto, Abel Ferres, Jessica Matas, Alberto Prats-Galino, Joaquim Enseñat, and Luigi Maria Cavallo

A. Di Somma
Department of Neurological Surgery, Institut Clínic de Neurociències (ICN), Hospital Clínic de Barcelona, Universidad de Barcelona, Barcelona, Spain

Laboratory of Surgical Neuroanatomy, Universitat de Barcelona, Barcelona, Spain

Institut d'Investigacions Biomèdiques August Pi i Sunyer (IDIBAPS), Barcelona, Spain

M. Codes · A. Mosteiro · A. Ferres
Department of Neurological Surgery, Institut Clínic de Neurociències (ICN), Hospital Clínic de Barcelona, Universidad de Barcelona, Barcelona, Spain

G. Guizzardi
Department of Neurological Surgery, Institut Clínic de Neurociències (ICN), Hospital Clínic de Barcelona, Universidad de Barcelona, Barcelona, Spain

Laboratory of Surgical Neuroanatomy, Universitat de Barcelona, Barcelona, Spain

R. Tafuto · L. M. Cavallo (✉)
Division of Neurosurgery, Department of Neuroscience and Reproductive and Odontostomatological Sciences, Università degli Studi di Napoli "Federico II", Naples, Italy

J. Matas
Department of Ophthalmology, Hospital Clínic de Barcelona, Universidad de Barcelona, Barcelona, Spain

A. Prats-Galino
Laboratory of Surgical Neuroanatomy, Universitat de Barcelona, Barcelona, Spain

Institut d'Investigacions Biomèdiques August Pi i Sunyer (IDIBAPS), Barcelona, Spain

J. Enseñat
Department of Neurological Surgery, Institut Clínic de Neurociències (ICN), Hospital Clínic de Barcelona, Universidad de Barcelona, Barcelona, Spain

Institut d'Investigacions Biomèdiques August Pi i Sunyer (IDIBAPS), Barcelona, Spain

© The Author(s), under exclusive license to Springer Nature Switzerland AG 2024
W. A. Azab (ed.), *Endoscope-controlled Transcranial Surgery*, Advances and Technical Standards in Neurosurgery 52,
https://doi.org/10.1007/978-3-031-61925-0_14

14.1 Introduction and History

Although transorbital surgery has recently gained notoriety, the use of this avenue was already pervasive throughout the twentieth century by multiple disciplines for both clinical and experimental purposes [1–4].

The evolution of this technique has been intriguing, going from being a medically and ethically controversial surgical procedure to becoming an attractive route for selected skull base pathologies. This progression reflects the impact of microsurgery, the advancement of technology (especially in visualization), and the importance of a multidisciplinary approach.

Before explaining the transorbital approach and its intracranial objectives, a brief historical excursus is conferred.

14.1.1 Past History of the Transorbital Route to the Intracranial Space

The evolution of ophthalmic surgery toward more expansive procedures was the beginning of transorbital surgery in the late 1800s [5]. Indeed, Hermann Knapp, an ophthalmologist, described the anterior orbitotomy for the first time in 1874 for the treatment of optic sheath carcinoma through a superior eyelid/eyebrow or transconjunctival/inferior eyelid incision [5]. More than 70 years later, this technique gained popularity because of its use by William Benedict to resect lesions of the anterior two-thirds of the orbit [6].

At the same time, the neurosurgical community was pushing the boundaries of interconnected cranial and orbital pathology looking for improved routes with greater exposure involving the posterior orbit. In 1886, Rudolf Krönlein described the lateral orbitotomy for excision of orbital dermoid cysts, used for the treatment of retrobulbar tumors, with no evidence of this technique being used for pathologies involving intracranial structures [7].

In 1922, Walter Dandy proposed that orbital tumors were best dealt with a transcranial approach, claiming superiority over transorbital surgery, in terms of localization, surgical exposure, and operative technique [8, 9]. Conversely, Raynold Berke continued to advocate for the ophthalmological transorbital approach [10].

Given the contradictory opinions between Berke and Dandy, the transorbital approach was limited to eye-related pathologies for the following years, until new surgical techniques gave it the focus of attention once again.

Amarro Fiamberti introduced the original transorbital prefrontal lobotomy in 1937 as a minimally invasive procedure for the treatment of schizophrenia and psychosis as an alternative to electroconvulsive shock therapy [11]. Walter Freeman and James Watts followed the study of leucotomy surgery by the transorbital approach, becoming widely accepted within the psychiatric community [12, 13].

However, after a few years, the paucity of evidence to support the intervention among the psychosocial and ethical issues associated with the procedure led to expulsion of Freeman and the transorbital approach from practice. All of this made a huge new setback for the transorbital approach.

In 1951, Toyoji Wada and Masateru Toyota described the transorbital route for a ventricular access to perform pneumoventriculography [14]. Given the limited results of pneumoventriculography, the technique never gained prestige or acceptance.

The development of the microscope and micro instrumentation allowed minimally invasive techniques with greater intracranial exposure addressing the new concerns like minimizing retraction injuries, incision sites, cosmetic defects, and surgical recovery time.

As the microscopic technique developed, so did the neurosurgical skull base approaches. The incorporation of the orbit was necessary for the expansion of those approaches, gaining a better visualization of the anterior and middle fossa.

In 1982, Jane and coworkers described the supraorbital approach [15]. A few years later in 1986, Akira Hakuba developed the orbitozygomatic infratemporal approach, incorporating Krönlein's lateral orbital osteotomy with the classical frontotemporal craniotomy [16]. This extended craniotomy allowed the management of intracranial lesions in parasellar region and interpeduncular fossa, including medial-third sphenoid wing meningiomas, petroclival meningiomas, trigeminal neuromas, and basilar tip aneurisms.

From that time on, the fusion of orbitotomy and craniotomy for the approach of the skull base was a regular practice.

14.1.2 The Endoscope in Transorbital Surgery

The idea of endoscopic assistance revolutionized the intracranial surgical field. It emerged from the need to obtain appropriate illumination, magnification, and visualization to control the structures of the field in small surgical corridors.

Gerard Guiot, in 1963, first published a neurosurgical trial of skull base endoscopy [17]. Regarding the first endoscopic-assisted orbital surgery, it was performed by John Norris and Gilbert Cleasby in 1981, with the aim of removing foreign bodies and to biopsy orbital tumors [18]. This confirmed that the retraction of the eyeball was possible and allowed direct access to anterior and middle cranial fossa.

Early collaboration between otolaryngologists and neurosurgeons using cranial endoscopy allowed the development of endonasal endoscopic surgery with the aim of successfully reaching anatomical targets previously considered problematic through the open transcranial approach.

In this way a new subspecialty was created, endoscopic skull base surgery, giving rise to new endonasal approaches in the early 2000s. Endonasal surgery became popular allowing great advances in skull base surgery [19–22].

In this novel and active scenario, the role of transorbital endoscopic surgery arose as a complementary route to the highly developed endonasal approach, in order to overcome its anatomical limitations for skull base lesions that extend laterally or that encompass broader intracranial parameters.

Kris Moe, in 2007, first introduced the concept of transorbital neuroendoscopic surgery (TONES), at the 91st Annual Meeting of the Pacific Coast Oto-Ophthalmological Society, later published in *Neurosurgery* [23]. The first procedures with this technique were performed for anterior cranial fossa pathologies, such as CSF leaks, optic nerve decompression, skull base fracture repair, and skull base tumor removal.

From this turning point, the number of publications and citations related to the transorbital approach has been increasing, from anatomical articles to the publication of the different case series [24–36].

The indications for TONES have also been expanding, and the surgical technique has been perfected, allowing the use of this corridor to address much more extensive pathologies of the skull base localized in the anterior, middle, and even posterior cerebral fossa [37–39].

The importance of a multi-perspective view of the intracranial spaces has also led to the emergence of combined approaches (transorbital and transnasal), initially described by Dallan and coworkers in 2015 [40, 41].

Hence, after this brief historical *excursus*, the transorbital approach will be explained below, from its initial cutaneous phase to the different intracranial areas accessible through this corridor.

14.2　Skin Incisions for Transorbital Approach

The transorbital endoscopic approaches involve various surgical pathways.

A thorough understanding of the anatomy of the eyelid is essential in order to avoid function compromise of the structures involved.

Different skin incisions can be performed in order to use the orbit cavity as a gate to the skull base, in particular, a superior eyelid crease (SLC), precaruncular approach (PC), lateral retrocanthal (LRC) approach, and preseptal lower eyelid (PS) skin incision. SLC is the only approach performed through the skin of the upper eyelid, while the others are carried out behind the palpebral structures (PC, PS, and LRC). Since SLC is the most widely used technique, and also the one used in our department, we will focus on describing this technique below [23, 42, 43].

14.2.1　Superior Eyelid Crease

The skin incision is made in the crease of the upper eyelid or supratarsal fold, as done in an upper eyelid blepharoplasty. It is usually planned at 8–10 mm from the horizontal palpebral fissure in females and 6–8 mm in males. Dissection is continued through the orbicularis oculi muscle at the junction between the pre-tarsal and preseptal plane, to subsequently lift a skin-muscle flap in a superolateral direction toward the lateral orbital rim. Stitches can be placed in order to keep in place firm the skin-muscle flap.

The identification of the orbital septum is crucial in order to avoid dissecting into the pre-levador fat pad which might cause a lesion of the levator aponeurosis resulting in ptosis.

After identifying the orbital rim, the periosteum is then incised at the inferior border, and the dissection is further progressed in a surgical plane between the periosteum and the periorbita.

At this point, the inferior orbital fissure (IOF) can be identified, being the first and most important landmark in achieving adequate orientation for further dissection.

The zygomaticofacial and zygomaticotemporal branches of the maxillary nerve entering the zygomatico-orbital foramina can also be identified on the orbital surface of the zygomatic bone, together with corresponding arteries, that can be spared. These are useful landmarks, even if not constant, in order to identify the IOF [44].

A malleable retractor can be introduced to slightly separate orbital contents medially, obtaining enough space to insert the endoscope and proceed with the creation of adequate working space (Fig. 14.1).

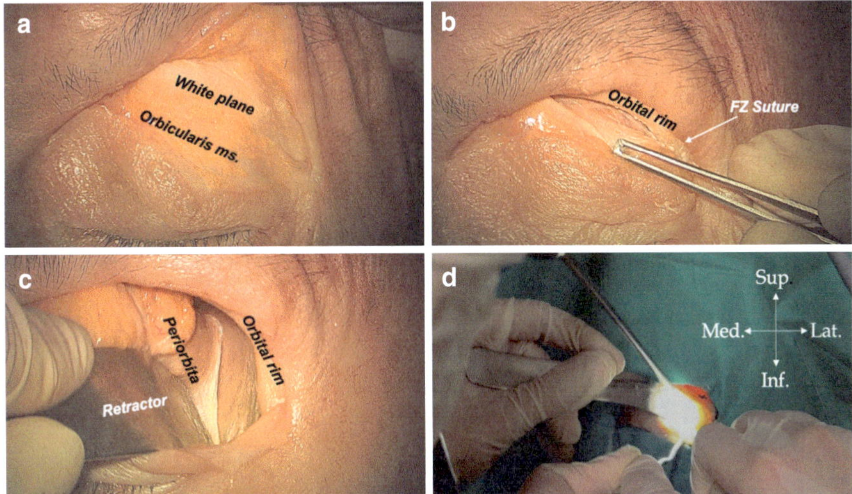

Fig. 14.1 **Anatomic dissection of left transorbital approach showing the skin phase.** A superior eyelid skin incision is performed at 8 mm from the palpebral fissure. (**a, b**) The palpebral portion of the orbicularis oculi muscle is then incised, and the fibers are spared laterally until visualization of the superolateral orbital rim. (**c**) Periosteum is incised in order to create the surgical space between the Periorbita medially and the orbital rim laterally. (**d**) Hand placement in the transorbital endoscopic approach
Orbicularis ms. Orbicularis oculi muscle; white plane (superior tarsus, orbital septum, and levator palpebrae muscle tendon); *FZ suture* Frontozygomatic suture, *Sup* Superior, *Inf* Inferior, *Med* Medial, *Lat* Lateral

14.3 Working Space: Creating Room for Surgery

Once the skin phase has been carried out, enough space must be created within the orbital cavity to allow working with the endoscope and thus be able to reach the target areas to treat the corresponding pathologies [42].

The placement of a malleable retractor in order to separate the orbital contents medially from the posterolateral wall of the orbit allows creating room for further dissection and also protecting the periorbita. The superior and inferior orbital fissures represent the limit of medial mobilization of the orbital contents [45].

At this point, the endoscope must be inserted to obtain better visualization of the anteriorly mentioned structures such as the orbital fissures, being paramount for adequate orientation.

The initial step to create adequate exposure and gain appropriate maneuverability is the drilling of the body of the zygoma. The craniectomy should start drilling the orbital surface of the body of the zygoma in the lateral wall of the orbit until the temporalis deep fascia is exposed. Subsequently, the ventral and vertical aspects of the greater sphenoid wing should also be drilled until the temporal dura mater is seen.

As more lateral space is created, the retractor should follow the long axis of the IOF, to allow gentle medialization and protection of the periorbita. The greater sphenoid wing is drilled until a "V" shape is identified. The vertex of this "V" shape points at the IOF, the base is represented by the lesser sphenoid wing, medially SOF, and periorbita can be found, while laterally temporal muscle/fascia can be observed. The central portion of the "V" corresponds to the temporal dura, while superiorly the frontal dura can be shown when further drilling is performed (Fig. 14.2).

Removal of the orbital rim has also been described as an option that allows further surgical space [46].

From this point, the procedure is tailored according to the targeted area and the underlying pathology.

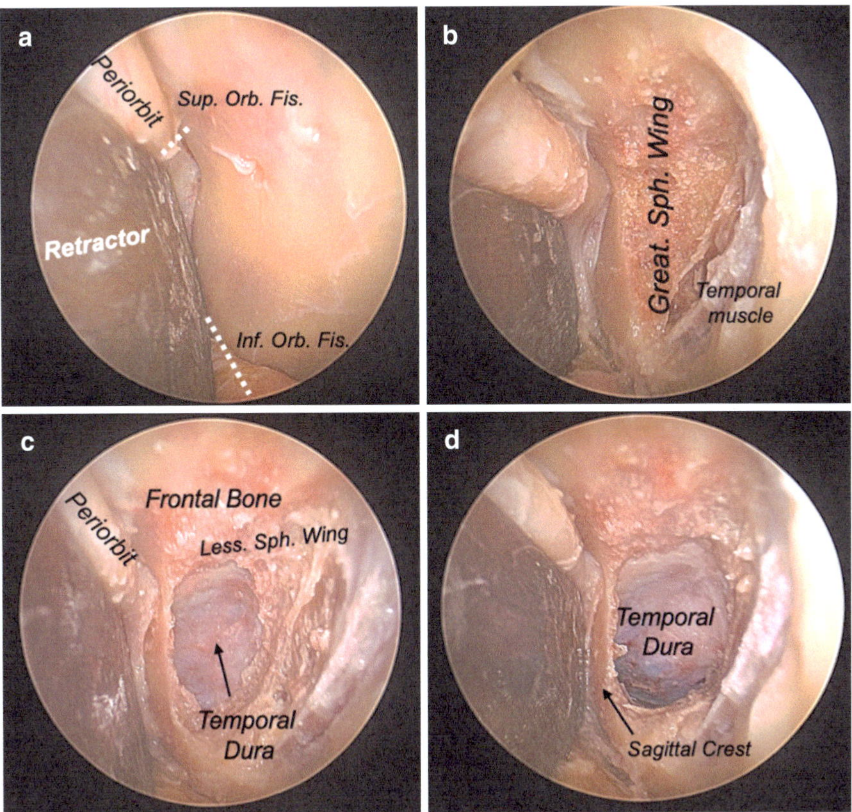

Fig. 14.2 Anatomic dissection of left transorbital approach showing the working space phase (**a**) Placement of malleable retractor in order to separate the orbital contents medially from the posterolateral wall of the orbit until visualization of superior and inferior orbital fissures. (**b**) Drilling of the orbital surface of the body of the zygoma until the temporalis deep fascia is exposed. (**c**) Drilling of the great sphenoid wing until the temporal dura mater is seen. (**d**) Visualization of the sagittal crest

Sup.Orb.Fis Superior orbital fissure, *Inf.Orb.Fis* Inferior orbital fissure, *Great.Sph.Wing* Greater sphenoid wing, *Less. Sph. Wing* Lesser sphenoid wing

14.4 Transorbital Bone Pillars and Intracranial Targets

From a didactic perspective, four main bone structures of the lateral skull base can be described related to the transorbital avenue that led to different intracranial areas. These are anterior clinoid and lesser sphenoid wing, sagittal crest, middle fossa floor, and petrous apex (Fig. 14.3). Each of them will be defined in the following sections.

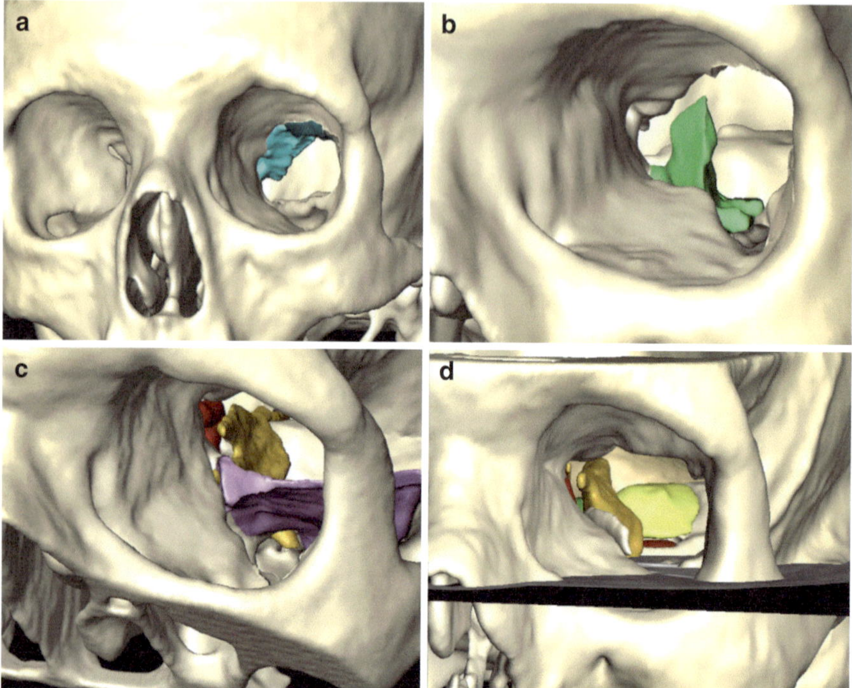

Fig. 14.3 Amira software three-dimensional reconstruction of the four bone targets described in the transorbital approach
Reconstruction of the four bone targets in the transorbital endoscopic approach described in the chapter from a didactic perspective. (**a**) Lesser sphenoid wing; (**b**) sagittal crest; (**c**) middle fossa floor (purple) with gasserian ganglion (yellow) and internal carotid artery (red); (**d**), petrous apex (yellow)

14.4.1 Anterior Clinoid and Lesser Sphenoid Wing: Optocarotid Region and Frontal Lobe, Sylvian Cistern, and Middle Cerebral Artery

Lesser sphenoid wing (LSW) and anterior clinoid (AC) will be discussed as one target since the latter represents the medial end of the LSW. After the initial phase of creating a good working space, the dura mater of both the temporal pole and frontal lobe has to be exposed.

Once this exposure is achieved, LSW must be drilled from lateral to medial; afterward, a dissector can be placed both superiorly and inferiorly in order to detach the dura from the LSW. Hence, with Kerrison rongeur removal of the LSW can be obtained. When dissection proceeds more medially, the identification of a strong dural band named the meningo-orbital band (MOB) in the lateral edge of SOF (its superolateral margin) is mandatory. This dural band joins the periosteal layer of the frontotemporal basal dura mater to the Periorbita and makes inferior medial retraction of the orbital content difficult, so it must be dissected in order to improve the field of view, especially in the optocarotid region. Drilling the upper and lateral edge of the SOF enables to peel off the MOB, gaining the desired working room. However, in order to achieve adequate exposure of the MOB also, the most superior part of the sagittal crest should be removed (see next paragraph).

Blunt dissection can then be continued medially through the SOF roof in a horizontal plane allowing the inferior displacement of the orbit content.

Once this point of the dissection has been reached, it is possible to identify the triangular-shaped area of the anterior clinoid process (ACP) base on the posterior wall projecting posteriorly from the medial end of the LSW.

The removal of the ACP is a relevant surgical procedure for the access and management of neurovascular and tumoral pathology involving the central skull base. It still remains a significant challenge due to the proximity of neurovascular structures and variability of anatomic features in the surrounding area [47].

The ACP base is bounded by three anatomic sites of attachment delineated as follows: laterally, the bone overlying the upper border of the superior orbital fissure and, medially, existing two roots—the anterior root extending from the upper wall of the optic canal to the lesser sphenoid wing forming the roof of the optic canal and the posterior root formed by the floor of the optic canal extending toward the medial part of the superior orbital fissure to form the optic strut [31]. The optic strut is a bony pillar extending lateromedially from the inferior surface of the anterior clinoid process to the lateral wall of the sphenoid body, which forms the floor of the optic canal, dividing it from the superior orbital fissure.

The lines connecting each landmark define the ACP triangular base delimited laterally by the SOF and medially by the roof of the optic canal.

After MOB dissection and protection of the orbital content shifting it inferomedially, the drilling and dissection can proceed in order to expose the anterior clinoid and the optic canal. The drilling continues medially through the SOF roof in a horizontal plane until correct visualization and unroofing of the optic canal, to later proceed deeply and posteriorly toward the center of the ACP base until careful detachment from the surrounding dura and its complete removal. The optic nerve (located superomedial to ACP) and the oculomotor nerve (located inferolateral to ACP) can be dissected from ACP under direct visualization [47]. However, because the internal carotid artery is hidden by the ACP and the optic strut, the dissection of the dura at this point from the posterior surface of the ACP has to be done extremely carefully [31].

This dissection allows the removal of ACP extradurally by finally twisting gently the posterior root or optic strut or progressive drilling. The limits of the obtained pyramidal dural pocket are as follows: laterally, the dura covering the superior surface of LSW; superiorly, the dura covering the superior surface of the LSW and attaching to the lateral edge of the planum sphenoidale; medially, at the unroofed optic nerve with the falciform ligament covering its proximal part; and inferiorly, the dural boundary at the floor of the optic canal, the anterior part of the distal dural ring of the internal carotid artery [47].

The opening of the dura mater and the subsequent intracranial exploration of this area shows the optocarotid region as well as the intracranial portion of the optic nerve running posteriorly and medially to form the optic chiasm. The clinoid portion of the internal carotid artery can also be seen, covered by a dural layer at the posterior surface of OS. The clinoid portion of the internal carotid artery is limited by two leaflets of dura mater emerging from the inferior and superior surfaces of the anterior clinoid process, the proximal and distal dural ring, respectively.

On the other hand, opening the dura superiorly to the optocarotid region discovers the fronto-basal lobe as well as the olfactory tract.

Removal of the LSW (and ACP, if most medial vascular exposure is needed) also allows the exposure of the Sylvian fissure. Dural incision at this location and opening the Sylvian cistern can be performed until correct visualization of superficial middle cerebral artery branches such as the anterior temporal arteries which guide toward the main trunk of the sphenoidal segment (M1) of the middle cerebral artery. Dissection can be carried out medially toward the carotid cistern, with exposure of the carotid bifurcation as well as the site of origin of the middle cerebral artery and the anterior cerebral artery. The medial lenticulostriate branches originate from the superior-posterior wall of the M1 and are also visible during its course toward the anterior perforated substance. Lateral dissection, on the other hand, exposes the MCA bifurcation, the insular segment (M2), and its superior and inferior trunks and lateral lenticulostriate branches [48] (Fig. 14.4).

14.4.2   Sagittal Crest: Cavernous Sinus and Temporal Lobe

The novel described sagittal crest is a relevant bone structure that guides the transorbital dissection to the cavernous sinus area and to the temporal lobe. Once the superior and inferior orbital fissures are reached, the anterior portion of the greater wing of the sphenoid is exposed, as previously mentioned.

The medial edge of the greater wing of the sphenoid bone (GSW) must then be removed in a superolateral to inferomedial direction toward the lateral margin of the superior orbital fissure. After this initial drilling, the sagittal crest is identified which is an important landmark, represented by a triangular-shaped bony ridge constituted of the residual medial portion of the GSW, that constantly remains between the temporal dura medially, the periorbita laterally, and the foramen rotundum cranially [49]. This surgical landmark is created artificially during the approach per progressive drilling of the GSW.

The complete resection of this key landmark is mandatory in order to guide the next steps, normally accomplished by drilling the apical portion of the crest and then the base until the anterior aspect of foramen rotundum. The removal of this structure allows visualization and identification of the dura mater covering the temporal pole and the meningo-orbital band (MOB) [49].

Removal of the sagittal crest (SC) permits the dissection with an interdural peeling of the lateral wall of the cavernous sinus. The interdural space of the lateral wall of the cavernous sinus is composed of two dural layers: the outer layer (dura propria or meningeal dura) and the inner layer (true cavernous membrane). The inner layer is composed of the epineurium of cranial nerves and surrounding connective tissue

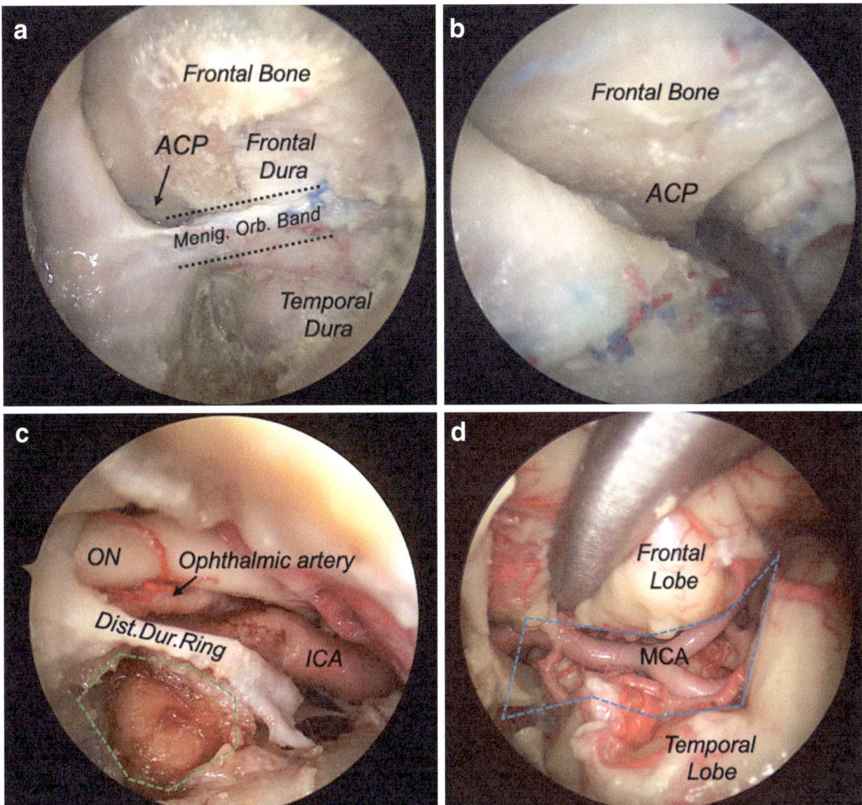

Fig. 14.4 Anatomic dissection of left transorbital approach showing the anterior clinoid process and lesser sphenoid wing bone targets along with the related intracranial areas (optocarotid region, frontal lobe, Sylvian cistern, and middle cerebral artery)
(**a**) Drilling of the upper and lateral portion of the lesser sphenoid wing to expose the base of the anterior clinoid process. (**b**) Visualization of the anterior clinoid process. (**c**) Optocarotid region from an orbital perspective. (**d**) Sylvian cistern with the middle cerebral artery
Mening.Orb.Band Meningo-orbital band, *ACP* Anterior clinoid process, *ON* Optical nerve, *ICA* Internal carotid artery, *Dist.Dur.Ring* Distal dural ring, *MCA* Middle cerebral artery. Green dotted line, anterior clinoid process removed exposing the internal carotid artery. Blue dotted line, Sylvian cistern

[50]. The identification of the sagittal crest represents the key anatomic point to split both layers and find a clear interdural plane [49].

This interdural surgical plane had already been described through a frontotemporal craniotomy [51].

Key structures can be observed after this dissection: oculomotor nerve, trochlear nerve, first two branches of the trigeminal nerve up to the gasserian ganglion, distal/plexiform portion of the trigeminal root posteriorly, and the mandibular branch of the trigeminal nerve and the middle meningeal artery laterally.

Additionally, MOB release permits the gentle and partial displacement of the medial part of the temporal lobe in an extradural plane [50].

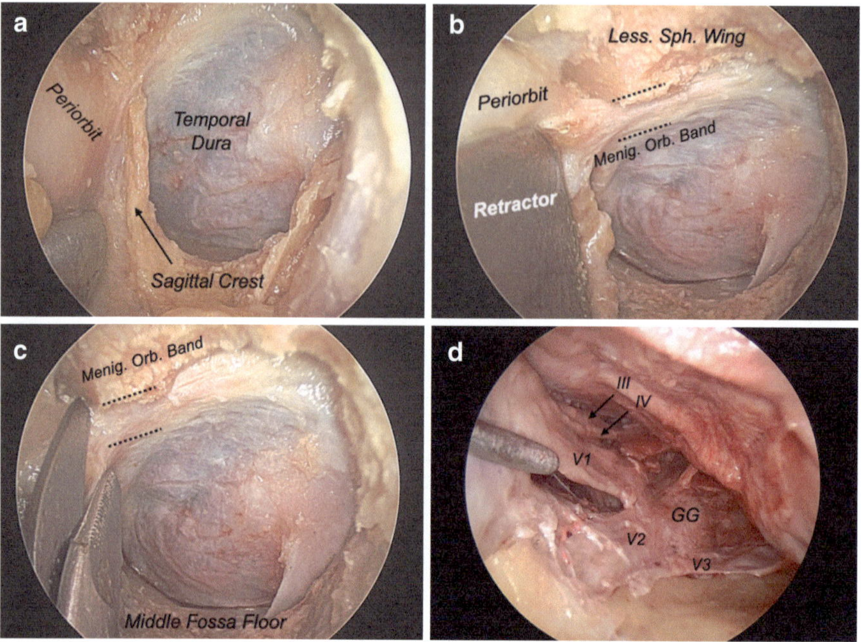

Fig. 14.5 Anatomic dissection of left transorbital approach showing the sagittal crest bone target along with the cavernous sinus interdural peeling
(**a**) Identification and drilling of the sagittal crest. (**b**, **c**) Exposition and cutting of the meningo-orbital band. (**d**) Exposure of the lateral wall of the cavernous sinus with an interdural dissection
Less. Sph. Wing Lesser sphenoid wing, *Mening.Orb.Band* Meningo-orbital band, *GG* Gasserian ganglion

The removal of the sagittal crest also improves the exposure of the dura mater covering the temporal pole, which can be opened in order to explore the temporal lobe and reach the temporomesial regions up to the temporal horn of the lateral ventricle. During intradural exposure of the temporal lobe, the Sylvian veins represent the most superior limit of the temporal exposure (Fig. 14.5).

14.4.3 Middle Fossa Floor: Infratemporal Fossa

The middle fossa floor is the third transorbital bone pillar that can be described. Before the middle fossa floor can be accessed, adequate exposure should be performed in order to gain maneuverability, by drilling the greater sphenoid until the temporal dura mater is seen.

The temporal lobe can then be elevated extradurally with a retractor until proper visualization of the middle meningeal artery exiting the spinous foramen, which must be cut to allow proper exposure of the entire floor of the middle cranial fossa.

The floor is composed of the horizontal portion of the greater sphenoid wing, the squama temporalis, and the petrous segment of the temporal bone. It has an oblique direction and inclines slightly from posterior to anterior. Once the entire floor of the middle cranial fossa has been exposed, the midsubtemporal ridge can be identified as a bony prominence that has to be drilled in order to obtain a flat middle fossa floor and proceed further with the dissection. This structure has been recently renamed as "crista ovale" [52].

The medial part corresponds to the parasellar area, where the limit for safe bone resection was represented by the lateral wall of the cavernous sinus. All three divisions of the trigeminal nerve should be visualized as well as the gasserian ganglion.

The lateral part is formed by the lateral aspect of the GSW and the squama temporalis, where the boundary for safe drilling was the limit of the squama temporalis.

The other safe limits for bone resection were the following: lateral pterygoid muscle covering the infratemporal fossa inferiorly; lesser sphenoid wing superiorly; greater superficial petrosal nerve, the petrous portion of the carotid artery, and the anterior surface of the petrous segment of the temporal bone posteriorly; and limits in between the ventral and vertical portion of the greater sphenoid wing anteriorly.

The removal of the middle cranial fossa floor respecting the anatomic boundaries described makes the communication of the middle fossa with the infratemporal fossa possible, allowing connections with other endoscopic approaches such as the endonasal and transmaxillary [37]. It also allows access to deep areas such as the clivus and the posterior cranial fossa through the transorbital route [53] (Fig. 14.6).

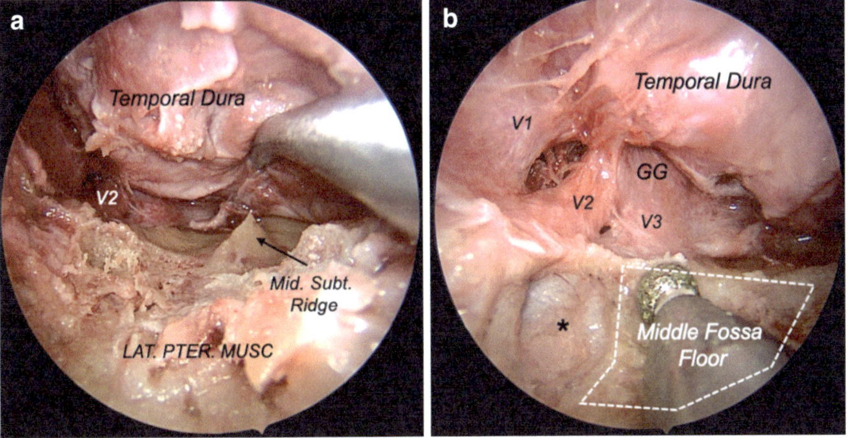

Fig. 14.6 Anatomic dissection of left transorbital approach showing the middle fossa floor bone target
(**a**) Extradural elevation of the temporal lobe with visualization of the middle fossa floor. (**b**) Drilling of the middle fossa floor to allow access to infratemporal fossa
Lat.Pter.Musc Lateral pterygoid muscle, *Mid.Subt.Ridge* Midsubtemporal ridge, *GG* Gasserian ganglion
* Sphenoid sinus mucosa

14.4.4 Petrous Apex: Internal Carotid Artery and Posterior Cranial Fossa

The petrous apex (PA) is the pyramid-shaped anteromedial part of the petrous part of the temporal bone, oriented obliquely in the skull base. It articulates with the posterior aspect of the GSW and occipital bones. PA remains one of the most challenging areas in skull base surgery because it is strictly related to critical neurovascular structure. The petrous apex is the deepest bone structure of the skull base that can be reached via a transorbital route, representing the fourth bone pillar of this approach. The removal of PA exposes the main neurovascular structures of the posterior fossa and allows complete description of the internal carotid artery. Accordingly, in this subparagraph, PA drilling will be explained as well as the course of ICA from a TO perspective along with all the neurovascular structures of the posterior fossa.

Once the temporal lobe is elevated extradurally and the middle cranial fossa floor is drilled and flattened as previously described, the following structures can be identified: Meckel's cave and third branch of the trigeminal nerve entering the foramen ovale and the middle meningeal artery exiting the spinous foramen. The middle meningeal artery is cut just lateral to the mandibular trigeminal branch entrance into the foramen ovale, uncovering the greater superficial petrosal nerve (GSPN). The localization of this nerve is a useful landmark for the position of the petrous region of the internal carotid artery (pICA) [54].

Trigeminal pore is then opened to obtain medial mobilization of the gasserian ganglion and the V3 branch, which allows correct visualization of the petrous apex and enough space to start its drilling [55].

The boundaries of safe bone removal are defined as follows [54]: inferiorly, the greater superficial petrosal nerve and the petrous internal carotid artery; medially, the lateral border of the mandibular division of the trigeminal nerve and the gasserian ganglion; laterally, the beginning of the inner ear, basal turn of the cochlea, and superior semicircular canal; and superiorly, the tentorium, the petrous ridge, and the superior petrosal sinus.

After recognition of key landmarks, the drilling of the petrous apex proceeds from medial to lateral direction, in order to recognize the internal acoustic canal and avoid damage to the basal cochlea and semicircular canals [56].

Dissection and subsequent resection of the petrous apex allow us to explore the course of the internal carotid artery (ICA) and the posterior cranial fossa, which are explained below [57].

A detailed knowledge of the course of the internal carotid artery (ICA) and its relationship with the main vulnerable neurovascular structures from the transorbital perspective is mandatory in order to avoid potential injuries.

As described earlier in this chapter, the transorbital approach can access the internal carotid artery from several points to access its different segments.

Once the final point of drilling is achieved and once all the previously named structures are identified, the ICA can be exposed in four different anatomical windows, named according to the corresponding triangle of the cavernous sinus.

The clinoidal window or Dolenc triangle is exposed after the anterior clinoidectomy and allows visualization of the clinoidal segment of the ICA, extended between the distal and proximal dural rings, corresponding to the C5 segment according to the ICA classification proposed by Bouthillier [58].

The infratrochlear window or Parkinson's triangle is exposed once the lateral wall of the cavernous sinus is visible, and the cavernous segment of the ICA is seen in the Parkinson's triangle. This triangle is delimited cranially by the lower margin of the trochlear nerve and caudally by the upper margin of the ophthalmic division of the trigeminal nerve. This ICA segment corresponds to the posterior bend of the cavernous ICA segment as established by Bouthillier [58]. Additional dissection of Parkinson's triangle allows access to the posteroinferior area of the cavernous sinus, where the lateral aspect of ICA becomes extensively visible in its horizontal, posterior bend, and posterior vertical portions. The origin of the meningo-hypophyseal trunk can also be recognized, among its arterial branches (tentorial, dorsal meningeal, and inferior hypophyseal arteries).

The anteromedial window or Mullan's triangle is exposed proceeding the dissection inferiorly between the ophthalmic nerve (V1) and the maxillary nerve (V2) once the cavernous sinus lateral wall is visible, in Mullan's triangle. This dissection exposes the distal portion of the cavernous segment of the ICA, corresponding to the C4 or cavernous segment described by Bouthillier, which is surrounded by sympathetic fiber bundles of carotid plexus [58]. The sixth cranial nerve running in posteroanterior direction can also be identified, after crossing Dorello's canal, underneath the petrosphenoidal ligament (Gruber's ligament) and entering the cavernous sinus.

The petrous window or Kawase's triangle is exposed after the drilling of the PA. The intrapetrous course of the ICA is referred to the segment in which the artery pierces the carotid foramen in exocranial surface of the petrous bone, passes within the carotid canal, crosses the foramen lacerum, and finally enters the cavernous sinus. This segment corresponds to C2 (petrous) and C3 (lacerum) segments described by Bouthillier [58]. From the transorbital perspective, it can be displayed within Kawase's triangle, delimited by the greater petrosal nerve, the lateral border of the mandibular nerve, and the arcuate eminence.

The extradural anterior petrosectomy also allows us to explore the posterior cranial fossa as mentioned above. The opening of the dura mater at this location permits the exploration of the following intradural spaces [57].

The cerebellopontine angle structures can be exposed through this approach. The anterolateral portion of the pons is identified in the center of the surgical field, with the petrous surface of the cerebellum more posterior.

The neural structures exposed by this approach are the origin of the trigeminal nerve, located medially, and the facial and vestibulocochlear nerves, located laterally. Regarding the important vascular structures in this area, the superior petrosal vein draining the superior petrosal sinus, as well as the AICA and labyrinthine arteries, can also be identified.

The middle incisural space located between the midbrain and tentorial edge can also be exposed. This incisural space opens upward into the ambient and crural cisterns and extends inferiorly into the anterior part of the cerebello-mesencephalic fissure.

If the superior petrosal sinus is ligated and the tentorium is elevated and cut, the dissection can proceed in a superior direction in order to reach this area. The antero-lateral portion of the mesencephalon is visualized at the center of the surgical field, surrounded by the superior cerebellar artery (SCA). If the dissection is continued medially, the oculomotor nerve at its cisternal segment can be identified, arising from the pontomesencephalic sulcus. More laterally, the trochlear nerve can be identified in the ambiens division of its cisternal segment, as it emerges from the dorsal brain stem and turns around the mesencephalon in close relation with the superior cerebellar artery and the free edge of the tentorium.

The ventral brain stem space is hardly accessible continuing the dissection, only by means of an angulated lens. The abducens nerve can be appreciated entering the cavernous sinus from Dorello's canal. The basilar trunk at the midline can also be identified, giving origin to the anterior inferior cerebellar artery (Fig. 14.7).

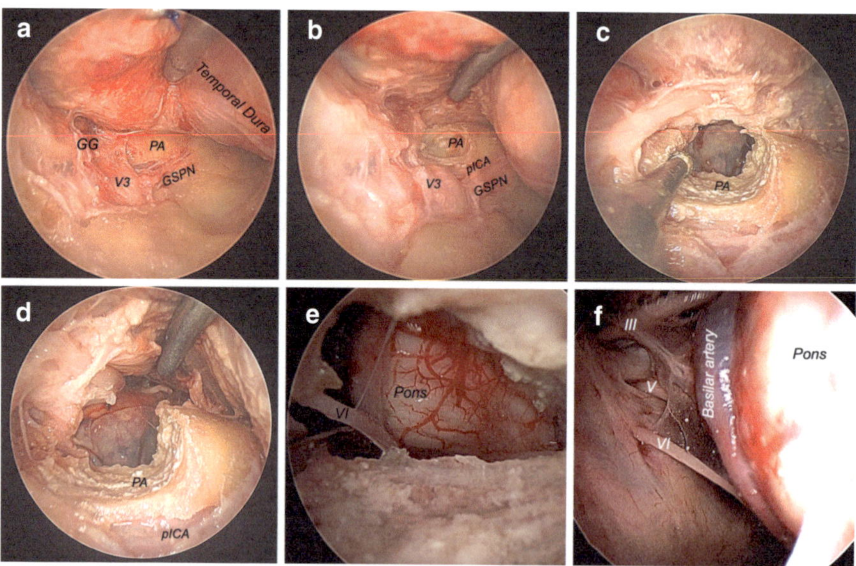

Fig. 14.7 Anatomic dissection of left transorbital approach showing the petrous apex bone target along with the posterior cranial
(**a**) Exposure of the petrous apex via the transorbital window and identification of the main anatomic boundaries. (**b**–**d**) Drilling of the petrous apex allowing the visualization of the posterior cranial fossa. (**e**, **f**) Posterior cranial fossa
GG Gasserian ganglion, *PA* Petrous apex, *GSPN* Greater superficial petrosal nerve, *pICA* Petrous internal carotid artery

14.5   Case Example

A 69-year-old man complaining of memory deficits and cognitive impairment was diagnosed with a left middle fossa/sphenoid wing meningioma (Fig. 14.8).

Accordingly, we proposed surgical treatment of the lesion via an endoscopic superior eyelid transorbital approach. Upon admission to our center for surgery, neurological examination showed no other deficits. Detailed preoperative 3D analysis has been performed as routine (Fig. 14.9).

The patient was placed supine under general anesthesia, with the head slightly elevated and fixed with the Mayfield head-holder. A protective antibiotic ointment was placed in both eyes. An endoscopic superior eyelid transorbital approach was performed; the lateral orbital rim was removed in this case. Proper exposure of the tumor was obtained; debulking, dissection, and satisfactory removal were obtained (Fig. 14.10).

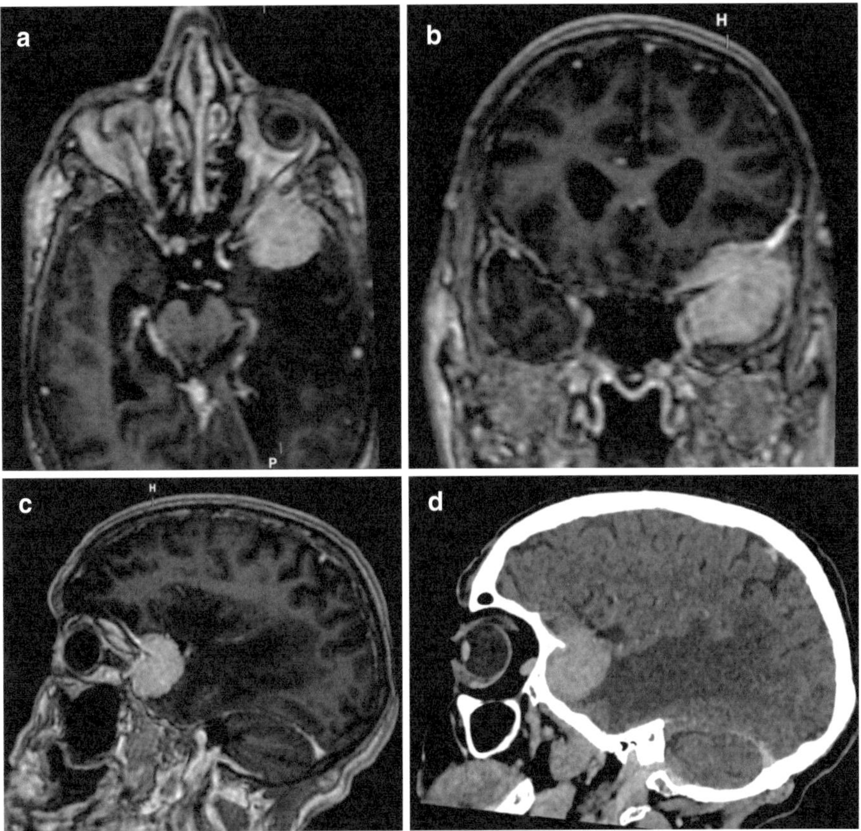

Fig. 14.8 Preoperative images of a middle fossa/sphenoid wing meningioma treated via a transorbital approach
(**a–c**) Axial, coronal, and sagittal MRI preoperative scan. (**d**) Sagittal CT scan

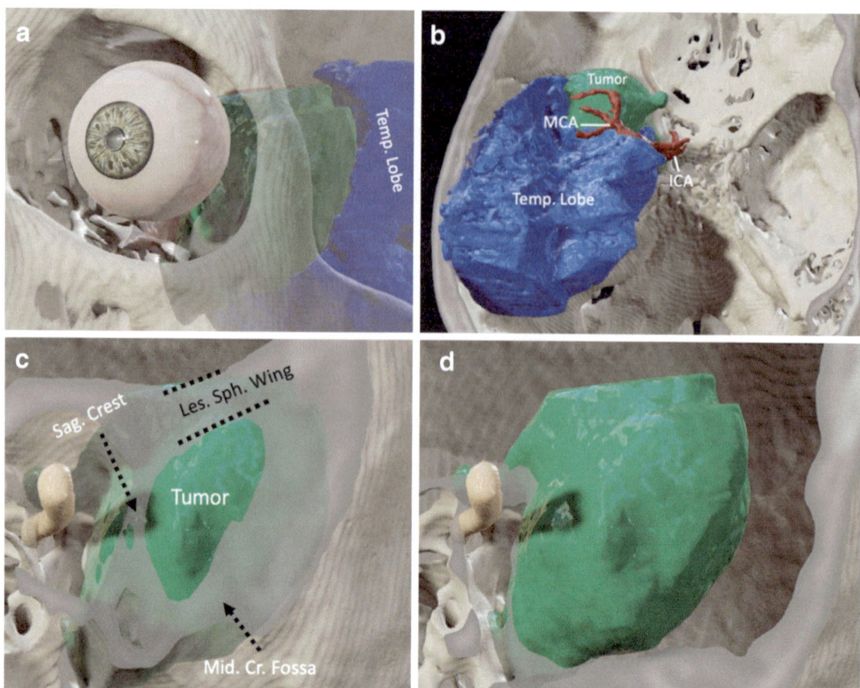

Fig. 14.9 Dedicated preoperative planning of the surgical case (**a–d**)
MCA Middle cerebral artery, *ICA* Internal carotid artery

The last part of the surgical procedure is the reconstruction of the osteodural skull base defect. Multilayer reconstruction with autologous materials is the technique of choice in our Skull Base Unit. Autologous fat graft was used to fill the surgical corridor, and it was fixed with fibrin glue. The lateral orbital rim was replaced. Finally, the superior eyelid skin approach was closed in different layers.

The postoperative period was favorable. Clinically, there was no new neurological deficit, with preserved eye movements and vision in his left eye. Post-op MRI was not performed for a renal insufficiency; however postoperative CT showed no complications with an adequate resection of the described lesion (Fig. 14.11).

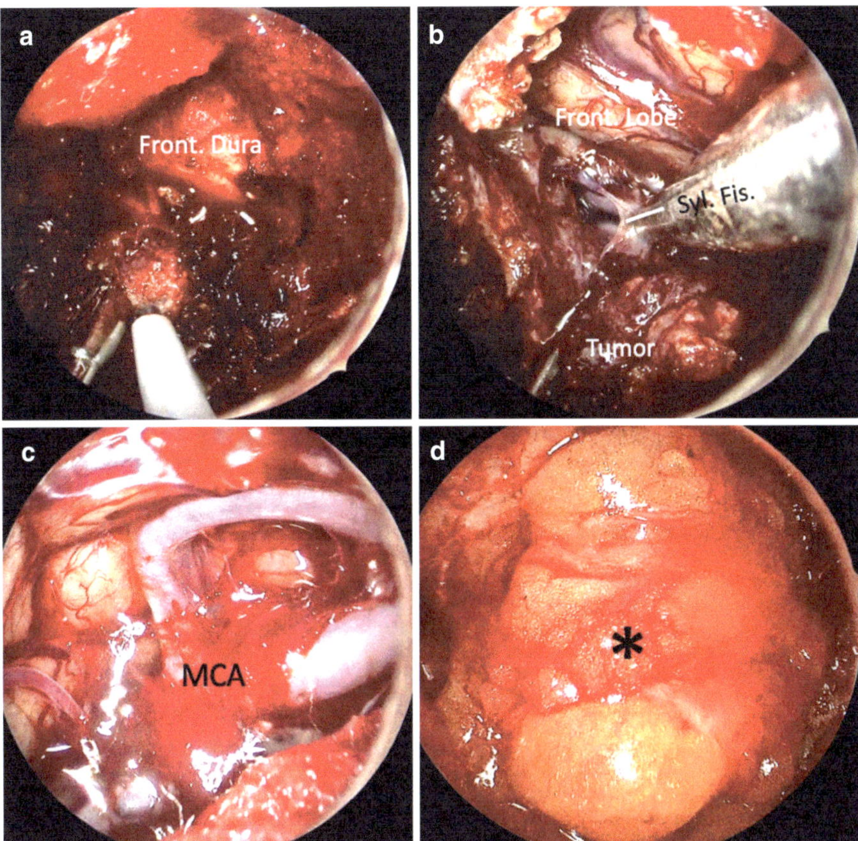

Fig. 14.10 Endoscopic superior eyelid transorbital surgery for a middle fossa/sphenoid wing meningioma
(**a–d**) Surgical steps of the removal of the meningioma *MCA* Middle cerebral artery, * Fat graft used for reconstruction

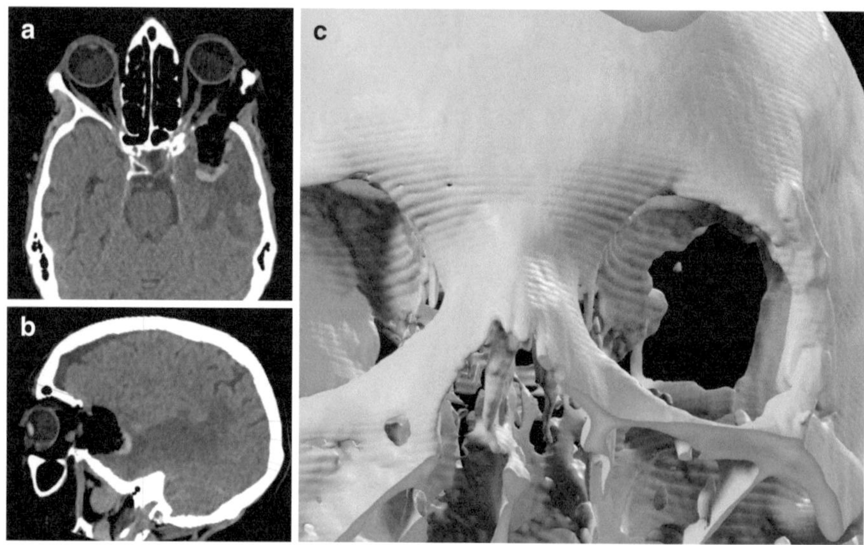

Fig. 14.11 Postoperative images of the surgical case
(**a**, **b**) Axial and sagittal CT scans of the surgical case showing no complications and adequate tumor removal. (**c**), 3D reconstruction demonstrating the bone removal obtained via the transorbital approach

14.6 Conclusions and Future Direction

The endoscopic transorbital approach has had a notorious evolution and has gained acceptance and popularity in recent years, proving to be an excellent route to access critical skull base regions. An extensive number of anatomical studies demonstrating its safeness and feasibility and the introduction of endoscopic assistance allowed its progressive growth leading to an increasing number of indications.

In this chapter, the anatomy of the transorbital approach in order to reach four described bone structures and multiple intracranial spaces has been described along with an illustrative case. It is our contention that this approach presents a valid and achievable minimally invasive option, either on its own or in conjunction with other surgical approaches, in order to reach pathologies in all the extent of the skull base.

The endoscopic transorbital approach requires a specific learning curve as well as a comprehensive understanding of neuroanatomy. Interdisciplinary cooperation among other specialists (ENT surgeons, ophthalmologists, and anesthesiologists) is mandatory to obtain satisfactory results.

References

1. Schwartz TH, et al. Endoscopic transorbital surgery: another leap of faith? World Neurosurg. 2022;159:54–5.
2. Kong DS, Moe KS. Editorial: endoscopic transorbital surgery for skull base tumors. Front Oncol. 2022;12:1042655.
3. Di Somma A, et al. Endoscopic transorbital surgery levels of difficulty. J Neurosurg. 2022:1–4.
4. Locatelli D, et al. Transorbital endoscopic approaches to the skull base: current concepts and future perspectives. J Neurosurg Sci. 2016;60(4):514–25.
5. Knapp H. A case of carcinoma of the outer sheath of the optic nerve, removed with preservation of the eyeball. Arch Ophthalmol Otol. 1874;4:323–54.
6. Benedict WL. Surgical treatment of tumors and cysts of the orbit. Am J Ophthalmol. 1949;Pt.1 32(6):763–73.
7. Krönlein RU. Zur Pathologie and operativen Behandlung der Dermoidcysten der Orbita. Beitr z Klin Chir Tubing. 1889;4:149–63.
8. Dandy WE. Prechiasmal intracranial tumors of the optic nerves. Am J Ophthalmol. 1922;5(3):169–88.
9. Dandy WE. Results following the transcranial operátive attack on orbital tumors. Arch Ophthalmol. 1941;25(3):191–216.
10. Berke RN. A modified Kronlein operation. AMA Arch Ophthalmol. 1954;51(5):609–32.
11. Fiamberti AM. Proposta di una tecnica operatoria modificata e semplificata per gli interventi alla Moniz sui lobi frontali in malati di mente. Raas Studi Psichiat. 1937;26:797.
12. Freeman W. Transorbital leucotomy. Lancet. 1948;2(6523):371–3.
13. Freeman W. Transorbital lobotomy in state mental hospitals. J Med Soc N J. 1954;51(4):148–50.
14. Wada T, Toyota M. Transorbital brain-ventricle puncture or a new method for pneumoventriculography. Tohoku J Exp Med. 1951;54(3):223–6.
15. Jane JA, et al. The supraorbital approach: technical note. Neurosurgery. 1982;11(4):537–42.
16. Hakuba A, Liu S, Nishimura S. The orbitozygomatic infratemporal approach: a new surgical technique. Surg Neurol. 1986;26(3):271–6.
17. Guiot J, et al. Intracranial endoscopic explorations. Presse Med. 1893;1963(71):1225–8.
18. Norris JL, Cleasby GW. Endoscopic orbital surgery. Am J Ophthalmol. 1981;91(2):249–52.
19. Kassam AB, et al. Endoscopic endonasal skull base surgery: analysis of complications in the authors' initial 800 patients. J Neurosurg. 2011;114(6):1544–68.
20. Cavallo LM, et al. The endoscopic endonasal approach for the management of craniopharyngiomas: a series of 103 patients. J Neurosurg. 2014;121(1):100–13.
21. Fraser JF, et al. Endoscopic endonasal transclival resection of chordomas: operative technique, clinical outcome, and review of the literature. J Neurosurg. 2010;112(5):1061–9.
22. Cavallo LM, et al. Endoscopic endonasal transsphenoidal surgery: history and evolution. World Neurosurg. 2019;127:686–94.
23. Moe KS, Bergeron CM, Ellenbogen RG. Transorbital neuroendoscopic surgery. Neurosurgery. 2010;67(3 Suppl Operative):ons16–28.
24. Ben Cnaan R, et al. Transorbital endoscopic-assisted management of intraorbital lesions: experience of 11 cases. Eur J Ophthalmol. 2023;33(3):1340–6.
25. Chibbaro S, et al. Endoscopic transorbital approaches to anterior and middle cranial fossa: exploring the potentialities of a modified lateral retrocanthal approach. World Neurosurg. 2021;150:e74–80.
26. Corvino S, et al. The feasibility of three port endonasal, transorbital, and sublabial approach to the petroclival region: neurosurgical audit and multiportal anatomic quantitative investigation. Acta Neurochir (Wien). 2023;
27. Dallan I, et al. Endoscopic-assisted transorbital surgery: Where do we stand on the scott's parabola? Personal considerations after a 10-year experience. Front Oncol. 2022;12:937818.
28. Di Somma A, et al. Endoscopic transorbital approach for the management of spheno-orbital meningiomas: literature review and preliminary experience. World Neurosurg. 2023;176:43–59.

29. Jung IH, et al. Endoscopic transorbital approach to the cavernous sinus: cadaveric anatomy study and clinical application ((double dagger)SevEN-009). Front Oncol. 2022;12:962598.
30. Kim EH, et al. Endoscopic transorbital approach to the insular region: cadaveric feasibility study and clinical application (SevEN-005). J Neurosurg. 2021;135(4):1164–72.
31. Lim J, et al. Endoscopic transorbital extradural anterior clinoidectomy: a stepwise surgical technique and case series study [SevEN-013]. Front Oncol. 2022;12:991065.
32. Noiphithak R, Yanez-Siller JC, Nimmannitya P. Transorbital approach for olfactory groove meningioma. World Neurosurg. 2022;162:66.
33. Polster SP, et al. The transcaruncular corridor of the medial transorbital approach to the frontal lobe: technical nuances and applications. Oper Neurosurg (Hagerstown). 2023;24(6):e458–62.
34. Radabaugh JP, et al. Transorbital-transsinus resection of sinonasal malignancy with extraconal orbital extension. Int Forum Allergy Rhinol. 2022;12(1):128–31.
35. Smith CS, et al. Transorbital debulking of sphenoid wing meningioma. J Craniofac Surg. 2022;33(3):859–62.
36. Yoo J, et al. Clinical applications of the endoscopic transorbital approach for various lesions. Acta Neurochir (Wien). 2021;163(8):2269–77.
37. Gerges MM, et al. Endoscopic transorbital approach to the infratemporal fossa and parapharyngeal space: a cadaveric study. J Neurosurg. 2019:1–12.
38. Almeida JP, et al. Transorbital endoscopic eyelid approach for resection of sphenoorbital meningiomas with predominant hyperostosis: report of 2 cases. J Neurosurg. 2018;128(6):1885–95.
39. Corvino S, et al. Functional and clinical outcomes after superior eyelid transorbital endoscopic approach for spheno-orbital meningiomas: illustrative case and literature review. Neurosurg Rev. 2022;46(1):17.
40. Dallan I, et al. Multiportal combined transorbital transnasal endoscopic approach for the management of selected skull base lesions: preliminary experience. World Neurosurg. 2015;84(1):97–107.
41. Di Somma A, et al. Combined and simultaneous endoscopic endonasal and transorbital surgery for a Meckel's cave schwannoma: technical nuances of a mini-invasive, multiportal approach. J Neurosurg. 2020;134(6):1836–45.
42. Di Somma A, et al. Endoscopic superior eyelid transorbital approach: how I do it. Acta Neurochir (Wien). 2022;164(7):1953–9.
43. Vural A, et al. Transorbital endoscopic approaches to the skull base: a systematic literature review and anatomical description. Neurosurg Rev. 2021;44(5):2857–78.
44. Martins C, Li X, Rhoton AL Jr. Role of the zygomaticofacial foramen in the orbitozygomatic craniotomy: anatomic report. Neurosurgery. 2003;53(1):168–72; discussion 172–3.
45. Di Somma A, et al. Endoscopic transorbital superior eyelid approach: anatomical study from a neurosurgical perspective. J Neurosurg. 2018;129(5):1203–16.
46. Lim J, et al. Extended endoscopic transorbital approach with superior-lateral orbital rim osteotomy: cadaveric feasibility study and clinical implications (SevEN-007). J Neurosurg. 2021:1–14.
47. Lopez CB, et al. Extradural anterior clinoidectomy through endoscopic transorbital approach: laboratory investigation for surgical perspective. Acta Neurochir (Wien). 2021;163(8):2177–88.
48. Almeida JP, et al. Transorbital endoscopic approach for exposure of the sylvian fissure, middle cerebral artery and crural cistern: an anatomical study. Acta Neurochir (Wien). 2017;159(10):1893–907.
49. Corrivetti F, et al. "Sagittal crest": definition, stepwise dissection, and clinical implications from a transorbital perspective. Oper Neurosurg (Hagerstown). 2022;22(5):e206–12.
50. Dallan I, et al. Endoscopic transorbital route to the cavernous sinus through the meningo-orbital band: a descriptive anatomical study. J Neurosurg. 2017;127(3):622–9.
51. Fukuda H, et al. The meningo-orbital band: microsurgical anatomy and surgical detachment of the membranous structures through a frontotemporal craniotomy with removal of the anterior clinoid process. J Neurol Surg B Skull Base. 2014;75(2):125–32.

52. Yanez-Siller JC, et al. The "crista ovale": a reliable anatomical landmark in transorbital endoscopic approaches to the middle cranial fossa. Oper Neurosurg (Hagerstown). 2023;24(3):e172–7.
53. Guizzardi G, et al. Endoscopic transorbital approach to the middle fossa: qualitative and quantitative anatomic study. Oper Neurosurg (Hagerstown). 2022;23(4):e267–75.
54. Di Somma A, et al. Endoscopic transorbital route to the petrous apex: a feasibility anatomic study. Acta Neurochir (Wien). 2018;160(4):707–20.
55. Lee WJ, et al. Endoscopic endonasal and transorbital approaches to petrous apex lesions. J Neurosurg. 2021:1–10.
56. Topczewski TE, et al. Endoscopic endonasal and transorbital routes to the petrous apex: anatomic comparative study of two pathways. Acta Neurochirurgica. 2020;162(9):2097–109.
57. De Rosa A, et al. Superior eyelid endoscopic transorbital approach to the tentorial area: a qualitative and quantitative anatomic study. Front Surg. 2022;9:1007447.
58. Bouthillier A, van Loveren HR, Keller JT. Segments of the internal carotid artery: a new classification. Neurosurgery. 1996;38(3):425–32; discussion 432–3.

Chapter 15
Purely Endoscopic Supracerebellar Infratentorial Approach to the Pineal Region in Pediatric Population

Sheena Ali ⓘ and Samer K. Elbabaa

15.1 Introduction

Pineal lesions are not only a surgical challenge, but their subsequent results including morbidity and mortality have almost always been poor [1]. While this structure has been studied over centuries scientifically, anatomically, and philosophically, the general apprehension toward approaching this disease is largely due to being an uncommon pathology and the challenging access due to the deep surgical field and associated critical neurovascular structures. Pineal tumors represent only 0.4–1% of all intracranial tumors [2–5]. They are more common in children than adults, accounting for 3–11% of all childhood brain tumors [6]. Among the various pathological entities encountered, pineocytomas, pineoblastomas, and primitive neuroectodermal tumors (PNETs) are the most prevalent [7–12]. Some other tumors encountered include neurocytomas [13, 14], glioblastomas [15, 16], meningiomas [9, 17], papillary tumors [18], metastatic tumors [19, 20], and vascular malformations [21]. Radical surgical resection is the main treatment for most of these lesions excluding pure germinomas and chemoradiotherapy-sensitive primary lymphoma [12, 22, 23]. In fact literature has proven repeatedly that radical resection yields better outcomes for both benign and malignant tumors [24–26] (Table 15.1).

Walter E. Dandy once stated that "Pineal tumors are perhaps the most dangerous of all intracranial tumors to attack surgically" [27]. While he was not entirely incorrect in his proclamation, the future had other plans in store. The first known pineal tumor resection was undertaken by Sir Victor Horsley in 1910 wherein he described

S. Ali · S. K. Elbabaa (✉)
Department of Pediatric Neurosurgery, Arnold Palmer Hospital for Children,
Orlando, FL, USA
e-mail: sheena.ali@orlandohealth.com; samer.elbabaa@orlandohealth.com

© The Author(s), under exclusive license to Springer Nature
Switzerland AG 2024
W. A. Azab (ed.), *Endoscope-controlled Transcranial Surgery*, Advances and
Technical Standards in Neurosurgery 52,
https://doi.org/10.1007/978-3-031-61925-0_15

Table 15.1 Review of literature

S. no.	Title	Authors	Results
1.	*Endoscopic Supracerebellar Infratentorial Retropineal Approach for Tumor Resection*	Tseng, Kuan-yin, ma, Hsin-I, Liu, Wei-Hsiu, and tang, chi-Tun (2012)	– Excellent illumination and magnification without sacrificing the inferior occipital sinus could be achieved with the aid of the endoscope with resultant complete excision – Postoperatively, the patient's diplopia resolved completely, and his hospital course was uneventful – This approach can be performed regardless of the size of the ventricle
2.	*Endoscopic surgery for tumors of the pineal region* via *a paramedian infratentorial supracerebellar keyhole approach (PISKA)*	Firas Thaher, Peter Kurucz, Lars Fuellbier, Markus Bittl, Nikolai J Hopf (2014)	- The first series of endoscopic procedures for lesions of the pineal region performed in the prone position using endoscope-assisted and endoscope-controlled technique -A single-institution series of 11 consecutive patients -Gross total resection was achieved in ten cases and subtotal resection in one case with no mortality
3.	*Pure Endoscopic Supracerebellar Infratentorial Approach to the Pineal Region: A Case Series*	Shane Shahrestani, Vignesh Ravi, Benjamin Strickland, Martin Rutkowski, Gabriel Zada (2020)	– Six patients who underwent pure endoscopic SCIT approach surgery in prone with 0- and 30° endoscopes – Gross total resection (GTR) was achieved in 5/6 patients, and NTR (near total resection) was achieved in 1/6 patients
4.	*Endoscopic supracerebellar infratentorial approach for pineal cyst resection: technical case report*	Pankaj A Gore, L Fernando Gonzalez, Harold L Rekate, Peter Nakaji (2008)	– Minimal brain retraction, poses no risk to the fornices – Visualization and avoidance of the Galenic veins, regardless of ventricular size
5.	*Extended endoscopic supracerebellar infratentorial (EESI) approach for a complex pineal region tumour—a technical note*	Saurabh Sinha, Elizabeth Culpin, and John McMullan (2018)	– The extra advantage gained by using the extended endoscopic supracerebellar infratentorial (EESI) with angled endoscopes is that pineal region lesions that extend beyond the midline can be seen and accessed without the potential need for a second approach

Table 15.1 (continued)

S. no.	Title	Authors	Results
6.	*Supracerebellar Infratentorial Endoscopic and Endoscopic-Assisted Approaches to Pineal Lesions: Technical Report and Review of the Literature*	Rita Snyder, Daniel R Felbaum, Walter C Jean, and Amjad Anaizi (2017)	– The purely endoscopic and endoscope-assisted paramedian supracerebellar infratentorial approach was successful in providing wide surgical navigability through a tight anatomical corridor
7.	*Fully Endoscopic Resection of Pineal Region Tumors*	Hrayr Shahinian, Yoon Ra (2013)	– 1 adult patient, operated on via this approach for a pineoblastoma – GTR was achieved with no complications – This technique combines the advantages and benefits of both open microsurgical resection and minimally invasive endoscopic surgeries
8.	*Endoscopic supracerebellar infratentorial approach to pineal and posterior third ventricle lesions in prone position with head extension: a technical note*	Spazzapan, P, Velnar, T, Bosnjak R. Neurol Res. 2020 Dec;42(12):1070–10	– All patients operated on had complete tumor excision with no complications in prone position with neck extension and head rotation and paramedian subtorcular craniotomy using a prone position, with neck extension and head rotation
9.	*Supracerebellar infratentorial endoscopically controlled resection of pineal lesions: case series and operative technique*	Uschold, T, Abla, AA, Fusco, D, Bristol, R & Nakaji, P (2011)	– A single-institution series of 9 consecutive patients – Gross total resection and/or adequate cyst fenestration was achieved in 8 cases with biopsy and conservative debulking -All patients had a stable or improved modified Rankin scale score
10.	*Pure endoscopic removal of pineal region tumors*	Sood, S, Hoeprich, M, Ham SD (2011)	– 2 patients (1 cystic, 1 solid tumor) operated in sitting position through a subtorcular approach – Endoscope was held in the left hand with suction tip extending beyond the tip through its instrument channel – Superior surgeon comfort – Complete resection was achieved in all cases

(continued)

Table 15.1 (continued)

S. no.	Title	Authors	Results
11.	*Paramedian supracerebellar approach in semi-sitting position for endoscopic resection of pineal cyst: 2-dimensional operative video*	Fernandez-Miranda JC (2019)	– Semi-sitting position provides excellent exposure of the pineal region secondary to gravity-based retraction of the cerebellum when head elevation is reduced to 30° and lower extremities are elevated – The paramedian supracerebellar approach is less invasive and faster than midline supracerebellar approach – Requires exposure of just 1 transverse sinus (nondominant for centered lesions) and avoids exposure of the torcula – The endoscopic technique improves the ergonomics of the approach when compared to the microscope-based technique and provides excellent visualization of all the neurovascular structures in the pineal region • Surgical resection was successfully performed with no complications and complete cyst resection
12.	*Keyhole Surgery of Pineal Area Tumors— Personal Experience in 22 Patients*	Zbigniew Kotwica, Agnieszka Saracen, Piotr Kasprzak (2017)	– No surgical complications in all 22 patients – No systemic complications of sitting position
13.	*Pure endoscopic resection of pineal region tumors through supracerebellar infratentorial approach with 'head-up' park-bench position*	Wei Hua, Hao Xu, Xin Zhang, Guo Yu, Xiaowen Wang, Jinsen Zhang, Zhiguang Pan & Wei Zhu (2022)	– This cohort included four patients with gross total resection (GTR) in all patients, with no morbidity – Relief from hydrocephalus among all patients
14.	*Purely endoscopic resection of pineal region tumors using infratentorial supracerebellar approach: How I do it*	Ye Gu, Fan Hu & Xiaobiao Zhang (2016)	– Purely endoscopic resection of pineal region tumors using infratentorial supracerebellar approach is feasible and safe alternative

a subtentorial infratentorial approach [28, 29]. Though this patient passed away from surgical complications, he deduced that his next case should be approached supratentorially. In 1913, Fedor Krause, a German surgeon, operated on a

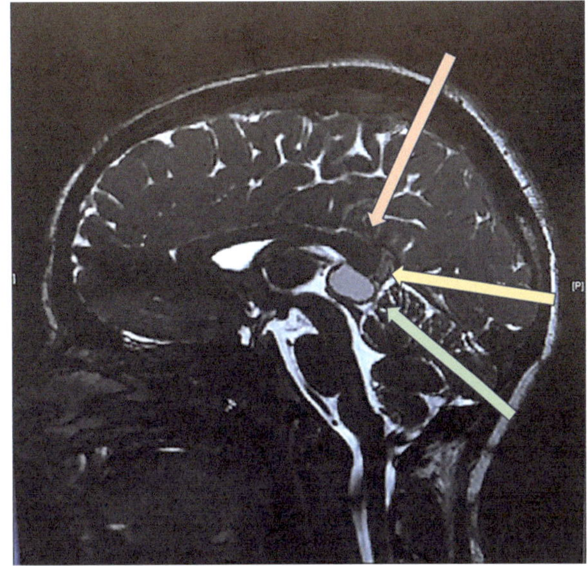

Fig. 15.1 Trajectories for supratentorial posterior transcallosal approach (Dandy) (orange arrow), occipital transtentorial approach (Poppen) (yellow arrow), and the infratentorial supracerebellar approach (Krause and Stein) (green arrow)

10-year-old boy with a pineal neoplasm via an infratentorial supracerebellar approach and achieved complete tumor resection, with resounding clinical success. Further success was noted via various other approaches like Dandy's parieto-occipital transcallosal approach (1921), Van Wagenen's transcortical transventricular approach (1931), and Poppen's occipital transtentorial approach. Hence, the 1960s adopted the infratentorial supracerebellar routes and the occipital transtentorial or transcallosal approaches, which require a wide surgical exposure for better visual access and orientation [30–33] (Fig. 15.1).

With the advent of the microscope and advances in stereotaxy and neuroimaging, the 1970s saw the introduction of safer, accessible lesion targeting. By 1971, Bennett M. Stein repopularized Krause's infratentorial supracerebellar approach and reported no perioperative mortality and morbidity [34]. Despite advancements in microneurosurgical techniques, the infratentorial supracerebellar approach is generally accepted as the standard approach to this area, even though it may require larger craniotomies.

The recent decade has seen novel minimally invasive procedures, wherein the use of the endoscope has helped to provide excellent visualization and illuminations and valuable close-up views of narrow working area corridors, and this has gained acceptance and reliability. The first purely endoscopic SCIT approach was described by Ruge et al. for the fenestration of a quadrigeminal arachnoid cyst [35]. Cardia et al. even demonstrated on cadaveric studies that endoscopy provides access not only to the pineal region but to the posterior third ventricle via a parapineal entry point [36]. Prior to this endoscopy to approach pineal tumors were via transventricular or extracerebral approaches sometimes as an adjunct to microscopic exposure [37, 38].

15.2   The Problem and Challenge

The pineal-tectal region is anatomically challenging as it is situated deep within the brain, bound by several critical neurovascular structures. This depth is almost equivalent in all surgical approaches. As pineal tumors are located in the midportion of the third ventricle and posteriorly compress the cerebellum, they usually arise from the undersurface of the velum interpositum, and rarely extend above it, but may extend into the foramen of Monro. It is bound by the superior cerebellar artery and the Galenic venous system, the fourth cranial nerve, the thalamus, and the midbrain. The tentorium is sharply upsloping with the tentorial cerebellar surface conformal to this slope, with the apex of the vermis tightly fitting in the apical tentorial cleft, blocking the simple access to the pineal region directly [39].

The pineal region marks the site of convergence of the deep venous drainage system, i.e., the internal cerebral veins, basal veins of Rosenthal, and the Galenic complex tributaries. The medial posterior choroidal arteries that arise from proximal posterior cerebral artery run forward beside pineal body in quadrigeminal cistern.

The SCIT approach is the most popular approach, which is flexible and simple to access; however, the long surgical corridor limits the maneuverability of surgical instruments; though the endoscope helps provide panoramic view and clear details, it has the shortcoming of 2D images and blind region in the proximity of the lens body, as any bleeding or unclear vision may cause. Hence, the learning curve is imperative [40]. Literature suggests that piecemeal resection is mandatory to avoid injury to the surrounding corridor of veins.

15.3   Endoscopic Surgical Freedom

The endoscopic approach is a relatively new method to access the posterior incisura space. Endoscopy reduces approach-related tissue disruption and brain retraction without compromising visualization. "Surgical freedom" is the maximal area via which a surgeon can move a hand holding dissector while moving the distal end of the instrument along the borders of the surgical field [41]. The wide panoramic endoscope allows increased visibility and illumination of the surgical field even in deep brain lesions. The compact nature of the endoscope allows minimally invasive and keyhole craniotomes. Moreover, endoscopic equipment is less expensive than surgical microscopes [42–44]. The SCIT approach is the most popular approach for pineal lesions due to the natural corridor between the tentorium and cerebellum. The SCIT approach has in fact evolved into the midline, paramedian, extreme lateral, and contralateral SCIT approaches, with endoscopy aiding in access to unseen corners.

Full endoscopic resection of a pineal tumor can be performed by a SCIT approach using the natural infratentorial corridor [45, 46], wherein it limits injury to bridging veins, cerebellomesencephalic vein (CMV), and Galenic veins [47, 48]. Due to the anatomically narrow corridor, instrument working angles and depth of exposure may be limited, which can be overcome by using the sitting position, flexing the neck, three-quarter prone position, or the Concorde position. Also, the rate of gross total resection (GTR) was significantly higher in the endoscopic surgery for pineal regions, and it contributed to a lower rate of postoperative complications [49].

Hasan et al. quantitatively measured surgical freedom in the endoscopic and microsurgical SCIT approaches and reported that, endoscopically, the far lateral approach provides the maximum surgical freedom with the most vertical attack angle, while the midline route provides the largest horizontal angle. They also reiterated how the endoscopic method required less cerebellar retraction without the need for sacrificing bridging veins [42]. Other studies further confirmed this, wherein it was observed that ipsilateral paramedian SCIT gives a shorter corridor distance and contralateral paramedian SCIT approach gives a better surgical view [50]. Thirty-degree and 70-degree endoscopes help visualize the tumors/lesions hidden behind the critical and delicate neurovascular structures [51]. Using 0° and 45° endoscopes provides a better view of the pineal gland, internal cerebral vein, and median posterior choroidal arteries [52].

15.4 Patient Selection and Indications

There are a variety of benign and neoplastic pineal region lesions, more than half of which are radiosensitive [53]. With advancements in radiogenomics, an anticipated pathology can help determine the surgical plan of action. But it may not reliably differentiate between the several histopathological subtypes. Imaging like a contrast MRI (magnetic resonance imaging) or CT (computed tomography) brain is essential for studying the anatomy and related neurovascular structures near the lesion and to plan a safe operative approach. So, the methods to approach these lesions will also depend upon presenting symptomatology, tumor markers, and chronicity of hydrocephalus.

Noninvasive methods to achieve a correct diagnosis must be attempted as much as possible, especially for the diagnosis of radiosensitive tumors. Serum or cerebrospinal fluid (CSF) studies suggestive of a raised beta-human chorionic gonadotropin (b-HCG) or alpha fetoprotein (AFP) can suggest a malignant germ cell tumor and deem the patient suitable for radiotherapy and chemotherapy without resection or a biopsy, and there is only a 15% sampling error [13, 54].

As these lesions are responsible for causing obstructive hydrocephalus, the chronicity must be noted. In an emergent situation, a bedside external ventricular drain (EVD) may be placed, till a definitive solution is planned. Usually, the ideal surgical plan would be to perform an endoscopic third ventriculostomy (ETV) and, if possible, biopsy the pineal lesion via the posterior third ventricle [55, 56].

The patient must receive cardiac clearance preoperatively, to rule out the possibility of any cardiac instability and patent foramen ovale (PFO). Another important aid for surgical success is the use of the transesophageal echocardiogram (TEE), which is a specialized cardiac ultrasound, involving the use of a probe that is inserted into the patient's esophagus as a real-time method to access the cardiac status and unpredictable events like embolisms, cardiac ventricular function, and the inferior vena cava status.

The treatment approach of pineal region tumors is a bit tricky. Literature states that the ideal surgical primary objective must be to establish an accurate diagnosis which can further aid in the ideal surgical strategy, adjuvant therapy, metastatic workup, its prognosis, and subsequent follow-up [23, 34, 55–57]. The secondary goal should be resection, irrespective of being partial or complete [23, 58–62].

This approach requires adequate planning, as one of the greatest dangers with an endoscope is the danger to strike critical structures in its blind spot, even though the SCIT approach trajectory is largely free of critical structures. The anticipated pathology must be analyzed as it can help determine the extent of resection and ideal approach and trajectory. Parenchymal tumors must undergo gross total excision as much as possible, compared to other cases like germ cell tumors and exophytic low-grade gliomas, which are ideal lesions for minimally invasive intervention.

15.5 Instrumentation

Neuronavigation, KARL STORZ endoscope (flexible and rigid; 0°, 30°), Mayfield or three-pin fixation, motor and sensory evoked potentials, transesophageal echocardiogram (TEE).

15.6 Positioning

Several approaches have been described and performed, the most common ones being prone, Concorde, and semi-sitting position with their own positives and drawbacks (Table 15.2, Fig. 15.2).

Once positioned as per the surgeon's choice, the neck is slightly flexed in a military "chin tuck" position. The head is fixed on a three-pin or Mayfield fixation, ensuring the body is in the reverse Trendelenburg position. The head should be midline with slight rotation away from specific side if lateral extension under tentorium is present.

The patient can be positioned in a lateral oblique with the upper body elevated 15° to benefit venous drainage and neck flexion to enhance surgeon's comfort. Motor and sensory evoked potentials (MEP and SSEP) can help confirm any over-flexion [46]. The anesthetists proceed to secure the transesophageal echocardiography (TEE) probe once the patient is induced.

Table 15.2 Positioning

S. no.	Position	Advantages	Drawbacks
1.	**Prone**	– Good surgical exposure – Alleviates need for retraction – Lower incidence of venous air embolism – As the head is elevated, venous bleeding is reduced	The exposure may not be as clear as that of semi-sitting position and park-bench position
2.	**Semi-sitting**	– Can be easily modified to reverse Trendelenburg position in case of suspected embolism – Improved venous and CSF drainage leading to a drier and less bloody field – Excellent visualization – No facial swelling – Face is exposed, making monitoring cranial evoked nerve easier – Cardiac Dopplers/ transesophageal echocardiograms (TEE) help detect small amounts of air within the venous system	– Risk of air embolisms – Contraindicated in those with cardiac instability and patent foramen ovale – Decreased preload and chances of hypotension
3.	**Park-bench**	– Head flexed, neck rotated to look at the floor – Better access and surgical exposure than prone position	– Neck rotation required, can cause venous congestion
4.	**Concorde or three-quarter prone**	– Combines prone and semi-sitting – Modified prone position with slight head flexion, tucked in arms and legs with flexion at knees – Chest is uncompressed – Minimal to no retraction needed – Good access to tentorial surface	– Trajectories and exposure require good surgical judgment and expertise

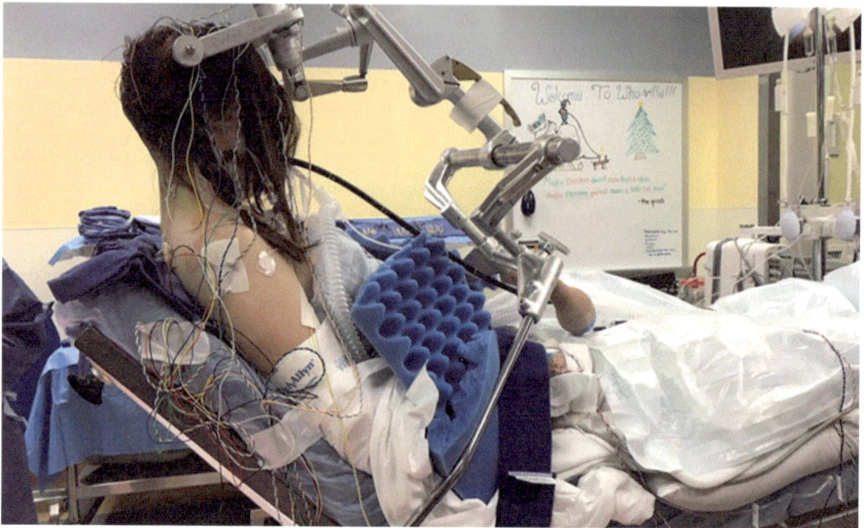

Fig. 15.2 Sitting position with head slightly flexed fixed on a three-pin or Mayfield retractor. The head is angulated to be flexed in order to flatten the tentorium

15.7 The Technique

The neuronavigation is registered and is used to determine the ideal "head up" angle. After the routine antiseptic preparation of the area of interest, a vertical occipital midline small incision is created (below the level of the transverse sinus) followed by a small craniotomy (3 × 3 cm). A U-shaped dural incision is made and brain relaxation is achieved by CSF release from the cisterna magna. With the combination of gravity and brain relaxation, a corridor between the cerebellum and tentorium could be easily opened (Fig. 15.3). The corridor is then inspected with a 0° scope, and the visualized superficial and deep drainage veins above the vermis were coagulated and transected, to release the cerebellum, using a single shaft minimally invasive bipolar forceps and microscissors (Fig. 15.4).

The endoscope can be held by an operative assistant or a fixed device, with the monitor in front of the operating surgeon. Additional dissection of the arachnoid and deep venous structures is then performed to expose the pineal region, posterior third ventricle, and colliculi (Fig. 15.5). The quadrigeminal cisternal space and some bridging veins between the superior surface of the cerebellum and tentorium were gradually sacrificed. Microdissection around the thickened and opaque arachnoid over the quadrigeminal cistern once opened via sharp dissection can uncover the precentral cerebellar vein, which can be sacrificed with impunity to further expose the tumor, so that a precise plane can be achieved between the neoplasm and healthy brain tissue which is clearly visible in most cases (Fig. 15.6). At this point, the samples can be collected for rapid frozen pathology. The vermian veins must not be divided or coagulated. Further devascularization can help obtain a clear view of

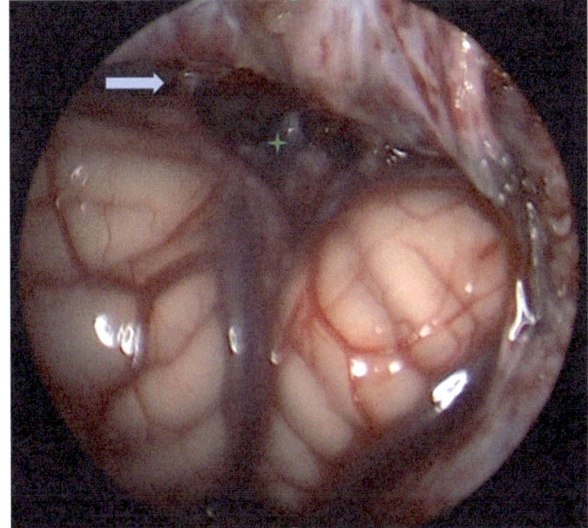

Fig. 15.3 The endoscope reveals the domes of the cerebellum below with the overlying precentral cerebellar vein (green star) and the small bridging veins of the upper cerebellar vermis above (blue arrow)

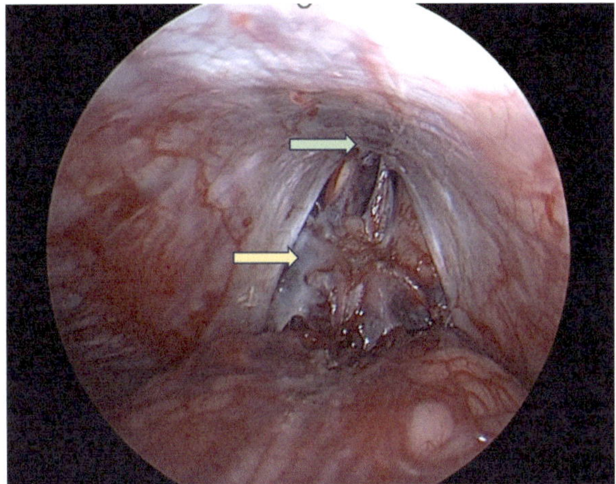

Fig. 15.4 On advancing the endoscope, the vein of Galen (green arrow) is seen pulsating above with the cystic pineal tumor (yellow arrow) immediately below surrounded by dense adhesions

the tumor. Once the tumor is identified, intracapsular debulking in a piecemeal manner must be done, dissecting it away from the adjacent neurovascular structures (Fig. 15.7).

Devascularization and disconnection bilaterally are of utmost importance as the pineal gland receives its blood supply from bilateral medial posterior choroidal arteries and the rostral stalk is connected to the bilateral habenula. Furthermore, if the tumor is vascular, one must attempt to devascularize the tumor as much as possible rather than debulking it. The CUSA could also be used if necessary.

If seen invading the third ventricle, the complete resection of the tumor and opening of the third ventricle are essential. A 30° scope could be used to observe the

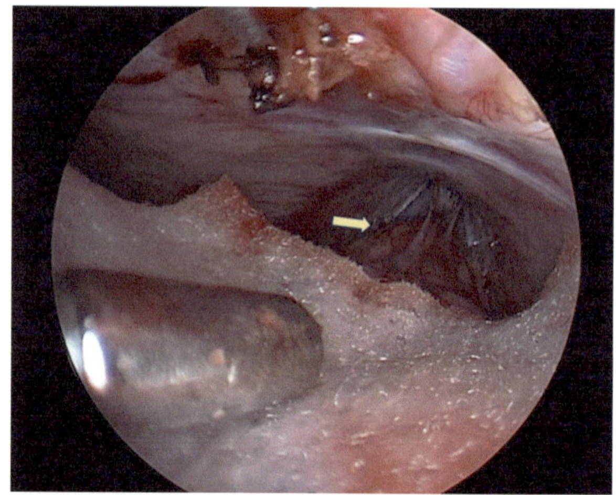

Fig. 15.5 Midline tethering adhesions are sharply dissected to mobilize the cerebellum, so cottonoids can be placed over its surface for maximal gravity-assisted retraction away from the tentorial surface, to visualize the tumor (yellow arrow)

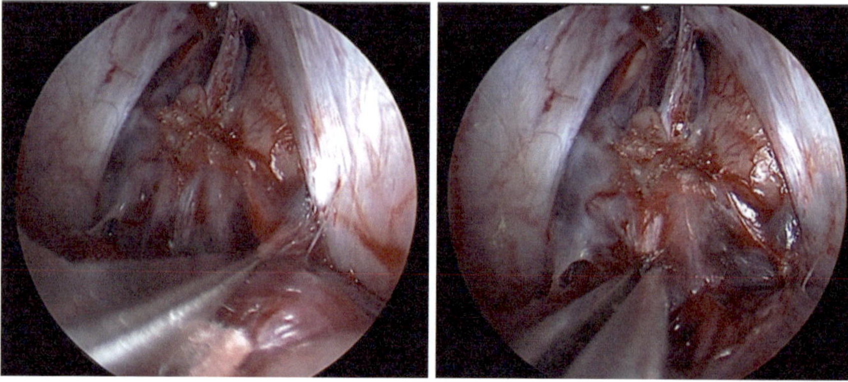

Fig. 15.6 Using sharp microscissors and minimally invasive bipolar forceps via a single endoscope shaft, dissection of the arachnoid, bordering tumor vasculature, and deeper venous structures is performed to expose the pineal tumor, posterior third ventricle, and colliculi. Sharp dissection off the quadrigeminal plate inferiorly and chasing the tumor into the third ventricle may be required

corners like the lateral thalamic or quadrigeminal cistern blocked by the vermis. A final sweep with a 0° or 30° scope is done to check for residuals and to do a final verification of complete tumor removal (Figs. 15.8 and 15.9). Thorough irrigation must be performed and retrieval of any clots near the aqueduct, to reduce any postoperative hydrocephalus. Watertight dural closure, bone flap fixation, and closure are then carried out. In acute setting with the presentation of hydrocephalus, an emergent EVD placement or ETV can be performed prior to a definitive surgery.

In an unfortunate event of excessive hemorrhage, the endoscope must be partially withdrawn to prevent soiling of the lens with a gradual increase in suction.

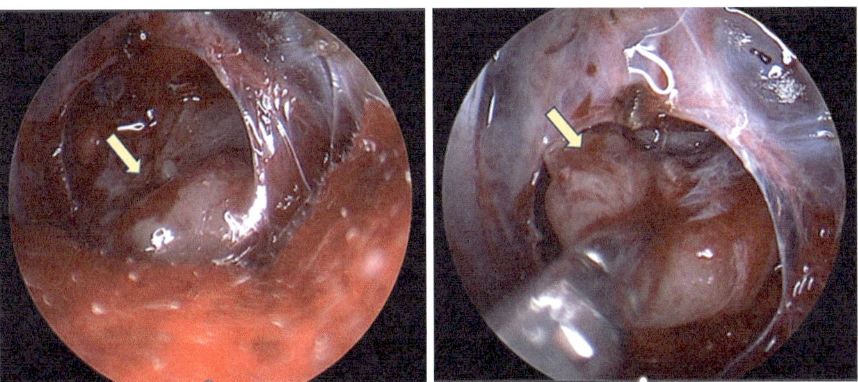

Fig. 15.7 The endoscope is docked superiorly against the tentorium while the yellowish-white tumor is extracted in a "piecemeal" manner

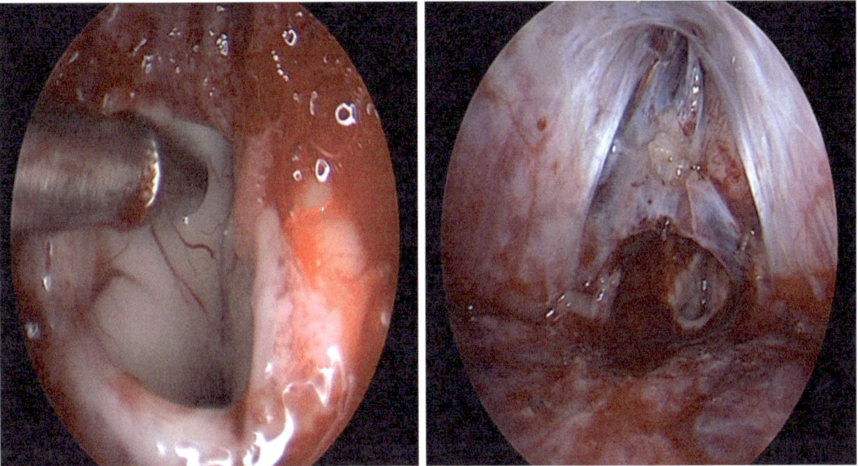

Fig. 15.8 The last inspection is done to visualize corners with the exposure of posterior third of the third ventricle to inspect for residual tumor and blood products (left, zoomed in; right, zoomed out)

Continuous warm saline irrigation and use of Gelfoam and a cottonoid can help secure the bleeding. Bayoneted bipolar forceps with angled tips can help achieve targeted coagulation. These steps can be repeated multiple times till a clear field is noted.

Postoperative imaging (Fig. 15.10) shows the gross total resection of the tumor mass with no evidence of any bleeding, infarcts, or hydrocephalus.

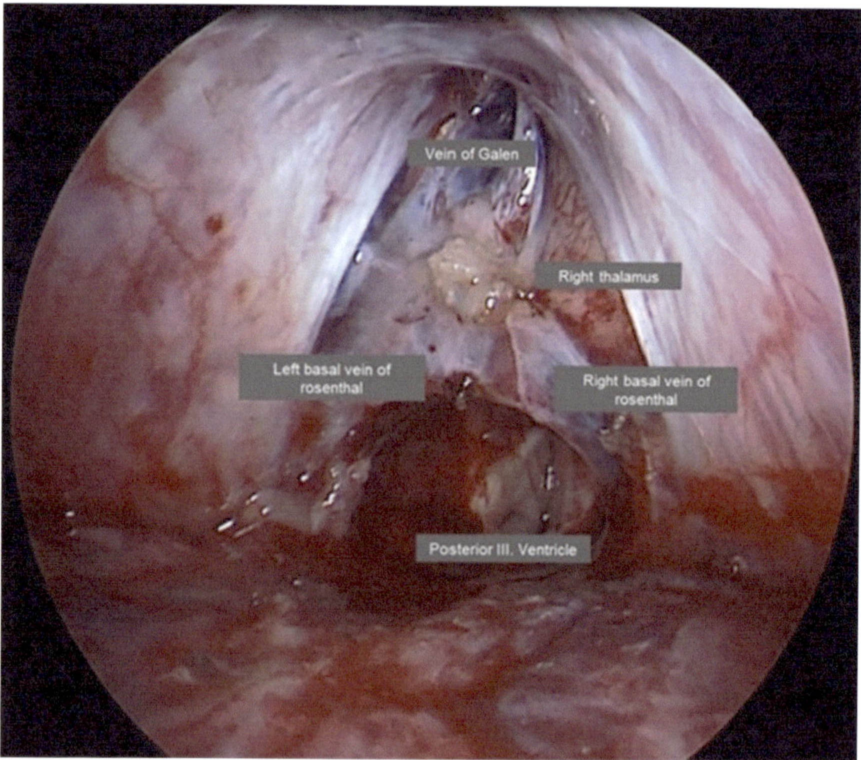

Fig. 15.9 The final view of the resected tumor bed at the end of the procedure, showing the surrounding labelled anatomical landmarks providing context, suggesting the gross total resection of the tumor

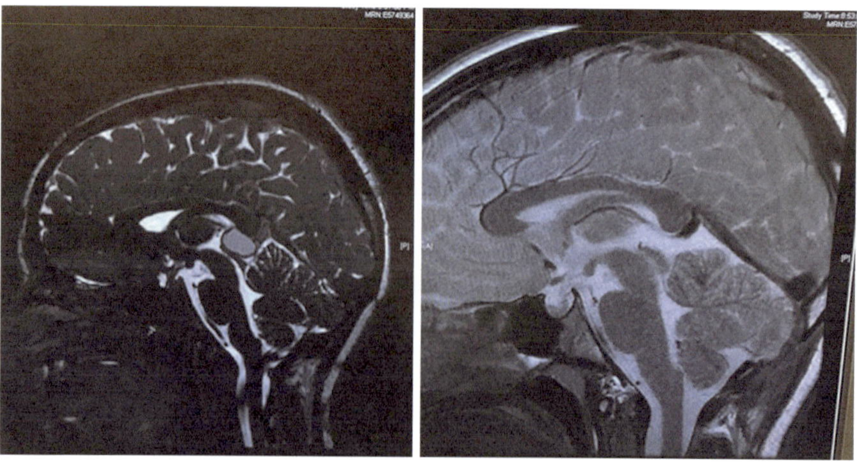

Fig. 15.10 The comparative preoperative (left) and postoperative (right) MRI brain show gross total resection of the pineal tumor

15.8 A Few Key Points

1. Choose the best approach based on the suspected pathology to dodge blind spots.
2. Ensure adequate bone opening to prevent transverse sinus injury.
3. Identify critical neurovascular anatomy in relation to the tumor, and avoid injury to deep veins by adequate dissection and skeletonization of vessels (veins) and their branches. This can prevent consequent edema.
4. Avoid sacrificing the superior vermian vein.
5. Maintain a clean plane of dissection within the cisternal planes while debulking the tumor capsule.
6. If the tumor is aggressive, infiltrating vital structures like the surrounding tectum or deep brain structures, one must be prepared to leave a residual.
7. Be aware of the different trajectories when using different positioning.
8. Allow good brain and cerebellar relaxation with adequate CSF release, good anesthetic monitoring with slight hyperventilation, and gravity, and avoid venous sacrifice as much as possible.
9. Use correct microsurgical instruments that are long limbed to assist in dissection and prevent unnecessary trauma.

15.9 The Technique and Variations

Several variations have been suggested for the following reasons:

1. The pineal gland is a midline deep-seated structure; the visualization is often hindered by the vermis, a paramedian approach can help counteract this, and it is ideal for lesions extending into the splenium of the corpus callosum.
2. The bridging veins can be preserved on moving more laterally, as they become progressively less prominent.
3. A shorter and more direct trajectory to the posterior incisura can be achieved further away from the midline, as it provides a more direct route to the superior colliculus and any inferiorly or laterally located lesions within the posterior incisura.

One may use image guidance with frameless navigation system to plan the craniotomy and the surgical targets and identify vital neurovascular structures.

15.10 Material and Methods

A literature search was performed using the PubMed search engine with combinations of Medical Subject Headings (MeSH) terms and text words. Combinations of the terms "pineal region" (MeSH), "pineal tumors" (text word), "purely endoscopic approach" (text word), "endoscope controlled" (text word), and "Supracerebellar infratentorial" (text word) were searched. References cited within relevant articles were also searched as additional sources of articles. Relevant articles were then searched for the keywords "purely endoscopic" or "supracerebellar infratentorial." Articles were excluded if the keywords were not mentioned in the text. Both articles that described purely endoscopic or endoscope-controlled supracerebellar infratentorial approach were used, and articles describing other endoscopic approaches, like "transventricular" and "transnasal," were excluded. "Endoscope assisted" articles were also excluded. Articles describing other corridors like the "Poppen's" or "occipital transtentorial" were also excluded. The relevant articles were not limited to each year, as this is a rather new procedure. However, all articles relevant to this review were published between 2008 and 2020. Only articles written in English were used. A total of 14 case reports and articles were analyzed.

15.11   Results

There were around 14 studies regarding purely endoscopic surgery to the pineal region (Table 15.1). It was comprised of 46 cases. Eleven studies comprising 38 cases underwent purely endoscopic SCIT approach resection of pineal region lesions. Other approaches involved slight modifications in trajectories. GTR was achieved in 33 cases and this population had an exceptionally low complication rate noted in only 7 patients. None of the cases reported any permanent morbidity or mortality. The most common position was the prone position wherein 60.9% of the cases were operated in the prone position, 30.4% in the sitting position, and 8.7% in semi-sitting position. The most common HPE were pineal cysts (13 cases). Other pathologies included germinomas (10.9%), five teratomas, three yolk sac tumors, three pineocytomas, and three gliomas.

One of the major challenges of the endoscopic approach faced by surgeons was the intraoperative bleeding and resultant loss of orientation. In larger and aggressively vascular lesions, accessing the main feeding artery is of utmost importance. This way, the endoscope provides excellent illumination and can help reduce the risk of any bleeding. The importance of positioning must be reiterated here, as gravity can help reduce pooling of blood within the operative field.

If one has access to neuronavigation, it must be utilized amply to identify important and surgically relevant landmarks to help guide in the resection. Making use of cerebellar relaxation and gravity can help provide the ideal surgical corridor irrespective of the trajectory used.

15.12   Discussion

Tseng, Kuan-Yin et al. performed this approach via two paramedian burr holes in one patient and observed that good excision could be achieved without sacrificing the occipital sinus, irrespective of the ventricular size. Clinically, the patient's symptomatic preoperative diplopia improved immediately postoperatively. Zbigniew et al.'s case series of 22 patients in 2017 showed excellent results wherein none of their patients experienced any mortality or morbidity when operated with a keyhole SCIT approach in the sitting position. Firas Thaher et al. used the "endoscope-assisted" and "endoscope-controlled" approach in prone position in their case series of 11 patients. While they achieved GTR in 10 out of 11 cases, they used the endoscope-only approach to achieve GTR in 1 patient. They note that there were no major morbidities or mortalities.

Kandregula et al. described the various approaches and the ones with the easiest accessibility to the pineal area via an endoscope. Shane et al. also performed this approach in the prone position using 0- and 30° scopes and were able to achieve GTR in five out of six patients and STR only in one, safely. Another cohort of four patients, by Wei Hua et al., described GTR in all patients and relief from hydrocephalus too. Comparable results were noted with long-term studies by Ali Ayyad et al. over 8 years, wherein they noted GTR in 19 out of 21 patients, with only 1 patient requiring a VP shunt postoperatively. Timothy Uschold's study noted improved long-term modified Rankin Scale scores in all his nine patients. Seven of his patients underwent concomitant third ventriculostomy into the quadrigeminal cistern.

Other studies certify that this approach provides wide surgical navigability through a tight anatomical corridor, with minimal brain retraction. It does not interfere with the deep venous system irrespective of any ventricular ballooning, but also claim that the supra- and infratentorial environments can be accessed easily by cutting the tentorium and the third ventricle could be easily accessed too, where needed. Other articles explain in detail the most gratifying routes and trajectories to achieve complete resection based on tumor morphology and location, using an endoscope, and which endoscope would be ideal. Joham Choque-Velasquez et al. explain a modified endoscopic supracerebellar infratentorial (eSCIT) approach using a laboratory-constructed "borescope" which provided excellent intraoperative visualization and claims to be an inexpensive aid while also acting as a medium for ideal surgical training for beginners, especially in economically backward countries [44]. Some upgrades like the use of the VITOM, a high-definition telescope modification, are some upgraded modifications of this technique that aids in maximal resectability of pineal tumors. Cadaveric studies further emphasize the importance of the trajectory and direction of craniotomies to help toward a good surgical outcome [42, 44] (Table 15.1).

Most studies also specify that endoscopic resection is ideal for tumors of a moderate size (<3 cm) [46, 63, 64] though there may be exceptions when it comes to highly vascular tumors or tumors with a firm to hard consistency. However, there are several case reports describing tumors larger than 3 cm with GTR achieved. Wei Hua et al. describe GTR in two tumors larger than 3 cm comprising of 50% of their cohort, wherein they all experienced symptom resolution after surgery [65].

15.13 Conclusion

In an appropriately selected group of patients, the endoscope is an excellent upgraded option to the larger craniotomies. Using the peculiar tight corridor to our advantage, we can successfully attain surgical navigability in a less invasive manner even to complex deep-seated lesions and reduce the chance of tumor residue in the ventricles. This is why even literature states that the GTR rate was significantly higher in the endoscopy group compared to the microneurosurgical group [49]. The dreaded complication of air embolisms can be simply counteracted upon by copious irrigation via a small burr hole. The smaller craniotomies, subsequent better wound healing, and shorter hospital stay are just a few more advantages [66].

This approach, if done correctly, would not require subsequent surgeries and can be used irrespective of the ventricular size. Choosing the right trajectory and choosing the corridor are key areas of discussion, and one must use utmost discretion in selecting the same with regard to suspected tumor pathology.

This has allowed future studies to elaborate further advantages and ideal approaches and study their long-term outcomes. With the assistance of cadaveric studies, we can further justify the importance of this beautiful approach.

Conflict of Interest All the authors declare that they have no conflicts of interest.

References

1. Ventureyra EC. Pineal region: surgical management of tumors and vascular malformations. Surg Neurol. 1981;16:77–84.
2. Villani V, Tomei G, Salvati M, et al. Pineal region tumors: surgical management, role of RT and review of literature. Clin Neurol Neurosurg. 2007;109(1):1–6. https://doi.org/10.1016/j.clinneuro.2006.08.015.
3. Motiei-Langroudi R, Sadeghian H, Soleimani MM, Seddighi AS, Shahzadi S. Treatment results for pineal region tumors: role of stereotactic biopsy plus adjuvant therapy vs. Open Resection Turk Neurosurg. 2016;26:336–40.
4. Sajko T, Kudelic N, Lupret V, Lupret V Jr, Nola IA. Treatment of pineal region lesions: our experience in 39 patients. Coll Antropol. 2009;33:1259–63.
5. Pettorini BL, Al-Mahfoud R, Jenkinson MD, Avula S, Pizer B, Mallucci C. Surgical pathway and management of pineal region tumors in children. Childs Nerv Syst. 2013;29:433–9.
6. Al-Hussaini M, Sultan I, Gajjar AJ, Abuirmileh N, Qaddoumi I. Pineal gland tumors: experience from the SEER database. J Neuro-Oncol. 2009;94:351–8.
7. Aboul-Enein H, El-Aziz Sabry AA, Hafez FA. Supracerebellar infratentorial approach with paramedian expansion for posterior third ventricular and pineal region lesions. Clin Neurol Neurosurg. 2015;139:100–9.
8. Lee J, Wakabayashi T, Yoshida J. Management, and survival of pineoblastoma: an analysis of 34 adults from the brain tor registry of Japan. Neurol Med Chir (Tokyo). 2005;45:132–42.
9. Biswas A, Mallick S, Purkait S, Roy S, Sarkar C, Bakhshi S, et al. Treatment outcome and patterns of failure in patients of non-pineal supratentorial primitive neuroectodermal tumor: review of literature and clinical experience form a regional cancer center in North India. Acta Neurochir. 2015;157:1251–66.

10. Yamamoto I. Pineal region tumor: surgical anatomy and approach. J Neuro-Oncol. 2001;54:263–75.
11. Thaher F, Kurucz P, Fuellbier L, Bittl M, Hopf NJ. Endoscopic surgery for tumors of the pineal region via a paramedian infratentorial supracerebellar keyhole approach (PISKA) Neurosurg. Rev. 2014;37:677–84.
12. Bruce JN, Ogden AT. Surgical strategies for treating patients with pineal region tumors. J Neuro-Oncol. 2004;69:221–36.
13. Chen CL, Shen CC, Wang J, Lu CH, Lee HT. Central neurocytoma: a clinical, radiological, and pathological study of nine cases. Clin Neurol Neurosurg. 2008;110:129–36.
14. Messing-Junger AM, Riemenschneider MJ, Reifenberger G. A 21-year-old female with a third ventricle tumor. Brain Pathol. 2006;16:87–8.
15. Stowe HB, Miller CR, Wu J, Randazzo DM, Ju AW. Pineal region glioblastoma, a case report and literature review. Front Oncol. 2017;12:123.
16. Sugita Y, Terasaki M, Tanigawa K, Ohshima K, Morioka M, Higaki K, et al. Gliosarcomas arising from the pineal gland region: uncommon localization and rare tumors. Neuropathology. 2016;36:56–63.
17. Maiti TK, Nagarjun MN, Arimappamagan A, Mahadevan A, Pandey P. Hemangiopericytoma of pineal region: case report and review. Neurol India. 2014;62:460–2.
18. Edson MA, Fuller GN, Allen PK, Levine NB, Ghia AJ, Mahajan A, et al. Outcomes after surgery and radiotherapy for papillary tumor of the pineal region. World Neurosurg. 2015;84:76–81.
19. Lassman AB, Bruce JN, Fetell MR. Metastases to the pineal gland. Neurology. 2006;10:1303–4.
20. Park JH, Hong YK. Primary malignant melanoma in the pineal region. J Korean Neurosurg Soc. 2014;56:504–8.
21. Sinson G, Zager EL, Grossman RI, Gennarelli TA, Flamm ES. Cavernous malformations of the third ventricle. Neurosurgery. 1995;37:37–42.
22. Azab WA, Nasim K, Salaheddin W. An overview of the current surgical options for pineal region tumors. Surg Neurol Int. 2014;5(1):39.
23. Konovalov AN, Pitskhelauri DI. Principles of treatment of the pineal region tumors. Surg Neurol. 2003;59(4):250–68.
24. Hernesniemi J, Romani R, Albayrak BS, et al. Microsurgical management of pineal region lesions: personal experience with 119 patients. Surg Neurol. 2008;70(6):576–83.
25. Qi S, Fan J, Zhang XA, et al. Radical resection of nongerminomatous pineal region tumors via the occipital transtentorial approach based on arachnoidal consideration: experience on a series of 143 patients. Acta Neurochir. 2014;156(12):2253–62.
26. Tate M, Sughrue ME, Rutkowski MJ, et al. The long-term postsurgical prognosis of patients with pineoblastoma. Cancer. 2012;118(1):173–9.
27. Dandy WE. Surgery of the brain, a monograph from Vol. XII, Lewis' practice of surgery. Hagerstown, MD: W. F. Prior Co., Inc; 1945.
28. Victor H. Discussion of paper by CMH Howell on tumors of the pineal body. Proc R Soc Med. 1910;3:77–8.
29. Pendl G. The surgery of pineal lesions—historical perspective. AE N. Diagnosis and treatment of pineal region tumors. Baltimore, MD: Williams & Wilkins; 1984. p. 139–54.
30. Isamat F. Tumors of the posterior part of the third ventricle: neurosurgical criteria. New York: Springer-Verlag; 1979.
31. Lazar ML, Clark K. Direct surgical management of masses in the region of the vein of Galen. Surg Neurol. 1974;2:17–21.
32. Page LK. The infratentorial-supracerebellar exposure of tumors in the pineal area. Neurosurgery. 1977;1:36–40.
33. Reid WS, Clark WK. Comparison of the infratentorial and transtentorial approaches to the pineal region. Neurosurgery. 1978;3:1–8.
34. Stein BM. The infratentorial supracerebellar approach to pineal lesions. J Neurosurg. 1971;35(2):197–202.

35. Ruge JR, Johnson RF, Bauer J. Burr hole neuroendoscopic fenestration of quadrigeminal cistern arachnoid cyst: technical case report. Neurosurgery. 1996;38(4):830–7.
36. Cardia A, Caroli M, Pluderi M, Arienta C, Gaini SM, Lanzino G, et al. Endoscope-assisted infratentorial-supracerebellar approach to the third ventricle: an anatomical study. J Neurosurg. 2006;104(6 Suppl):409–14.
37. Turtz AR, Hughes WB, Goldman HW. Endoscopic treatment of symptomatic pineal cyst: technical case report. Neurosurgery. 1995;37:1013–5.
38. Tirakotai W, Schulte DM, Bauer BL, Bertalanffy H, Hellwig D. Neuroendoscopic surgery of intracranial cysts in adults. Childs Nerv Syst. 2004;20:842–51.
39. Portillo ML, de Gonzalez CM, Sangines JB, et al. Pineal region tumors. Int Surg. 1982;67:329–33.
40. Hart MG, Santarius T, Kirollos RW. How I do it—pineal surgery: supracerebellar infratentorial versus occipital transtentorial. Acta Neurochir. 2013;155:463–7.
41. Elhadi AM, Zaidi HA, Hardesty DA, Williamson R, Cavallo C, Preul MC, Nakaji P, Little AS. Malleable endoscope increases surgical freedom when compared to a rigid endoscope in endoscopic endonasal approaches to the parasellar region. Neurosurgery. 2014;10:393–9.
42. Zaidi HA, Elhadi AM, Lei T, Preul MC, Little AS, Nakaji P. Minimally invasive endoscopic supracerebellar-Infratentorial surgery of the pineal region: anatomical comparison of four variant approaches. World Neurosurg. 2015. ISSN: 1878-8750.;84(2):257. https://doi.org/10.1016/j.wneu.2015.03.009.
43. Ferrer E, Santamarta D, Garcia-Fructuoso G, Caral L, Rumia J. Neuroendoscopic management of pineal region tumors. Acta Neurochir. 1997;139:12–20.
44. Choque-Velasquez J, Colasanti R, Collan J, Kinnunen R, Jahromi BR, Hernesniemi J. Virtual reality glasses and "eye-hands blind technique" for microsurgical training in neurosurgery. World Neurosurg. 2018;112:126–30.
45. Shahinian H, Ra Y. Fully endoscopic resection of pineal region tumors. J Neurol Surg B Skull Base. 2013;74(3):114–7.
46. Gu Y, Hu F, Zhang X. Purely endoscopic resection of pineal region tumors using infratentorial supracerebellar approach: how I do it. Acta Neurochir. 2016;158(11):2155–8.
47. Gu Y, Zhou Q, Zhu W, et al. The purely endoscopic supracerebellar infratentorial approach for resecting pineal region tumors with preservation of cerebellomesencephalic vein: technical note and preliminary clinical outcomes. World Neurosurg. 2019;128:e334–9.
48. Matsuo S, Baydin S, Gungor A, et al. Midline and off-midline infratentorial supracerebellar approaches to the pineal gland. J Neurosurg. 2016;126(6):1984–94.
49. Xin C, Xiong Z, Yan X, et al. Endoscopic-assisted surgery versus microsurgery for pineal region tumors: a single-center retrospective study. Neurosurg Rev. 2021;44(2):1017–22.
50. Cohen-Cohen S, Cohen-Gadol AA, Gomez-Amador JL, Alves-Belo JT, Shah KJ, Fernandez-Miranda JC. Supracerebellar infratentorial and occipital transtentorial approaches to the pulvinar: ipsilateral versus contralateral corridors. Oper Neurosurg (Hagerstown). 2019;16:351–9. https://doi.org/10.1093/ons/opy173.
51. Schroeder HW, Oertel J, Gaab MR. Endoscope-assisted microsurgical resection of epidermoid tumors of the cerebellopontine angle. J Neurosurg. 2004;101:227–32. https://doi.org/10.3171/jns.2004.101.2.0227.
52. Akiyama O, Matsushima K, Gungor A, Matsuo S, Goodrich DJ, Tubbs RS, et al. Microsurgical and endoscopic approaches to the pulvinar. J Neurosurg. 2017;127:630–45. https://doi.org/10.3171/2016.8.JNS16676.
53. Regis J, Bouillot P, Rouby-Volot F, et al. Pineal region tumors and the role of stereotactic biopsy: review of the mortality, morbidity, and diagnostic rates in 370 cases. Neurosurgery. 1996;39:907–12. [discussion: 912–4].
54. Choi JU, Kim DS, Chung SS, et al. Treatment of germ cell tumors in the pineal region. Childs Nerv Syst. 1998;14:41–8.
55. Bruce J. Pineal tumors. Winn H. Youman's neurological surgery. Philadelphia: WB Saunders Company; 2004. p. 1011–29.

56. Goodman RR. Magnetic resonance imaging-directed stereotactic endoscopic third ventriculostomy. Neurosurgery. 1993;32:1043–7.
57. Bruce JN, Stein BM. Surgical management of pineal region tumors. Acta Neurochir. 1995;134:130–5.
58. Dempsey PK, Kondziolka D, Lunsford LD. Stereotactic diagnosis and treatment of pineal region tumors and vascular malformations. Acta Neurochir. 1992;116:14–22.
59. Edwards MS, Hudgins RJ, Wilson CB, et al. Pineal region tumors in children. J Neurosurg. 1988;68:689–97.
60. Fauchon F, Jouvet A, Paquis P, et al. Parenchymal pineal tumors: a clinicopathological study of 76 cases. Int J Radiat Oncol Biol Phys. 2000;46:959–68.
61. Lapras C, Patet JD, Mottolese C, et al. Direct surgery for pineal tumors: occipital-transtentorial approach. Prog Exp Tumor Res. 1987;30:268–80.
62. Neuwelt EA. An update on the surgical treatment of malignant pineal region tumors. Clin Neurosurg. 1985;32:397–428.
63. Spazzapan P, Velnar T, Bosnjak R. Endoscopic supracerebellar infratentorial approach to pineal and posterior third ventricle lesions in prone position with head extension: a technical note. Neurol Res. 2020;42(12):1070–3.
64. Schonauer C, Jannelli G, Tessitore E, et al. Endoscopic resection of a low-grade ependymoma of the pineal region. Surg Neurol Int. 2021;12:279.
65. Hua W, Hao X, Zhang X, Guo Y, Wang X, Zhang J, Pan Z, Zhu W. Pure endoscopic resection of pineal region tumors through supracerebellar infratentorial approach with 'head-up' park-bench position. Neurol Res. 2023;45(4):354–62. https://doi.org/10.1080/01616412.2022.2146266.
66. Abecassis IJ, Hanak B, Barber J, et al. A single-institution experience with pineal region tumors: 50 tumors over 1 decade. Oper Neurosurg. 2017;13(5):566–75.

Chapter 16
Fully Endoscopic Retrosigmoid Approach for Cerebellopontine Angle Tumors

Mohamed Saied, Mustafa Najibullah, Zafdam Shabbir, Athary Saleem, Amjad Ali, and Waleed Abdelfattah Azab

16.1 Introduction

Advances in endoscopic technology have significantly contributed to the development and refinement of minimally invasive brain surgery. As a matter of fact, minimally invasive approaches are associated with lower complication profile, comparable or even better outcomes, better cosmetic results, and faster recovery times in comparison to the conventional approaches [1–3]. Fully endoscopic or endoscope-controlled approaches are essentially keyhole approaches in which rigid endoscopes are the sole visualization tools used during the whole procedure.

The term "keyhole surgery" was first coined in 1971 by Donald Wilson who elaborated on a variety of approaches for supratentorial pathologies in his technical note titled "Limited Exposure in Cerebral Surgery" that was then published in *Journal of Neurosurgery*. He employed small linear incisions and a 2-inch D'Errico trephine to create limited craniotomies that were yet sufficiently large to operate through. He pointed out that such operating methodology avoided unnecessary exposure of brain tissue and thus its potential damage [4]. Later, Axel Perneczky popularized the principle of keyhole surgery, especially the supraorbital keyhole approach, and demonstrated the importance of endoscopic assistance in these approaches through several published large series of vascular and tumor cases [1, 3, 5].

Endoscopic assistance in cranial surgery emerged out of the need to operate via small openings and yet obtain appropriate visualization and control of the structures

M. Saied
Neurosurgery Department, Ibn Sina Hospital, Al-Sabah Medical Area, Kuwait City, Kuwait

Neurosurgery Department, Faculty of Medicine, Benha University, Benha, Egypt

M. Najibullah · Z. Shabbir · A. Saleem · A. Ali · W. A. Azab (✉)
Neurosurgery Department, Ibn Sina Hospital, Al-Sabah Medical Area, Kuwait City, Kuwait

W. A. Azab (ed.), *Endoscope-controlled Transcranial Surgery*, Advances and Technical Standards in Neurosurgery 52,
https://doi.org/10.1007/978-3-031-61925-0_16

within the field—in other words, to perform a minimally invasive yet maximally effective surgery. At the early attempts of endoscope-assisted cranial surgery, it was noted that rigid endoscopes enabled overcoming the problem of suboptimal visualization when small exposures are used.

In 1974, Werner Prott, working then as an otosurgeon at the University of Würzburg, used a rigid endoscope to explore and operate within the cerebellopontine angle via a transpyramidal retrolabyrinthine approach through Trautmann's triangle. After a mastoidectomy, a bone flap with a diameter of 1 cm was made; then the endoscope was inserted through this narrow space between the sigmoid sinus, the superior petrosal sinus, the posterior semicircular canal, and the endolymphatic sac without damaging any functional structure of the inner ear or of the cerebellum [6]. In 1981, Falk Oppel and colleagues used a similar approach for sectioning the sensory root of trigeminal nerve, the glossopharyngeal nerve, and the cranial part of the vagus nerve to treat an intractable facial pain in a patient with recurrent upper jaw carcinoma [7]. Apuzzo and colleagues in 1977 described the use of Hopkins 70° and 120° side-viewing telescopes in a variety of approaches including intrasellar procedures by either the transsphenoidal or subfrontal routes to assist with visualization for complete gland ablation or total tumor excision. They also employed this endoscope-assisted strategy in aneurysm surgery while working in the vicinity of the circle of Willis, with particular emphasis on the assessment of adequacy and accuracy of clip placement, especially in lesions of the apex of the basilar artery [8].

Currently, the use of endoscopes in transcranial surgery can broadly be categorized into endochannel, endoscope-assisted, and endoscope-controlled or fully endoscopic approaches. In this chapter we present an overview of the literature and describe the surgical technique and nuances of the fully endoscopic retrosigmoid approach for cerebellopontine angle tumors.

16.2   Rationale for the Fully Endoscopic Technique

The technical specifications and design of the currently available rigid endoscopes are associated with a group of unique features that define the endoscopic view and lay the basis for its superiority over the microscopic view during brain surgery (Fig. 16.1).

When a rigid endoscope is inserted into the surgical field, a very highly illuminated area of interest is obtained because the light beam is completely brought inside the field without any loss of light energy at the edges of the craniotomy or cortical incision. Furthermore, the close proximity of the light source to the structures being viewed eliminates shadows within the field, adding to the extreme clarity of the endoscopic images. The superiority of the endoscopic view also

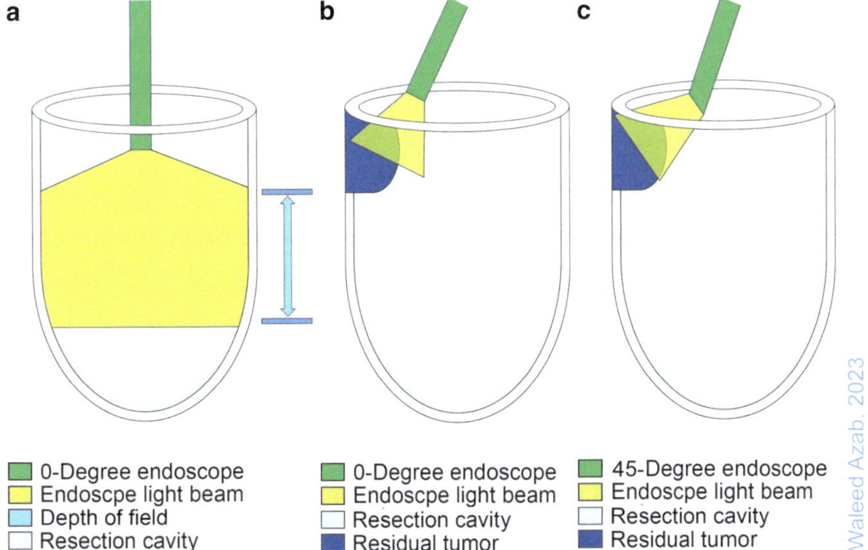

Fig. 16.1 The rationale for the purely endoscopic approach. (**a**) As the rigid endoscope is inserted into the surgical field, a very highly illuminated area of interest is obtained without any loss of light energy at the edges of the craniotomy. The proximity of the light source to the structures and greater depth of field adds to the extreme clarity of the endoscopic images. Angulating a 0° scope (**b**) and the use of angled scopes (**c**) bring concealed tumor remnants into view and obviate the need for retraction of neurovascular structures

results from the wide-angle view as well as the high color fidelity and image definition capabilities of today's state-of-the-art rigid endoscopes. In addition, rigid endoscopes are characterized by a greater depth of field. Therefore, the viewed objects remain in focus throughout a greater range of distances from the viewing lens. This means lesser need to adjust the focus of the endoscope during the procedure, and consequently a seamless operative workflow. The use of angled scopes also enables "looking around the corners" and thereby adds further to the efficacy and safety of the procedure as it brings concealed tumor remnants into view and obviates the need for retraction of neurovascular structures. On the contrary, the microscope in keyhole surgery requires frequent changing of the viewing angle to allow illumination and visualization of the area of interest deep in the surgical field, an inevitable consequence of the light source and the viewing lens being located outside the craniotomy. The loss of light energy at the edges of the small craniotomy and the dropped shadows on the structures within the field further contribute to the lesser quality of the microscopic view obtained during keyhole brain surgery [9].

The frequently raised concerns of endoscopic visualization include the lack of three-dimensionality, the need for familiarity with endoscopic devices, the need to develop eye–hand coordination, and the limitation of the operating range of movement of instruments [10]. These drawbacks are easily overcome by the surgeon's experience and are largely balanced by the superb image quality, increased radicality, and lower risk of complications that this form of surgery offers. In our opinion, rigid endoscopes are indispensable components of the array of surgical tools required to perform a keyhole brain surgery, and we firmly believe that they will eventually completely replace surgical microscopes for this type of surgery.

16.3   Endoscope-Controlled Surgery and the Cerebello-pontine Angle (CPA)

Several reports described the superior visualization of the neurovascular structures of the CPA with endoscopy compared with microscopy [11–14]. By carefully positioning the endoscope in the CPA, the anatomical features of the tumor, blood vessels, and nerves are clearly visualized. A wider surgical field, encompassing the supratentorial cistern, the cranial nerves, the surface between the tentorium and the cerebellum, and the contralateral field via the prepontine cistern, may be achieved by using different endoscopic viewing angles, rotating the endoscope, and adjusting its depth [14, 15]. A multitude of reports of endoscope-assisted CPA surgery demonstrated the success and benefits of this surgical philosophy in microvascular decompression [16–19], vestibular neurectomy [20, 21], and resection of various tumors such as epidermoid cysts [22], and vestibular schwannomas [23–25].

Notwithstanding, few series of purely endoscopic resection of CPA lesions are available in the literature [26–28]. From these series, the observed intraoperative benefits specifically pertinent to the endoscope-controlled retrosigmoid approach to CPA tumors will be summarized in the following paragraphs.

First, a clear advantage of using the endoscope during the circumferential extracapsular dissection of tumors was demonstrated. Angled optics enabled visualization of the "corners" and allowed dissection to proceed without the need for piecemeal removal necessary when using the surgical microscope. This advantage is even more important during dissection of the facial nerve from the tumor, since blunt and "blind" dissections are avoided [27, 29]. Second, the improved exposure of the entire tumor provided by the endoscope with minimal or no retraction reduces the risk of injury to the brain stem and the surrounding cranial nerves and results in a complete tumor removal. The more direct "keyhole" approach significantly decreases the time required for exposure of the tumor and the overall operative time [26, 27]. Third, an additional advantage of endoscopy is the "dynamic magnification" in which dynamic readjustments of the operative field are possible as the assistant surgeon holds and manipulates the angulation of the endoscope and its distance from the surgical target depending on the main surgeon's needs. This advantage is lost when the endoscope is fixed using a holder. One potential risk of utilizing dynamic magnification is that repetitive entry and exit of the endoscope into the CPA increases the risk of neurovascular injuries [29–31]. Fourth, angled endoscopes allow better visualization of the open mastoid cells, thus reducing the risk of inadvertent CSF fistula [32].

Notably, Setty et al. pointed out that endoscope alone, without the need for the operative microscope, can be safely used in hearing preservation surgery for vestibular schwannomas. In their report, facial nerve and hearing preservation were similar if not improved compared with other approaches while providing a smaller incision, lesser cranial opening, no cerebellar retraction, and less manipulation of the neurovascular structures [28]. Piloto et al. demonstrated that the fully endoscopic retrosigmoid keyhole approach achieved a greater degree of tumor resection and postoperative facial and auditory function preservation compared to the conventional approach. Facial paralysis was identified as the most frequent complication [33]. In a series of 44 patients, Parab et al. demonstrated that purely endoscopic keyhole retromastoid approach is feasible in addressing a variety of lesions in and around the CPA. Even large-sized tumors were resected with this approach. Out of 33 tumor cases, GTR and NTR were achieved in 97% of cases and STR was achieved in 3% of cases, with a facial nerve preservation rate of 90%. In all cases of MVD, facial nerve function was preserved [34]. A summary of the results achieved in various reports of endoscope-controlled retrosigmoid approach is presented in Tables 16.1 and 16.2.

We share the opinion of others pointing out that the improved visualization of the endoscope is ideal for operating in the intricate corridors of the CPA. It is imperative, however, that surgeons are very comfortable with the endoscope and CPA anatomy before attempting such a procedure [28].

Table 16.1 Endoscope-controlled retrosigmoid approach series: main outcome parameters

Ref.	No of cases	Pathology	Max. tumor diameter (cm)	EOR	Complications	Hearing preservation (Gardner–Robertson)	Facial nerve preservation (House–Brackmann)
Caballero-García et al. (2020)	40	31 VS (77.5%) 5 meningioma (12.5%) 2 cholesteatoma (5.0%) 2 metastases (5.0%)	3.4 cm (1.4–4.3)	GTR 28 (70.0%) NTR 9 (22.5%) STR 3 (7.5%)	– CSF fistula 1 (2.5%) – Surgical wound infection 1 (2.5%) – Pneumonia 1 (2.5%) – Hearing loss 3/8 patients (37.5%) – Facial nerve palsy 8 patients (20%)	5/8 (62.5%)	House–Brackmann grades I, II, and III (80.0%; 32/40)
Shahinian and Ra (2011)	527	VS	2.8 cm (0.3–5.8)	GTR 496 STR 31	– CSF leak 17 – Hydrocephalus/temporary ventricular catheter 1 – Exposure keratitis 9 – Recurrent/residual tumor 39 – Superficial wound infection 13	213/374 (57%)	House–Brackmann grades I and II (93%; 491/527) House–Brackmann grades III and IV (4%; 21/527) House–Brackmann grades V and VI (3%; 15/527)
Kabil and Shahinian (2006)	112	VS	2.6 cm (0.6–5.7)	GTR 106 STR 6	– CSF leak 3 – Hydrocephalus/temporary ventricular catheter 1 – Exposure keratitis 2 – Recurrence 1 – Superficial wound infection 3	59/101 (58%)	House–Brackmann grade I (87%; 97/112) House–Brackmann grade II (8%; 9/112) House–Brackmann grade III (5%; 6/112)

Setty et al. (2015)	12	VS	1.5 cm (1.0–2.0)	GTR 12 (100%)	– Recurrence 1 – Hearing deterioration 4/12 (33%)	8/12 (67%)	House–Brackmann grade I (92%; 11 of 12) House–Brackmann grade III (8%; 1/12)
Hu et al. (2016)	30	EP	NA	GTR (30) (100%)	– Communicating hydrocephalus 1 – Facial nerve paralysis 1 – Abducens nerve palsy 1	NA	NA
Parab et al. (2019)	44	Tumors 33 VS 14 LCNS 1 TS 1 EP 14 Meningioma 1 MCP cavernoma 1 Medulloblastoma 1 Vascular loop 11	3.47 cm (2–5)	GTR 20 NTR 12 STR 1	– CSF leak with meningitis 1 – New-onset facial paresis 12 – Transient facial hypoesthesia 2 – Transient abducens paresis 4 – Transient lower cranial nerve paresis 3 – Pseudomeningocele 1	30/33 11	NA NA

No switch to surgical microscope took place in any series

Table 16.2 Additional outcome parameters

Ref.	Mean operative time (min)	Average intraoperative bleeding (mL)	Hospital stay (days)
Caballero-García et al, (2020)	286.5	286.5	7.5
Shahinian and Ra (2011)	193	NA	2.4
Kabil and Shahinian (2006)	132	NA	2.2
Setty et al. (2015)	261.6	56.3	3.6
Hu et al. (2016)	2.61 h	96.8	7.5
Parab et al. (2019)	NA	NA	NA

16.4 Surgical Technique

16.4.1 Operating Room Setup

The operating room setup is illustrated in Fig. 16.2 and is geared toward achieving an unobstructed line of view of the endoscope monitor by the surgical team and ergonomically appropriate working space around the patient's head.

16.4.2 Endoscopic Equipment Setup and Ergonomics

The rigid endoscope (0°, 30°, or 45°) is connected to a 4K endoscopic camera and inserted into the suction–irrigation sheath. The assembly is fixed to a holding mechanical arm (KARL STORZ, Germany) or to an intuitively movable manual support arm (ENDOFIX exo, AKTORmed, Germany). The endoscope holding arm is fixed opposite to the surgeon across the operating table. The endoscope tower and monitor are positioned on one side of the operating table so that a straight line of view by the operating surgeon is established (Fig. 16.2). At the initial phase of the procedure, the endoscope is fixed in an exoscopic position and is later inserted through the craniotomy as tumor resection proceeds. At some points, the endoscope is held free hand by the assistant surgeon.

16.4.3 Positioning

The patient is positioned in lateral or three-quarter prone position with the head elevated 30° above the level of the heart and fixed in three-pin head clamp (Fig. 16.2).

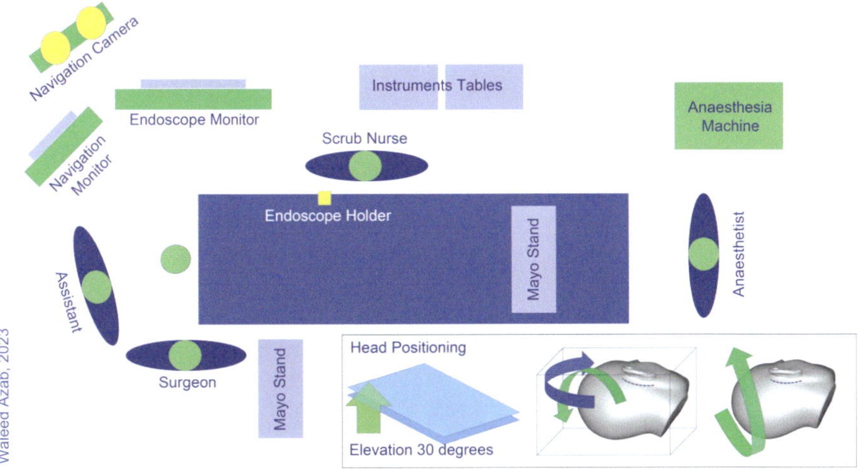

Fig. 16.2 The operating room setup for purely endoscopic retrosigmoid approach

16.4.4   Scalp Incision and Craniotomy

A 4–5 cm retroauricular incision is performed down to the bone. Fish-hook retractors are used to retract the scalp. The use of fish-hooks is very important because of its low profile which helps achieving much less crowded field and allows more space for endoscope shaft and instrument manipulation. Using the asterion as a bony landmark, a craniotomy flap is performed at the confluence of the sigmoid and transverse sinuses in the standard fashion, taking care to benefit maximally from the confines of the scalp incision.

16.4.5   Tumor Resection

A standard microsurgical technique is followed for tumor resection, hemostasis, and closure. Many of these technical aspects are demonstrated in the following representative case.

16.5   Representative Case

A 45-year-old female patient presented with 1-year history of progressively severe headaches, unsteady gait, hoarseness of voice, and dysphagia. She was treated 7 months earlier at another institution where an attempt of resection of a lesion

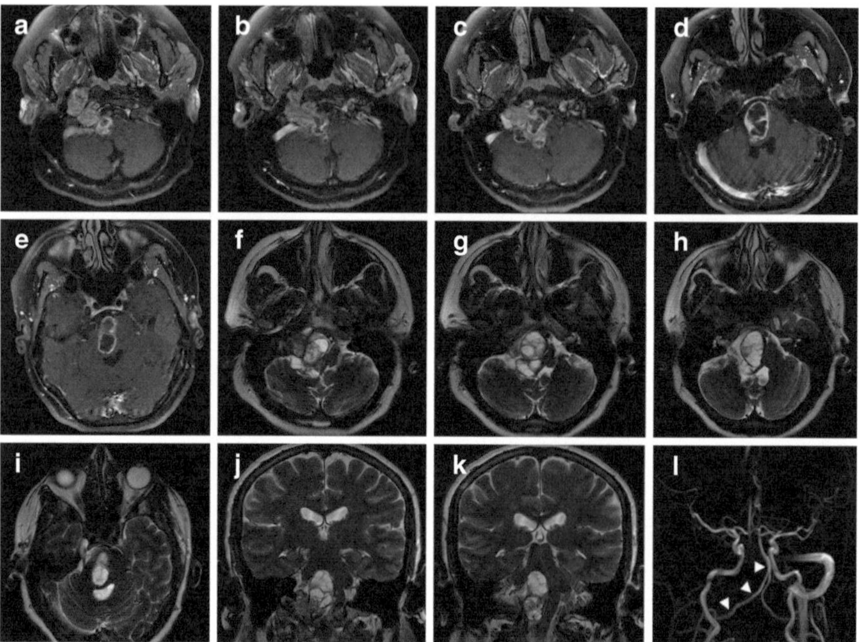

Fig. 16.3 Representative case. Preoperative MRI in a case of right hypoglossal schwannoma. Serial axial T1-weighted FSPGR post-contrast MR images revealed a large partially cystic mass occupying both the cerebellomedullary and cerebellopontine cisterns on the right side. The mass traverses the right hypoglossal canal and exerts significant compression of the brain stem (**a–e**). Serial axial (**f–i**) and coronal (**j, k**) T2-weighted MR images demonstrate similar findings along with evidence of hemorrhage within the cystic components. MRA demonstrated displacement of the right vertebral artery, vertebrobasilar junction, and proximal basilar artery (arrowheads, **l**). (Modified from Azab W, 2022 [35] with permission)

occupying the right cerebello-pontine and cerebello-medullary angles was unsuccessful and a ventriculoperitoneal shunt was inserted for associated hydrocephalus. Neurological exam revealed right cranial nerves IX through XII palsies and bilaterally exaggerated deep tendon reflexes more on the left side. Right upper limb intention tremor and horizontal nystagmus were also detected. Preoperative MR images (Fig. 16.3) revealed a large partially cystic hypoglossal schwannoma occupying both the cerebellomedullary and cerebellopontine cisterns on the right side. The mass traversed the right hypoglossal canal with significant compression of the brain stem. An endoscope-controlled right retrosigmoid approach was performed to excise the intracranial part of the tumor. Intraoperative images of the procedure are demonstrated in Figs. 16.4, 16.5, and 16.6. An operative case report of the procedure was previously published by our group [35]. Postoperative MRI is shown in Fig. 16.7.

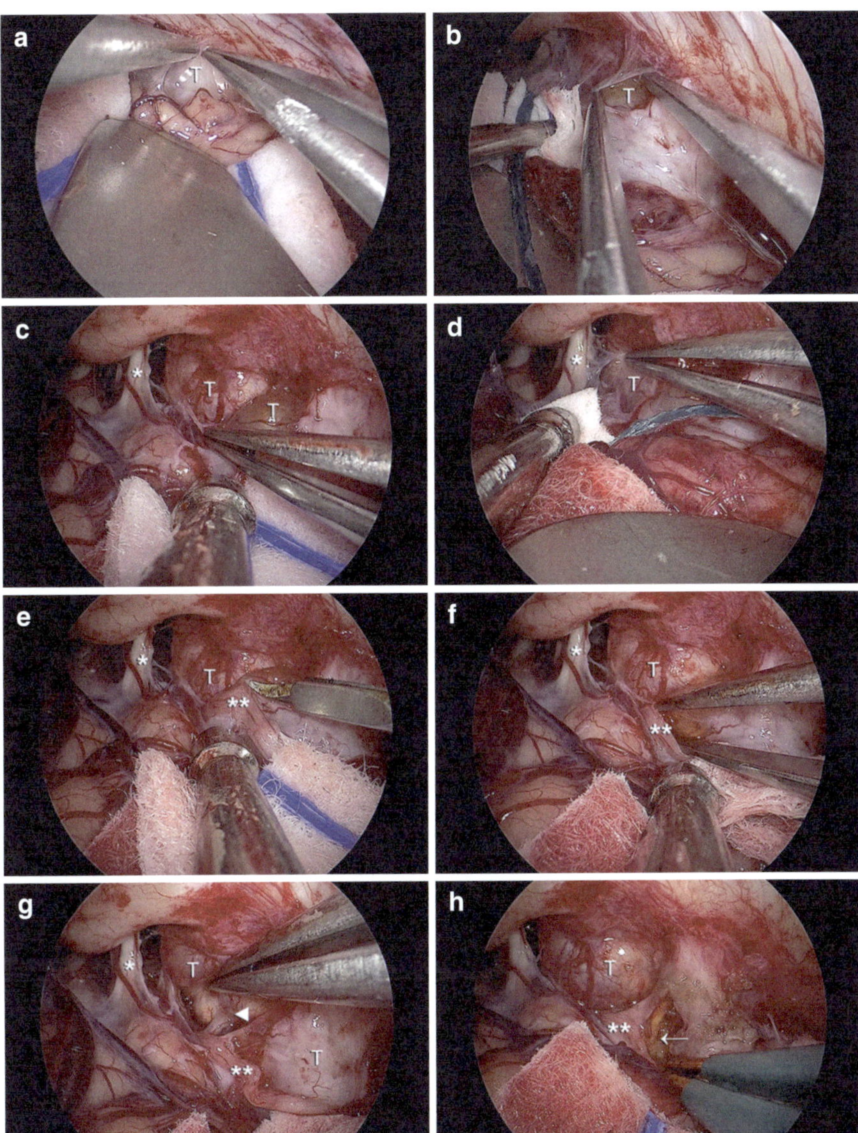

Fig. 16.4 Representative case. Initial tumor exposure at the right CP angle. The arachnoid is dissected off the tumor surface in (**a–c**) and from CN VII–VIII (**d**). The spinal accessory nerve is sharply dissected from the tumor capsule (**e, f**). The spinal accessory nerve is seen dipping into the tumor substance (arrowhead, **g**). One cystic component of the tumor is open, its content (arrow) is evacuated, and the capsule is bipolar coagulated (**h**). (Modified from Azab W, 2022 [35] with permission)

(*T* Tumor; *asterisk*, CN VII–VIII; *double asterisk*, spinal accessory nerve)

M. Saied et al.

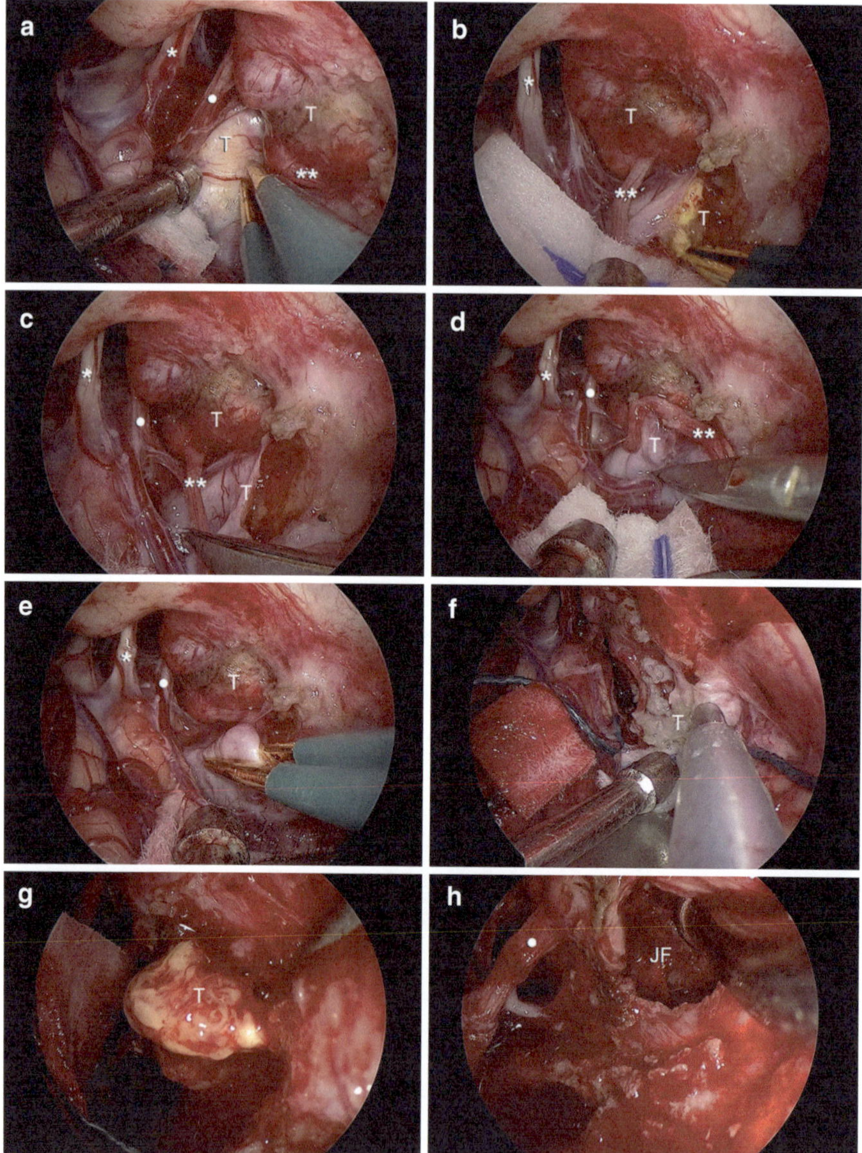

Fig. 16.5 Representative case. Tumor dissection and debulking are further continued (**a–h**) with further exposure of CN IX–X and resection of the tumor components within the jugular foramen. (Modified from Azab W, 2022 [35] with permission)
(*T* Tumor; *asterisk*, CN VII–VIII; *double asterisk*, spinal accessory nerve; *JF* Jugular foramen; *white circle*, CN IX–X)

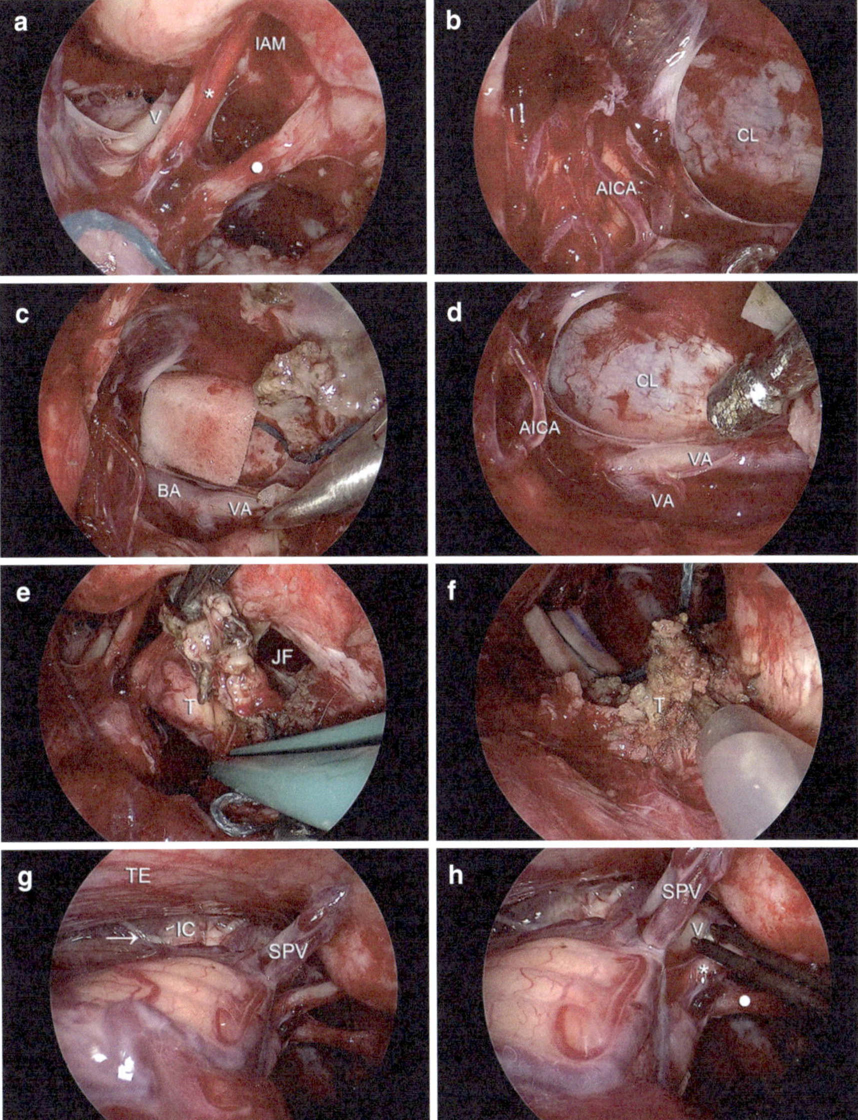

Fig. 16.6 Representative case. Final stages of tumor resection (**a–h**). Panoramic views of the cranial nerves IV to IX–X and vertebrobasilar junction are demonstrated as tumor excision is finalized. (Modified from Azab W, 2022 [35] with permission)
(*AICA* Anterior inferior cerebellar artery; *BA* Basilar artery, *CL* Clivus, *IAM* Internal acoustic meatus, *IC* Inferior colliculus, *TE* Tentorium, *V* Trigeminal nerve, *VA* Vertebral artery, *T* Tumor, *asterisk*, CN VII–VIII; *white circle*, CN IX–X)

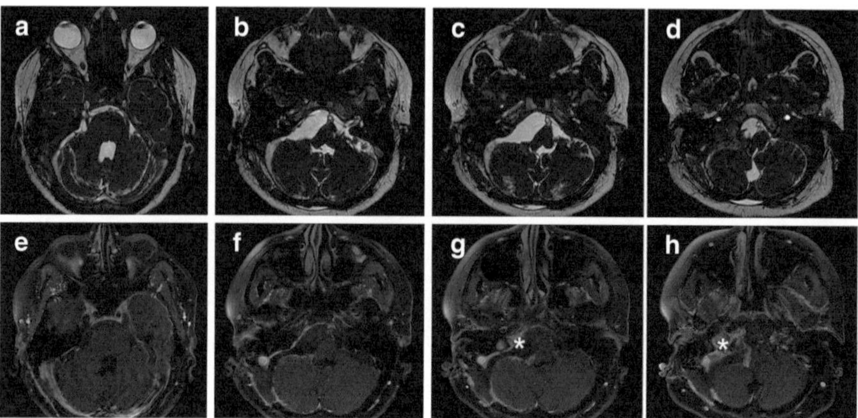

Fig. 16.7 Representative case. Postoperative axial T2-weighted (**a–d**) and axial FSPGR post-contrast images (**e–h**) demonstrating resection of the intracranial tumor except for the tumor adherent to the transverse sinus (asterisk). (Modified from Azab W, 2022 [35] with permission)

References

1. van Lindert E, Perneczky A, Fries G, Pierangeli E. The supraorbital keyhole approach to supratentorial aneurysms: concept and technique. Surg Neurol. 1998;49:481–90.
2. Ottenhausen M, Rumalla K, Alalade AF, Nair P, La Corte E. Decision-making algorithm for minimally invasive approaches to anterior skull base meningiomas. Neurosurg Focus. 2018;44(4):E7. https://doi.org/10.3171/2018.1.FOCUS17734.
3. Perneczky A, Müller-Forell W, van Lindert E, Fries G. Keyhole concept in neurosurgery: with endoscope-assisted microsurgery and case studies. 1st ed. Stuttgart: Thieme Medical Publishers; 1999.
4. Wilson DH. Limited exposure in cerebral surgery: technical note. J Neurosurg. 1971;34:102–6. https://doi.org/10.3171/jns.1971.34.1.0102.
5. Fries G, Perneczky A. Endoscope-assisted brain surgery—part 2—analysis of 380 procedures. Neurosurgery. 1998;42(2):226–32.
6. Prott W. Cisternoscopy—endoscopy of the cerebellopontine angle. Acta Neurochir. 1974;31:105–13. https://doi.org/10.1007/BF01432786.
7. Oppel F, Mulch G, Brock M. Endoscopic section of the sensory trigeminal root, the glossopharyngeal nerve, and the cranial part of the vagus for intractable facial pain caused by upper jaw carcinoma. Surg Neurol. 1981;16(2):92–5. https://doi.org/10.1016/0090-3019(81)90102-6.
8. Apuzzo ML, Heifetz MD, Weiss MH, Kurze T. Neurosurgical endoscopy using the side-viewing telescope. J Neurosurg. 1977;46(3):398–400. https://doi.org/10.3171/jns.1977.46.3.0398.
9. Azab WA, Elmaghraby MA, Zaidan SN, Mostafa KH. Endoscope-assisted transcranial surgery for anterior skull base meningiomas. Mini-invasive. Surgery. 2020;4:88.
10. Linsler S, Fischer G, Skliarenko V, Stadie A, Oertel J. Endoscopic assisted supraorbital keyhole approach or endoscopic endonasal approach in cases of tuberculum sellae meningioma: which surgical route should be favored? World Neurosurg. 2017;104:601–11. https://doi.org/10.1016/j.wneu.2017.05.023.
11. Borucki L, Szyfter W, Leszczyńska M. Microscopy and endoscopy of the cerebellopontine angle in the retrosigmoid approach [in Polish]. Otolaryngol Pol. 2004;58(3):509–15.
12. Cappabianca P, Cavallo LM, Esposito F, de Divitiis E, Tschabitscher M. Endoscopic examination of the cerebellar pontine angle. Clin Neurol Neurosurg. 2002;104(4):387–91.

13. Takemura Y, Inoue T, Morishita T, Rhoton AL Jr. Comparison of microscopic and endoscopic approaches to the cerebellopontine angle. World Neurosurg. 2014;82(3–4):427–41.
14. Van Rompaey J, Bush C, McKinnon B, Solares AC. Minimally invasive access to the posterior cranial fossa: an anatomical study comparing a retrosigmoidal endoscopic approach to a microscopic approach. J Neurol Surg A Cent Eur Neurosurg. 2013;74(1):1–6.
15. Hu Z, Guan F, Kang T, et al. Whole course neuroendoscopic resection of cerebellopontine angle epidermoid cysts. J Neurol Surg A Cent Eur Neurosurg. 2016;77(5):381–8. https://doi.org/10.1055/s-0035-1558818.
16. Broggi M, Ferroli P, Acerbi F, Tringali G, Franzini A, Broggi G. The value of endoscopy in microvascular decompression procedures. Neurosurgery. 2012;71(2):E564.
17. Chen MJ, Zhang WJ, Yang C, Wu YQ, Zhang ZY, Wang Y. Endoscopic neurovascular perspective in microvascular decompression of trigeminal neuralgia. J Craniomaxillofac Surg. 2008;36(8):456–61.
18. Duntze J, Litré CF, Eap C, et al. Adjunctive use of endoscopy during microvascular decompression in the cerebellopontine angle: 27 case reports [in French]. Neurochirurgie. 2011;57(2):68–72.
19. El-Garem HF, Badr-El-Dine M, Talaat AM, Magnan J. Endoscopy as a tool in minimally invasive trigeminal neuralgia surgery. Otol Neurotol. 2002;23(2):132–5.
20. Miyazaki H, Deveze A, Magnan J. Neuro-otologic surgery through minimally invasive retrosigmoid approach: endoscope assisted microvascular decompression, vestibular neurotomy, and tumor removal. Laryngoscope. 2005;115(9):1612–7.
21. Cutler AR, Kaloostian SW, Ishiyama A, Frazee JG. Two-handed endoscopic-directed vestibular nerve sectioning: case series and review of the literature. J Neurosurg. 2012;117(3):507–13.
22. Schroeder HWS, Oertel J, Gaab MR. Endoscope-assisted microsurgical resection of epidermoid tumors of the cerebellopontine angle. J Neurosurg. 2004;101(2):227–32.
23. Goksu N, Bayazit Y, Kemaloglu Y. Endoscopy of the posterior fossa and endoscopic dissection of acoustic neuroma. Neurosurg Focus. 1999;6(4):e15.
24. Magnan J, Chays A, Cohen JM, Caces F, Locatelli P. Endoscopy of the cerebellopontine angle. Rev Laryngol Otol Rhinol (Bord). 1995;116(2):115–8.
25. Wackym PA, King WA, Poe DS, et al. Adjunctive use of endoscopy during acoustic neuroma surgery. Laryngoscope. 1999;109(8):1193–201.
26. Shahinian HK, Eby JB, Ocon M. Fully endoscopic excision of vestibular schwannomas. Minim Invas Neurosurg. 2004;47:329–32.
27. Kabil MS, Shahinian HK. A series of 112 fully endoscopic resections of vestibular schwannomas. Minim Invas Neurosurg. 2006;49:362–8.
28. Setty P, D'Andrea KP, Stucken EZ, Babu S, LaRouere MJ, Pieper DR. Endoscopic resection of vestibular schwannomas. J Neurol Surg B Skull Base. 2015;76(3):230–8. https://doi.org/10.1055/s-0034-1543974.
29. Caballero-García J, Morales-Pérez I, Michel-Giol-Álvarez A, Aparicio-García C, López-Sánchez M, Huanca-Amaru J. Endoscopic retrosigmoid keyhole approach in cerebellopontine angle tumors. A surgical cohort. Neurocirugia (Astur:Engl Ed). 2020:S1130-1473(20)30127-5. English, Spanish. https://doi.org/10.1016/j.neucir.2020.10.001.
30. de Divitiis O, Cavallo LM, Dal Fabbro M, Elefante A, Cappabianca P. Freehand dynamic endoscopic resection of an epidermoid tumor of the cerebellopontine angle: technical case report. Neurosurgery. 2007;61:E239–40.
31. Dubernard X, Kleiber J-C, Makeieff M, Bazin A, Chays A. Drilling and control of the internal auditory canal by fixed endoscope. Eur Ann Otorhinolaryngol Head Neck Dis. 2019;136:37–9. https://doi.org/10.1016/j.anorl.2018.09.005.
32. Cohen NL. Retrosigmoid approach for acoustic tumor removal. Otolaryngol Clin N Am. 1992;25:295–310.
33. Piloto OL, Hernández TM, Barreto GT, Flores CD, Ayala OL, Garcia ET. Endoscopic keyhole and microsurgery approach to cerebellopontine angle tumors: surgical outcomes. Mathews J Case Rep. 2020;5(2):65.

34. Parab A, Khatri D, Singh S, et al. Endoscopic keyhole retromastoid approach in neurosurgical practice: ant-man's view of the neurosurgical marvel. World Neurosurg. 2019;126:e982–8. https://doi.org/10.1016/j.wneu.2019.02.203.
35. Azab WA. Purely endoscopic retrosigmoid approach for excision of a large multicystic hypoglossal schwannoma. World Neurosurg. 2022;168:133. https://doi.org/10.1016/j.wneu.2022.09.108.

Chapter 17
Endoscopic Microvascular Decompression

Sonia Ajmera, Rachel Blue, and John Y. K. Lee

17.1 History of Microvascular Decompression

Microvascular decompression for cranial neuropathy was first described in the 1920s by Walter Dandy. Dandy postulated that the lancinating facial pain of trigeminal neuralgia, formerly titled "tic douloureux" by Nicolas André in 1756, resulted from proximal compression of the trigeminal nerve near the root entry zone and thus decompression at this location could offer relief. His theory was controversial and met with much skepticism during his time, but the work was ultimately carried forward in the 1950s by Palle Taarnhøj in Denmark and by W. James Gardner at the University of Pennsylvania. Gardner also performed the first decompression for hemifacial spasm. Decompressions were performed without the use of the microscope, which changed when Peter Jannetta performed the first microscopic retromastoid craniotomy for trigeminal neuralgia at Harbor General Hospital in 1957 [1]. Since then, microvascular decompression (MVD) has been recognized as an effective treatment not only for trigeminal neuralgia but also for hemifacial spasm, genicular neuralgia, glossopharyngeal neuralgia, and other associated

S. Ajmera (✉)
Department of Neurosurgery, Hospital of the University of Pennsylvania,
Philadelphia, PA, USA

Department of Neurosurgery, University of Pennsylvania, Perelman Center for Advanced
Medicine, Philadelphia, PA, USA
e-mail: sonia.ajmera@pennmedicine.upenn.edu

R. Blue · J. Y. K. Lee
Department of Neurosurgery, Hospital of the University of Pennsylvania,
Philadelphia, PA, USA
e-mail: rachel.blue@pennmedicine.upenn.edu; john.lee3@pennmedicine.upenn.edu

© The Author(s), under exclusive license to Springer Nature
Switzerland AG 2024
W. A. Azab (ed.), *Endoscope-controlled Transcranial Surgery*, Advances and
Technical Standards in Neurosurgery 52,
https://doi.org/10.1007/978-3-031-61925-0_17

cranial pain syndromes. The most common arterial sources of compression are the supracerebellar artery for trigeminal neuralgia, the anterior inferior cerebellar artery for hemifacial spasm and geniculate neuralgia, and the posterior inferior cerebellar artery for glossopharyngeal neuralgia.

17.2 Microscopic Approach

Classically, MVDs have been performed using a microscope, a surgical adjunct with which neurosurgeons are very familiar. The microscope offers a wide, three-dimensional view of the surgical field; however, visualization of the target area requires direct line of sight. As such, if intracranial structures, such as the petrous tubercle, are obstructing the view of the nerve of interest, manipulation of these tissues may be necessary intraoperatively to obtain the optimal view. In contrast, the endoscope allows visualization "around" obstructing structures without removal. Furthermore, when using the microscope, the depth of field (what is in focus from proximal to distal) becomes increasingly smaller as magnification increases, an issue commonly encountered when visualizing deep structures such as the root entry zones of cranial nerves. In contrast, the endoscope provides superior depth of field with more critical structures in focus throughout the surgery. Given the limitations of the microscope, the endoscope has been employed with increasing success for microvascular decompression.

17.3 Introduction of the Endoscope

Endoscopy has been widely implemented in anterior skull base and ventricular surgery as a minimally invasive visual augmentation tool. Described by Magnan in 1994, the distal light and panoramic view offered by endoscopes allow expansion of visualization without as much tissue manipulation necessary to obtain the direct line of sight needed by the microscope [2]. Furthermore, the use of angled scopes introduces the possibility of accessing structures that are difficult or impossible to see using the microscope [3]. In the late 1990s and early 2000s, several reports of combined endoscopic and microscopic (aka endoscope-assisted) approaches for MVD for trigeminal neuralgia and hemifacial spasm were described [4–7]. These experiences noted the utility in endoscopic confirmation of microscopic findings and, more importantly, the identification of vascular compression sites that were missed by views offered by the microscope. In 2008, Chen and colleagues found that almost 15% of sites of neurovascular compression were being missed with microscopic use and subsequently caught with endoscopic assistance [7]. Furthermore, cleavage planes between nerves were more easily identified, while cerebellar and brain stem retraction was minimal [8]. Fully endoscopic MVD without the use of a microscope was pioneered by several independent neurosurgeons. In 2001, one of the first reports of fully endoscopic microvascular decompression (E-MVD) was described by Eby and Shahinian, who used the endoscope alone in patients with hemifacial spasm [9]. Dr. Shahinian in Los Angeles continued to publish his results in a series of papers, including reports on endoscopic decompression of the trigeminal and glossopharyngeal nerves [10, 11]. In 2005, a comparative retrospective analysis was conducted by Kabil and Shahinian, showing endoscopic decompression offered higher rates of neuralgia relief secondary to improved visualization and lower rates of complications compared to microscopic decompressions [12]. In 2008, Pieper and colleauges in Michigan described a large series of MVDs performed in conjunction with otolaryngologists at the Michigan Ear Institute [13]. Dr. Hae-Dong Jho collaborated with Dr. Peter Jannetta in Pittsburgh to perform E-MVDs; however his series was not published. The first large series of fully endoscopic MVDs performed at an academic center by a neurosurgeon was by Dr. John Lee at the University of Pennsylvania [3, 14–16]. The views offered by endoscopy allow for smaller incisions and craniotomies, with increased surgeon experience allowing even more reduction of the exposure necessary [17, 18]. E-MVD patients have also been reported to have reduced lengths of stay and lower rates of post-operative headaches at 1 month [13, 14].

Based on the success of individual surgeons at individual centers, meta-analysis reviews have been conducted confirming the benefits of fully endoscopic MVD. A 2008 meta-analysis by Zagzoog highlighted shortened operative times, lower rates of hearing loss and facial paralysis, lower rates of recurrence, and smaller craniotomies in E-MVD patients [19]. In a 2021 meta-analysis conducted by Zhao and colleagues, E-MVD had significantly higher rates of detection of compressive vasculature, lower complication rates including hearing loss and facial paralysis, and lower neuralgia recurrence rates [20]. Several studies have shown that when surgeons are comfortable with endoscopy, E-MVD can have superior outcomes compared to MVD for treatment of proximal cranial nerve vascular compression [21–25].

Despite E-MVD's advantages, limitations do exist. The loss of three-dimensional depth perception offered by endoscopy is a major limitation compared to the microscope, and surgeon experience will dictate comfort with manipulation of the endoscope in the lateral skull base. Furthermore, the visual field offered by the endoscope is limited to the structures anterior to the tip of the scope, necessitating caution when introducing or removing instruments from the field to avoid injury to tissues outside of the field of view. The endoscope is susceptible to condensation when in the surgical cavity, an issue not encountered with microscopes. Depending on surgical technique, maneuverability can be limited using the endoscope.

17.4 Endoscopic Microvascular Decompression: Operative Technique and Post-operative Care

The technique described is utilized at the authors' institution [15], with alternative reported techniques noted as well.

17.4.1 Positioning

The patient is placed in a lateral position. At our institution, rigid fixation with a Mayfield head clamp is not utilized, although use of a Mayfield clamp is traditional for cranial fixation for E-MVD. Once in the lateral position, the patient's head is placed on a donut pillow with the vertex extended 10°. The head is circumferentially secured with silk tape. The ipsilateral shoulder is pulled caudally away from the operative area and taped in place [26]. Neuromonitoring of the cranial nerves is utilized throughout the case [16, 27]. The bed is turned 90°, with the endoscope monitor placed across from the surgeon next to anesthesia. A pneumatic arm is attached to the bed (at the head of the bed superior to the arm board) to hold the endoscope in place during the endoscopic portion of the case, freeing both of the surgeon's hands for microsurgical dissection.

17.4.2 Incision and Craniotomy

A postauricular 4 cm linear incision is planned based on key anatomic landmarks: transverse and sigmoid sinuses, the insertion of the digastric muscle, and the tip of the mastoid process. The fascia and muscle are dissected down to the bone. A burr hole is centered inferior and posterior to the transverse-sigmoid junction and expanded until the inferior transverse and posterior sigmoid borders are identified. Mastoid air cells are opacified with bone wax during the exposure to prevent cerebrospinal fluid (CSF) leak post-operatively. Hemostasis is achieved prior to dural opening.

17.4.3 Dural Opening and Endoscope Setup

A 1-cm-wide C-shaped dural opening is made and reflected anteriorly toward the sigmoid sinus. Some centers opt for a cruciate dural opening [18]. The dura is held in place with a tack-up suture. The endoscope is attached to the pneumatic arm and introduced into the field. The 2.7 mm 0° endoscope (KARL STORZ; El Segundo, CA, USA) is preferred by the authors for its smaller diameter. Angled scopes are also readily available and used if needed. The endoscope is kept at the superior vertex of the surgeon's working corridor, allowing inferolateral entry of instruments on either side. This triangular orientation is maintained to prevent instruments from clashing into the endoscope. If needed, the endoscope can be removed from the pneumatic arm and held in one hand, allowing instrumentation with the other.

17.4.4 Intracranial Exposure

A cottonoid patty is placed on a piece of Duraprene glove to protect the cerebellum during exposure. The endoscope is introduced in the dural opening and the patty and glove are advanced with gentle cerebellar retraction. The suction is held in the non-dominant hand with microinstruments held in the dominant hand. Sharp arachnoid dissection is performed to expose the cerebellopontine and cerebellomedullary cisterns. Enough CSF is released to allow brain relaxation and minimize retraction; aggressive drainage should be avoided to prevent brain sag and stretch on neurovascular elements. Small blood vessels should be dissected away and carefully coagulated using low bipolar cautery only when necessary, taking care to avoid surrounding nerves. Commonly encountered obstacles in adequate exposure to the trigeminal nerve include the suprameatal tubercle, which the endoscope can be advanced to see around or alternatively can be drilled for enhanced visualization, and the superior petrosal vein [28]. The safety of sacrificing the superior petrosal vein has been previously published; however, it should be protected when able [18, 29]. The endoscopic lens is susceptible to obscuring by surgical debris or condensation and should be cleaned as needed.

17.4.5 Identification and Treatment of Vascular Compression

As arachnoid dissection is performed, the vestibulocochlear and facial nerve complex is typically the first to be identified, with the trigeminal nerve being medial and cranial to this complex, closer to the tentorium. The glossopharyngeal, vagus, and accessory nerves are found more caudally. Once the cranial nerve of interest is identified, microdissecting instruments are used to explore sites of vascular compression. The offending vessel(s) should be mobilized off the nerve. A Teflon pad is placed between the vessel(s) and nerve. If no offending vessel is identified, neurolysis is performed. Hemostasis is ensured prior to closure.

17.4.6 Closure

Given the risk of CSF leak in the posterior fossa, tight dural closure is achieved using primary repair, muscle patches, a dural graft such as DuraGen (Integra; Plainsboro, NJ, USA), and a dural sealant such as Adherus (Stryker; Durham, NC, USA). Bone cement such as CRANIOS REINFORCED Fast Set Putty (DePuy Synthes; West Chester, PA, USA) is used to repair the craniotomy defect. Titanium mesh is an alternative option [18]. The wound is copiously irrigated. A multilayer muscular, facial, subcutaneous, and dermal closure is performed.

17.4.7 Bailouts

The surgeon must ensure the craniotomy is advanced to the inferior aspect of the transverse sinus and the posterior aspect of the sigmoid sinus. Doing so allows further dural opening if increased exposure is needed. Subsequently, additional CSF drainage from the cisterns can provide cerebellar relaxation and open the surgical corridor further. Angled scopes should be available if the view is limited using a 0° scope [30]. If technical difficulties are encountered using the endoscope, the surgeon can convert to the microscope. Hemostasis should be meticulously maintained throughout the case and hemostatic agents should be readily available if needed.

17.4.8 Complications

Possible post-operative complications are similar to those encountered with use of the microscope, including the following: hemorrhage, infection, cerebrospinal fluid leak, pseudomeningocele, wound breakdown, transient or permanent cranial neuropathy, cerebellar injury, stroke, or death.

17.4.9 Post-Operative Care

In uncomplicated cases, patients are monitored on the neurosurgical floor or intensive care unit, depending on support staff comfort and resources, with frequent initial neurological examinations. No post-operative imaging is obtained unless there is clinical concern. Typical post-operative symptoms can include headache, incisional pain, neck stiffness, muscle spasms, nausea, and vomiting, which are all managed medically. Physical and occupational therapy consultations occur on post-operative day 1. Patients are typically discharged on post-operative day 2 or 3.

17.5 Conclusion

Endoscopy is a safe and effective tool for microvascular decompression of cranial nerves at the brain stem. The visualization offered by the panoramic views of the endoscope can reveal sources of cranial nerve compression not otherwise seen with microscope use. If comfortable with endoscope use, surgeons can achieve excellent outcomes with better identification of compressive vessels, minimal brain stem and cerebellar retraction, smaller incisions and craniotomies, and minimal post-operative complications.

References

1. Patel SK, Markosian C, Choudhry OJ, Keller JT, Liu JK. The historical evolution of microvascular decompression for trigeminal neuralgia: from Dandy's discovery to Jannetta's legacy. Acta Neurochir. 2020;162(11):2773–82. https://doi.org/10.1007/s00701-020-04405-7. Epub 2020 Jun 9.
2. Magnan J, Chays A, Lepetre C, Pencroffi E, Locatelli P. Surgical perspectives of endoscopy of the cerebellopontine angle. Am J Otol. 1994;15(3):366–70.
3. Halpern CH, Lang S, Lee JYK. Fully endoscopic microvascular decompression: our early experience. Minim Invasive Surg. 2013;2013:739432.
4. Abdeen K, Kato Y, Kiya N, Yoshida K, Kanno T. Neuroendoscopy in microvascular decompression for trigeminal neuralgia and hemifacial spasm: technical note. Neurol Res. 2000;22(5):522–6. https://doi.org/10.1080/01616412.2000.11740712.
5. Caces F, Chays A, Locatelli P, Bruzzo M, Epron JP, Fiacre E, Magnan J. Décompression neuro-vasculaire dans le spasme de l'hémiface: résultats anatomiques, électrophysiologiques et thérapeutiques à propos de 100 cas [Neuro-vascular decompression in hemifacial spasm: anatomical, electrophysiological and therapeutic results apropos of 100 cases]. Rev Laryngol Otol Rhinol (Bord). 1996;117(5):347–51. French.
6. Jarrahy R, Berci G, Shahinian HK. Endoscope-assisted microvascular decompression of the trigeminal nerve. Otolaryngol Head Neck Surg. 2000;123(3):218–23. https://doi.org/10.1067/mhn.2000.107451.
7. Chen MJ, Zhang WJ, Yang C, Wu YQ, Zhang ZY, Wang Y. Endoscopic neurovascular perspective in microvascular decompression of trigeminal neuralgia. J Craniomaxillofac Surg. 2008;36(8):456–61. https://doi.org/10.1016/j.jcms.2008.05.002. Epub 2008 Jul 10.
8. King WA, Wackym PA, Sen C, Meyer GA, Shiau J, Deutsch H. Adjunctive use of endoscopy during posterior fossa surgery to treat cranial neuropathies. Neurosurgery. 2001;49(1):108–15; discussion 115–6. https://doi.org/10.1097/00006123-200107000-00017.
9. Eby JB, Cha ST, Shahinian HK. Fully endoscopic vascular decompression of the facial nerve for hemifacial spasm. Skull Base. 2001;11(3):189–97. https://doi.org/10.1055/s-2001-16607.
10. Jarrahy R, Cha ST, Eby JB, Berci G, Shahinian HK. Fully endoscopic vascular decompression of the glossopharyngeal nerve. J Craniofac Surg. 2002;13(1):90–5. https://doi.org/10.1097/00001665-200201000-00021.
11. Jarrahy R, Eby JB, Cha ST, Shahinian HK. Fully endoscopic vascular decompression of the trigeminal nerve. Minim Invasive Neurosurg. 2002;45(1):32–5. https://doi.org/10.1055/s-2002-23586.
12. Kabil MS, Eby JB, Shahinian HK. Endoscopic vascular decompression versus microvascular decompression of the trigeminal nerve. Minim Invasive Neurosurg. 2005;48(4):207–12. https://doi.org/10.1055/s-2005-870928.
13. Artz GJ, Hux FJ, Larouere MJ, Bojrab DI, Babu S, Pieper DR. Endoscopic vascular decompression. Otol Neurotol. 2008;29(7):995–1000. https://doi.org/10.1097/MAO.0b013e318184601a.
14. Lee JYK, Pierce JT, Sandhu SK, Petrov D, Yang AI. Endoscopic versus microscopic microvascular decompression for trigeminal neuralgia: equivalent pain outcomes with possibly decreased postoperative headache after endoscopic surgery. J Neurosurg. 2017;126(5):1676–84. https://doi.org/10.3171/2016.5.JNS1621. Epub 2016 Jul 29.
15. Piazza M, Lee JY. Endoscopic and microscopic microvascular decompression. Neurosurg Clin N Am. 2016;27(3):305–13. https://doi.org/10.1016/j.nec.2016.02.008.
16. Flanders TM, Blue R, Roberts S, McShane BJ, Wilent B, Tambi V, Petrov D, Lee JYK. Fully endoscopic microvascular decompression for hemifacial spasm. J Neurosurg. 2018;131(3):813–9. https://doi.org/10.3171/2018.4.JNS172631.
17. Mostafa BE, El Sharnoubi M, Youssef AM. The keyhole retrosigmoid approach to the cerebellopontine angle: indications, technical modifications, and results. Skull Base. 2008;18(6):371–6. https://doi.org/10.1055/s-0028-1087220.

18. Pak HL, Lambru G, Okasha M, Maratos E, Thomas N, Shapey J, Barazi S. Fully endoscopic microvascular decompression for trigeminal neuralgia: technical note describing a single-center experience. World Neurosurg. 2022;166:159–67. https://doi.org/10.1016/j.wneu.2022.07.014. Epub 2022 Jul 8.
19. Zagzoog N, Attar A, Takroni R, Alotaibi MB, Reddy K. Endoscopic versus open microvascular decompression for trigeminal neuralgia: a systematic review and comparative meta-analysis. J Neurosurg. 2018;131:1–9. https://doi.org/10.3171/2018.6.JNS172690. Epub ahead of print.
20. Zhao Z, Chai S, Xiao D, Zhou Y, Gan J, Jiang X, Zhao H. Microscopic versus endoscopic microvascular decompression for the treatment of hemifacial spasm in China: a meta-analysis and systematic review. J Clin Neurosci. 2021;91:23–31. https://doi.org/10.1016/j.jocn.2021.06.034. Epub 2021 Jun 28.
21. Jiang H, Zou D, Wang P, Zeng L, Liu J, Tang C, Zhang G, Tan X, Wu N. Case report: Fully endoscopic microvascular decompression for trigeminal neuralgia. Front Neurol. 2023;13:1090478. https://doi.org/10.3389/fneur.2022.1090478.
22. Jiang H, Zhou D, Wang P, Zeng L, Liu J, Tang C, Zhang G, Tan X, Wu N. Case report: fully endoscopic microvascular decompression for glossopharyngeal neuralgia. Front Surg. 2023;9:1089632. https://doi.org/10.3389/fsurg.2022.1089632.
23. El Refaee E, Matthes M, Schroeder HWS. Value of endoscopic visualization during the sling-transposition technique for microvascular decompression of the facial nerve in a case with hemifacial spasm. World Neurosurg. 2022;163:4. https://doi.org/10.1016/j.wneu.2022.03.117. Epub 2022 Apr 2.
24. Wang P, Li Q, Wang C, Li C. Complete neuroendoscopic *versus* microscopical trigeminal neuralgia microvascular decompression (MVD) in primary trigeminal neuralgia (PTN). Am J Transl Res. 2021;13(11):12,905–12.
25. Sun Z, Wang Y, Cai X, Xie S, Jiang Z. Endoscopic vascular decompression for the treatment of trigeminal neuralgia: clinical outcomes and technical note. J Pain Res. 2020;13:2205–11. https://doi.org/10.2147/JPR.S268441.
26. Blue R, Alexis M, Mensah-Brown K, Yang AI, Spadola M, Ajmera S, Lee JYK. Endoscopic microvascular decompression without the use of rigid head fixation. J Clin Neurosci. 2022;106:213–6. https://doi.org/10.1016/j.jocn.2022.10.030. Epub 2022 Nov 10.
27. Al Menabbawy A, El Refaee E, Elwy R, Shoubash L, Matthes M, Schroeder HWS. Preemptive strategies and lessons learned from complications encountered with microvascular decompression for hemifacial spasm. J Neurosurg. 2023;140:1–12. https://doi.org/10.3171/2023.4.JNS23557. Epub ahead of print.
28. Rennert RC, Brandel MG, Stephens ML, Rodriguez A, Morris TW, Day JD. Surgical relevance of the suprameatal tubercle during superior petrosal vein-sparing trigeminal nerve microvascular decompression. Oper Neurosurg (Hagerstown). 2021;20(6):E410–6. https://doi.org/10.1093/ons/opab046.
29. Blue R, Li C, Spadola M, Saylany A, McShane B, Lee JYK. Complication rates during endoscopic microvascular decompression surgery are low with or without petrosal vein sacrifice. World Neurosurg. 2020;138:e420–5. https://doi.org/10.1016/j.wneu.2020.02.142. Epub 2020 Mar 4.
30. Luzzi S, Del Maestro M, Trovarelli D, De Paulis D, Dechordi SR, Di Vitantonio H, Di Norcia V, Millimaggi DF, Ricci A, Galzio RJ. Endoscope-assisted microneurosurgery for neurovascular compression syndromes: basic principles, methodology, and technical notes. Asian J Neurosurg. 2019;14(1):193–200. https://doi.org/10.4103/ajns.AJNS_279_17.

Chapter 18
Fully Endoscopic Resection of Frontal Osteomas

Waleed Yousef, Mustafa Najibullah, Zafdam Shabbir, Shayma Shamo, and Waleed Abdelfattah Azab

18.1 Introduction

Osteomas are the most common primary bone tumors of the calvaria, with an incidence of less than 0.5% [1]. They are benign, slow growing, firm immobile masses which commonly occur in the cranial vault, mastoid, paranasal sinuses, and the mandible. Osteomas can be divided into conventional classic, periosteal, and medullary types. The conventional classic type is the most common and is usually found in the craniomaxillofacial region [2]. In skull vault osteomas, the exostotic form that grows from the outer table is more common than the enostotic ones which arise from the inner table and grow intracranially [3].

Histopathologically, they consist of osteoid tissue within osteoblastic tissue, surrounded by reactive bone. Radiologically they appear well demarcated and arising most commonly from the outer table and are homogeneous and very radiodense on CT.

Osteomas of the forehead are very noticeable and disfiguring; patients usually seek medical advice for cosmetic reasons. Occasionally, pain can be the chief complaint [4]. Forehead osteomas were traditionally excised via either a direct incision over the lesion using the naturally occurring creases or a conventional bicoronal flap. Both techniques have their own disadvantages. Direct incision obviously results in a visible scar on the forehead and carries the risk of damage to the nerves of the forehead. Although the conventional bicoronal flap is done behind the hairline with subcutaneous dissection [5], it requires thorough dissection of the subcutaneous tissue and is therefore associated with potential risks including injury to the frontal branch of the facial nerve, injury to the supraorbital or the supratrochlear nerves which run perpendicular to the incision, and a visible larger scar even though it is located behind the hairline.

W. Yousef · M. Najibullah · Z. Shabbir · S. Shamo · W. A. Azab (✉)
Neurosurgery Department, Ibn Sina Hospital, Al-Sabah Medical Area, Kuwait City, Kuwait

© The Author(s), under exclusive license to Springer Nature Switzerland AG 2024
W. A. Azab (ed.), *Endoscope-controlled Transcranial Surgery*, Advances and Technical Standards in Neurosurgery 52,
https://doi.org/10.1007/978-3-031-61925-0_18

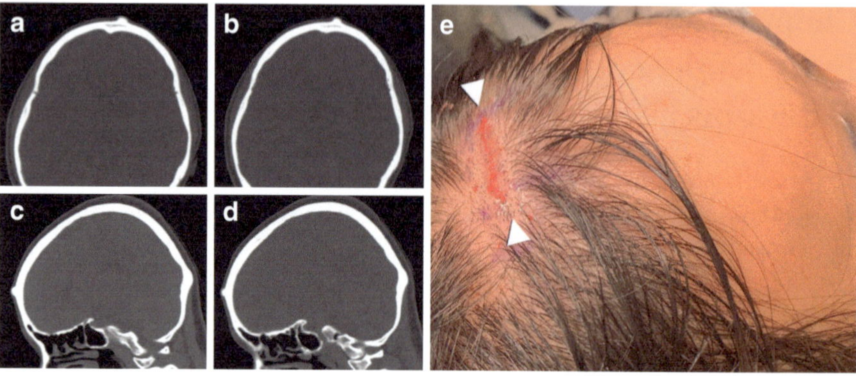

Fig. 18.1 Preoperative consecutive CT images in axial (**a**, **b**) and sagittal (**c**, **d**) planes of a case of frontal osteoma and a postprocedure demonstration of the cosmetic result in the same patient (**e**). The closed skin incision is seen (arrowheads) in (**e**)

Onishi et al. were the first to describe an endoscopic approach for excision of a frontal osteoma in 1995. They used a 30° endoscope and two 5–7 mm incisions. The first incision was utilized for the endoscope and the other for the instruments [6]. The results were very encouraging and the technique was adopted by many groups worldwide yet with many technical variations [2, 3, 7, 8].

The endoscopic technique has many advantages over the conventional procedures because the design of the rigid endoscope allows obtaining a very detailed view of the osteoma through an incision distant from the forehead region and completely far away from the nerves, vessels, and frontalis muscle fibers as the approach is performed in a subperiosteal plane. The fully endoscopic approach for the excision of forehead osteomas in our experience has proven to be less time-consuming, efficient, and minimally invasive with excellent cosmetic results (Fig. 18.1).

In this chapter we elaborate on the surgical technique of fully endoscopic resection of frontal osteomas.

18.2 Surgical Technique

Under general anesthesia, the patient is positioned supine with head on a horseshoe head rest. A point 1 cm behind the hairline is chosen as a center of the incision and placed so that the shortest working distance from the incision to the osteoma is obtained. Limited hair trimming of 3 to 4 mm breadth is performed along the planned incision, and a local injection of lidocaine 2% with adrenaline (epinephrine) 1:200,000 mixture is injected at the incision site. A 3 cm scalp incision is performed down to the bone (Fig. 18.2a). The periosteum is then dissected using a periosteal elevator. A small handheld Langenbeck retractor is used to elevate the

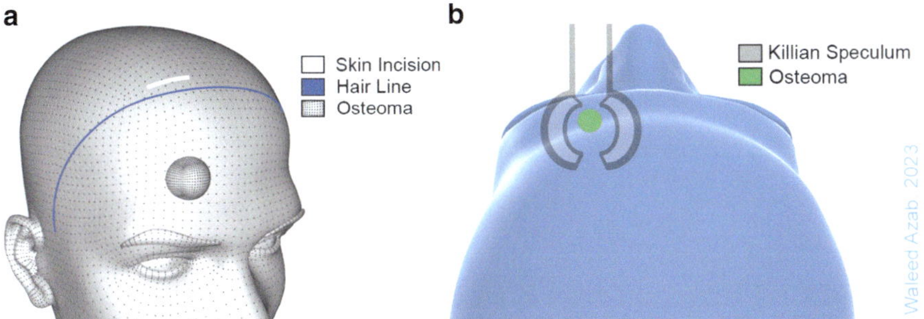

Fig. 18.2 Scalp incision and surgical corridor planning. (**a**) The scalp incision is 1 cm behind the hairline and is placed so that the shortest working distance from the incision to the osteoma is obtained. (**b**) Killian transsphenoidal speculum is inserted down to the osteoma and is opened to develop the working corridor

scalp, and a Killian transsphenoidal speculum is inserted down to the osteoma and is opened so as to develop the working corridor (Fig. 18.2b).

A 0° rigid endoscope with irrigation sheath is connected to a 4K endoscopic camera and monitor. The operative steps under endoscopic view are demonstrated in Fig. 18.3a–f. The endoscope is held by the assistant surgeon and inserted down the corridor at the 12 o'clock position until the osteoma is clearly seen. Further adjustment of the speculum blades is performed under endoscopic vision. A dissector is at times needed to dissect the periosteum from the osteoma at the deepest part of the corridor. Smudging of the endoscope lens can be easily cleared by injecting saline and aspirating the last drop of fluid by the syringe held by the assistant surgeon. A suction tube is most of the time kept at the lower corner of the corridor. The suction tube may also serve as a retractor at the depth in addition to its other function of clearing the irrigation fluid, bone dust during drilling, and smoke when cautery is used.

The next step is to use a long-angled drill with a slim-profile handle to remove the osteoma. A 4 mm sharp diamond drill bit is usually used, although a smaller bit may be needed at the final stages of osteoma removal.

At times a 30° or 45° endoscope is used to gain better visualization. Keeping the endoscope shaft away from the center of the corridor is important to save space for instrument manipulation. Dynamic insertion and withdrawal movements of the endoscope shaft and instruments through the working corridor are crucial for a seamless performance of the procedure. This surgical harmony of the team is developed with more work and cooperation of the members of the surgical team.

Eventually, few drilling movements are performed after the osteoma has been drilled in order to smoothen the surface of the outer table. Copious irrigation of the cavity is then performed and closure in the standard fashion is done to conclude the procedure.

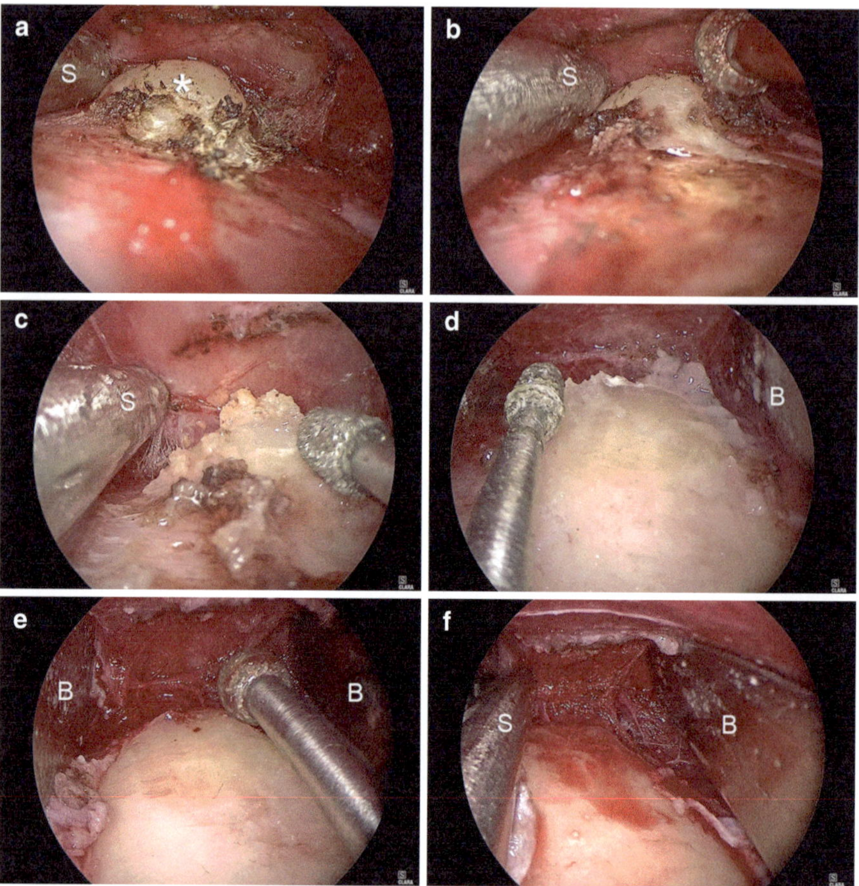

Fig. 18.3 (**a**) The endoscope is inserted down the corridor until the osteoma is clearly seen. (**b**) The osteoma has been partially drilled. Note that the suction tube is most of the time kept at the lower corner of the corridor and additionally serves as a retractor at the depth. (**c**, **d**) Further drilling of the osteoma is performed. A smaller drill bit is used for drilling the very last part of the osteoma (**d**). (**e**) Smoothening of the outer table surface after the osteoma has been drilled is then performed. (**f**) A final view of the operative field is seen. *B* Blade of the speculum, *S* Suction tube

References

1. Izci Y. Management of the large cranial osteoma: experience with 13 adult patients. Acta Neurochir. 2005;147:1151–5.
2. Oyer SL, Patel KG. Endoscopic brow approach for frontal osteoma in a pediatric patient. Int J Pediatr Otorhinolaryngol. 2012;76(8):1211–3. https://doi.org/10.1016/j.ijporl.2012.04.011.
3. Lai CH, Sun IF, Huang SH, Lai CS, Lin SD. Forehead osteoma excision by endoscopic approach. Ann Plast Surg. 2008;61(5):533–6. https://doi.org/10.1097/SAP.0b013e31816d829a.
4. Foustanos A, Zavrides H. Endoscopic resection of forehead osteomas. Br J Oral Maxillofac Surg. 2007;45(5):392–5.

5. Kim JS, Lee JH, Kim NG, Lee KS. Forehead osteoma excision by anterior hairline incision with subcutaneous dissection. Arch Craniofac Surg. 2016;17(1):39–42. https://doi.org/10.7181/acfs.2016.17.1.39.

6. Onishi K, Maruyama Y, Sawaizumi M. Endoscopic excision of forehead osteoma. J Craniofac Surg. 1995;6(6):516–8. https://doi.org/10.1097/00001665-199511000-00021.

7. Papay FA, Stein JM, Dietz JR, Luciano M, Morales L Jr, Zins J. Endoscopic approach for benign tumor ablation of the forehead and brow. J Craniofac Surg. 1997;8(3):176–80. https://doi.org/10.1097/00001665-199705000-00007.

8. da Costa MDS, Suzuki FS, Biló JP, Cavalheiro S. Endoscopic approach for resection of frontal forehead osteoma: technical case report instruction. World Neurosurg. 2023;175:11. https://doi.org/10.1016/j.wneu.2023.03.135.

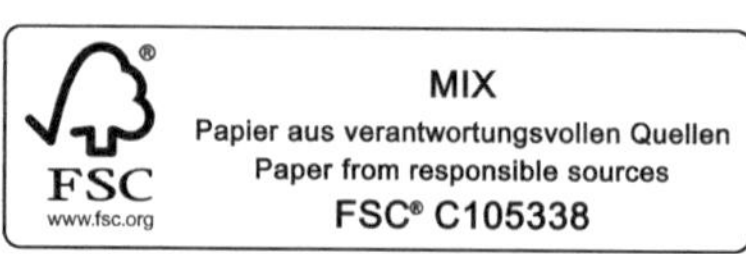
MIX
Papier aus verantwortungsvollen Quellen
Paper from responsible sources
FSC® C105338
FSC
www.fsc.org